Chronic Viral Hepatitis

CLINICAL GASTROENTEROLOGY

George Y. Wu, SERIES EDITOR

Chronic Viral Hepatitis: Diagnosis and Therapeutics, edited by Raymond S. Koff and George Y. Wu, 2001.

Diseases of the Gastroesophageal Mucosa: The Acid-Related Disorders, edited by James W. Freston, 2001.

Chronic Viral Hepatitis

Diagnosis and Therapeutics

Edited by

Raymond S. Koff, MD
University of Massachusetts Medical School, Worcester, MA

and

George Y. Wu, MD, PhD
University of Connecticut Health Center, Farmington, CT

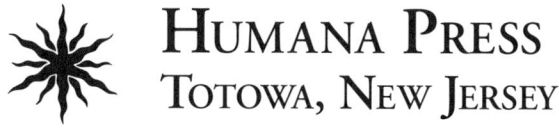

Humana Press
Totowa, New Jersey

© 2002 Humana Press Inc.
999 Riverview Drive, Suite 208
Totowa, New Jersey 07512
humanapress.com

For additional copies, pricing for bulk purchases, and/or information about other Humana titles, contact Humana at the above address or at any of the following numbers: Tel: 973-256-1699; Fax: 973-256-8341; E-mail: humana@humanapr.com or visit our Website at http://humanapress.com

All rights reserved. No part of this book may be reproduced, stored in a retrieval system, or transmitted in any form or by any means, electronic, mechanical, photocopying, microfilming, recording, or otherwise without written permission from the Publisher.

All articles, comments, opinions, conclusions, or recommendations are those of the author(s), and do not necessarily reflect the views of the publisher.

Due diligence has been taken by the publishers, editors, and authors of this book to ensure the accuracy of the information published and to describe generally accepted practices. The contributors herein have carefully checked to ensure that the drug selections and dosages set forth in this text are accurate in accord with the standards accepted at the time of publication. Notwithstanding, as new research, changes in government regulations, and knowledge from clinical experience relating to drug therapy and drug reactions constantly occurs, the reader is advised to check the product information provided by the manufacturer of each drug for any change in dosages or for additional warnings and contraindications. This is of utmost importance when the recommended drug herein is a new or infrequently used drug. It is the responsibility of the health care provider to ascertain the Food and Drug Administration status of each drug or device used in their clinical practice. The publisher, editors, and authors are not responsible for errors or omissions or for any consequences from the application of the information presented in this book and make no warranty, express or implied, with respect to the contents in this publication.

This publication is printed on acid-free paper. ∞
ANSI Z39.48-1984 (American National Standards Institute)
Permanence of Paper for Printed Library Materials.

Cover design by Patricia F. Cleary.

Production Editor: Mark J. Breaugh.

Photocopy Authorization Policy:
Authorization to photocopy items for internal or personal use, or the internal or personal use of specific clients, is granted by Humana Press Inc., provided that the base fee of US $10.00 per copy, plus US $00.25 per page, is paid directly to the Copyright Clearance Center at 222 Rosewood Drive, Danvers, MA 01923. For those organizations that have been granted a photocopy license from the CCC, a separate system of payment has been arranged and is acceptable to Humana Press Inc. The fee code for users of the Transactional Reporting Service is: [0-89603-880-7/02 $10.00 + $00.25].
Printed in the United States of America.   10 9 8 7 6 5 4 3 2 1

Chronic viral hepatitis : diagnosis and therapeutics / edited by Raymond S. Koff and George Y. Wu
    p. ; cm. -- (Clinical gastroenterology)
  Includes bibliographical references and index.
  ISBN 0-89603-880-7 (alk. paper)
  1. Hepatitis, Viral. I. Koff, Raymond S. (Raymond Steven), 1939- II. Wu, George Y., 1948- III. Series.
  [DNLM: 1. Hepatitis, Viral, Human--diagnosis. 2. Hepatitis, Viral, Human--therapy. 3. Chronic Disease. WC 536 c55725 2001]
  RC848.H43 C48 2001
  616.3'623--dc21   2001024307

Dedication

This book is dedicated to the memory of Herman Lopata, and to his family who have been so generous with their support of our research on viral hepatitis.

G. Y. W.

Preface

Forty years ago, just prior to the discovery of the hepatitis B surface antigen, the concept that chronic liver disease could be a sequel to infection by any agent of acute viral hepatitis was controversial and hotly debated. With the development of specific and sensitive serologic and virologic markers of infection by the bloodborne and enterically transmitted hepatitis viruses, the linkage of the former agents with chronic hepatitis, cirrhosis, end-stage liver disease, and hepatocellular carcinoma was established beyond doubt. The enterically transmitted viruses, in contrast, elicit self-limited infections without chronic sequelae. In addition, it is now recognized that chronic viral hepatitis is the predominant liver disease throughout the world and although the role of the hepatitis D virus has diminished dramatically in recent years, hepatitis B and C viruses continue to be the most common causes of persistent viremia in the United States, as well as elsewhere. At least 10 million individuals have been infected by these two agents in the United States alone, and over 3 million have active infection. On a global basis, over 2 billion people have been infected by the bloodborne hepatitis viruses and 500 million may have chronic infection; annually, over one million deaths have been attributed to these chronic infections. End-stage liver disease arising from chronic viral hepatitis is the single most common indication for liver transplantation and the rising incidence of hepatocellular carcinoma in this country and elsewhere has been attributed to chronic hepatitis B and C infections.

The prevalence and morbidity and mortality of chronic viral hepatitis underscore the necessity to provide clear and accurate information to healthcare professionals who encounter affected patients. Enormous progress has been made in diagnosis and in understanding the epidemiology and natural history of infection, its associated liver disease, and factors affecting rates of progression. Therapeutic interventions now permit clearance of virus, interruption of disease progression, and restoration of health-related quality of life, and life expectancy, in a substantial and growing number of patients. Yet much remains unknown. Continuing research will be necessary to ensure that infection rates decline through expanded use of hepatitis B vaccine, the development of a hepatitis C vaccine, and education about the dangers of high-risk behaviors. It will also be essential to develop new therapies for those with established infections and to improve the benefits of current therapies by finding optimal regimens for viral clearance and reversal of liver injury.

Chronic Viral Hepatitis: Diagnosis and Therapeutics will provide the reader with a comprehensive overview of the field of chronic viral hepatitis arising from the hepatitis B and C viruses, with a focus on epidemiology, natural history, the problem of co-infections, and a number of facets of patient management. The latter include contributions on developing the therapeutic plan, supporting the patient during treatment, alternative treatment, the use of drugs in chronic viral hepatitis, liver transplantation, and pregnancy in chronic viral hepatitis. In each instance, the authors are leading scientists, clinicians, and clinical investigators who bring to each chapter an extensive review of the available literature, a critical understanding of the state-of-the-art, as well as a broad experience in clinical trials and the management of patients with chronic viral hepatitis.

It has been a pleasure to participate with this outstanding group of contributors in the creation of this book. I hope it will serve as a useful guide for the reader and set the stage for understanding future advances in this field.

Raymond S. Koff, MD

CONTENTS

Preface .... *vii*

List of Contributors .... *xi*

1 **Molecular Virology of Hepatitis B and C:**
   Clinical Implications 1
   Robert M. Smith and George Y. Wu

2 **Epidemiology of Hepatitis B and Hepatitis C** 25
   Robert L. Carithers, Jr.

3 **Natural History of Hepatitis B Virus Infection** 41
   David G. Forcione, Raymond T. Chung,
   and Jules L. Dienstag

4 **Natural History of Hepatitis C** 59
   Gregory T. Everson

5 **Hepatitis C and HIV Co-Infection** 95
   Michael A. Poles and Douglas T. Dieterich

6 **HBV and HCV Co-Infection** 109
   Terence L. Angtuaco and Donald M. Jensen

7 **Treatment of Chronic Hepatitis B** 123
   Eng-Kiong Teo and Anna Suk-Fong Lok

8 **Treatment of Chronic Hepatitis C Infection** 145
   Manal F. Abdelmalek and Gary L. Davis

9 **Treatment of Chronic Viral Hepatitis in Patients
   with Autoimmune Diseases** 169
   Gehad Ghaith and Stuart C. Gordon

10 **Developing Therapeutic Plans for the Patient
    with Chronic Hepatitis B or C:**
    A Practical Approach 189
    Robert Reindollar

11 **Supporting the Patient with Chronic Hepatitis
    During Treatment** 211
    Nezam H. Afdhal and Tiffany Geahigan

12 **Complementary and Alternative Treatment of Liver Disease** *233*
Ken Flora and Kent Benner

13 **Drugs and Chronic Viral Hepatitis** *251*
Ajay Batra, Richard W. Lambrecht, and Herbert L. Bonkovsky

14 **Chronic Viral Hepatitis and Liver Transplantation** *273*
Aijaz Ahmed and Emmet B. Keeffe

15 **Viral Hepatitis and Pregnancy** *291*
Rene Davila and Caroline A. Riely

16 **Prevention and Immunoprophylaxis of Chronic Viral Hepatitis** *305*
Raymond S. Koff

Index *325*

Contributors

Manel F. Abdelmalek, MD • *Section of Hepatobiliary Diseases, University of Florida College of Medicine, Gainesville, FL*
Nezam H. Afdhal, MD • *Liver Center, Beth Israel Deaconess Medical Center, Boston, MA*
Aijaz Ahmed, MD • *Division of Gastroenterology and Hepatology, Department of Medicine, Stanford University Medical Center, Stanford, CA*
Terence L. Angtuaco, MD • *Section of Hepatology, Rush-Presbyterian-St. Luke's Medical Center, Chicago, IL*
Ajay Batra, MD • *Division of Digestive Disease and Nutrition, University of Massachusetts Memorial Medical Center, Worcester, MA*
Kent Benner, MD • *Division of Gastroenterology and Hepatology, Oregon Health Sciences University, Portland, OR*
Herbert L. Bonkovsky, MD • *Division of Digestive Disease and Nutrition, University of Massachusetts Memorial Medical Center, Worcester, MA*
Robert L. Carithers, MD • *Department of Medicine, Hepatology Section, University of Washington Medical Center, Seattle, WA*
Raymond T. Chung, MD • *Department of Medicine and Gastrointestinal Unit, Massachusetts General Hospital, Boston, MA*
Rene Davila, MD • *Department of Medicine, Division of Gastroenterology and Hepatology, The University of Tennessee Health Science Center, Memphis, TN*
Gary L. Davis, MD • *Section of Hepatobiliary Diseases, University of Florida College of Medicine, Gainesville, FL*
Jules L. Dienstag, MD • *Department of Medicine and Gastrointestinal Unit, Massachusetts General Hospital, Boston, MA*
Douglas T. Dieterich, MD • *Division of Gastroenterology and Hepatology, Cabrini Medical Center, and Department of Medicine, NYU School of Medicine, New York, NY*
Gregory T. Everson, MD • *Section of Hepatology, Division of Gastroenterology and Hepatology, Department of Medicine, University of Colorado School of Medicine, Denver, CO*
Ken Flora, MD • *Division of Gastroenterology and Hepatology, Oregon Health Sciences University, Portland, OR*

DAVID G. FORCIONE, MD • *Department of Medicine and Gastrointestinal Unit, Massachusetts General Hospital, Boston, MA*
TIFFANY GEAHIGAN, PA-C • *Liver Center, Beth Israel Deaconess Medical Center, Boston, MA*
GEHAD GHAITH, MD • *Gastroenterology–Hepatology Section, William Beaumont Hospital, Royal Oak, MI*
STUART C. GORDON, MD • *Gastroenterology–Hepatology Section, William Beaumont Hospital, Royal Oak, MI*
DONALD M. JENSEN, MD • *Section of Hepatology, Rush-Presbyterian-St. Luke's Medical Center, Chicago, IL*
EMMET B. KEEFFE, MD • *Division of Gastroenterology and Hepatology, Department of Medicine, Stanford University Medical Center, Stanford, CA*
RAYMOND S. KOFF, MD • *Department of Medicine, University of Massachusetts Medical School, Worcester, MA*
RICHARD W. LAMBRECHT, PHD • *Division of Digestive Disease and Nutrition, University of Massachusetts Memorial Medical Center, Worcester, MA*
ANNA SUK-FONG LOK, MD • *Division of Gastroenterology, University of Michigan Medical Center, Ann Arbor, MI*
MICHAEL A. POLES, MD • *Division of Digestive Diseases, UCLA Center for Health Sciences, Los Angeles, CA*
ROBERT REINDOLLAR, MD • *Carolina Center for Liver Disease, Charlotte, NC*
CAROLINE A. RIELY, MD • *Department of Medicine, Division of Gastroenterology and Hepatology, The University of Tennessee Health Science Center, Memphis, TN*
ROBERT M. SMITH, BS • *Division of Gastroenterology–Hepatology, University of Connecticut Health Center, Farmington, CT*
ENG-KIONG TEO, MB, BS • *Division of Gastroenterology, University of Michigan Medical Center, Ann Arbor, MI*
GEORGE Y. WU, MD, PhD • *Division of Gastroenterology–Hepatology, University of Connecticut Health Center, Farmington, CT*

1 Molecular Virology of Hepatitis B and C
Clinical Implications

Robert M. Smith, BS
and George Y. Wu, MD, PHD

CONTENTS
INTRODUCTION
HEPATITIS B VIRUS
HEPATITIS C VIRUS
CONCLUSION: FUTURE TREATMENT STRATEGIES
REFERENCES

INTRODUCTION

Despite fundamental differences in genome structure, hepatitis B (HBV) and C (HCV) viruses use many of the same strategies to achieve high-level replication and persistence of infection in hepatocytes. The limited genome size of these viruses necessitates an efficient use of host-cell machinery to carry out viral gene expression. This strong dependence on virus–host interactions restricts HBV- and HCV-cell tropism to the hepatocytes of higher primates and precludes their reliable and reproducible propagation in cell culture. Recent studies have begun to overcome this experimental limitation, so as to permit a more complete understanding of the molecular basis for viral replication, and the concomitant induction or evasion of the host antiviral immune response. Some of the important molecular biological properties of these viruses, as well as how they are reflected in the clinical manifestations of viral infection, are presented below.

From: *Clinical Gastroenterology: Diagnosis and Therapeutics*
Edited by: R. S. Koff and G. Y. Wu © Humana Press Inc., Totowa, NJ

HEPATITIS B VIRUS

HBV is a member of the hepadnavirus family, a group of hepatotropic mammalian and avian DNA viruses, which replicate via reverse transcription of a genomic RNA intermediate *(1)*. Human HBV strains have been classified into nine different serologic subtypes, determined by surface antigen immunogenicity, and, more recently, into seven genotypes (A–G), based on DNA sequence comparison. Each of the various genotypes exhibits a characteristic serotype profile and geographical distribution, allowing an evaluation of HBV phylogenetic evolution and possible genotypic influence on the natural course of HBV infection *(2)*. The sequencing of clinical isolates has even been used as an epidemiological marker to trace routes of transmission.

HBV infection is highly cell-type and species-specific: hepatocytes of the great apes are the only confirmed site of HBV replication. Reported infection of other cell types, e.g. lymphocytes, is controversial, and generally thought to be of little clinical relevance. Neither hepatocyte-derived cell lines nor transgenic mice support the full HBV replication cycle. Fortunately, other hepadnaviruses, particularly duck and woodchuck hepatitis viruses, provide convenient model systems for HBV infection and associated liver disease.

Replication Cycle

HBV commonly achieves infection in virtually 100% of the hepatocyte population. Following entry into the host cell, the 3.2 kilobase (kb) partially double-stranded (pdsDNA) HBV genome is transported to the nucleus, and converted to a covalently-closed circular (cccDNA) template, from which all viral mRNAs are transcribed by host RNA polymerase activity (Fig. 1). The viral pregenomic RNA transcript, encompassing the entire genome sequence, is subsequently encapsidated and reverse-transcribed into the pdsDNA form by a virus-encoded polymerase. Although direct cytopathic liver injury is seen under conditions of very high viral load—as in fibrosing cholestatic hepatitis, a rare condition observed in some patients with recurrent post-transplantation hepatitis B—the virus itself is generally noncytolytic. Rather, HBV-associated injury is attributed to lysis of infected hepatocytes by the host immune response *(3)*.

Cellular Entry

Virion endocytosis, uncoating, and nuclear transport of the pdsDNA genome remain poorly understood, although the host-cell contribution to these events is believed to be a major determinant of HBV-cell tropism.

Chapter 1 / Molecular Virology of Hepatitis B and C

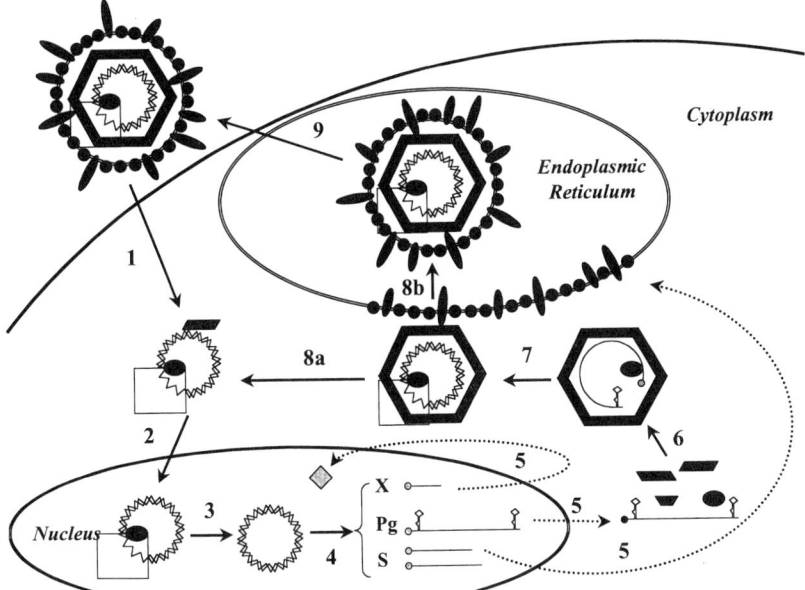

Fig. 1. HBV Replication Cycle. The events of hepatocellular HBV infection are indicated: (**1**) endocytosis and uncoating, (**2**) nuclear import of partially-double-stranded DNA, (**3**) formation of covalently-closed circular DNA, (**4**) transcription, (**5**) translation, (**6**) encapsidation of pregenomic (Pg) RNA and polymerase, (**7**) reverse transcription, (**8a**) replenishment of the nuclear DNA pool, (**8b**) budding, (**9**) secretion.

Increasing evidence suggests that the N-terminal domain of the large HBV envelope protein is responsible for attachment to hepatocytes. The cell surface receptor(s) mediating viral entry has not yet been identified, though studies with duck hepatitis B virus suggest the involvement of a carboxypeptidase receptor. Nuclear import of pdsDNA may be facilitated by the covalently-attached HBV polymerase, or by the noncovalently associated capsid protein, which bears a nuclear localization signal. Host components involved in this nucleocytoplasmic transport have yet to be determined. Interestingly, the translocation event does not occur in transgenic mouse models of HBV infection, despite the ability of mouse hepatocytes to support subsequent steps in HBV replication.

cccDNA

The mechanism by which HBV pdsDNA is converted to covalently-closed circular form is not known, but presumably involves host-cell DNA-repair pathways. Once formed, the cccDNA does not undergo

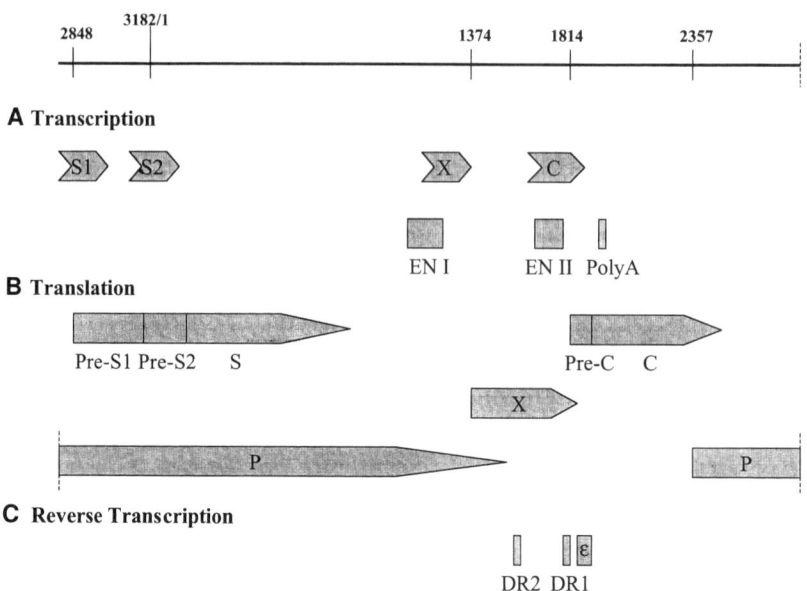

Fig. 2. HBV Genomic Organization. The compactness of the HBV genome is manifested in the alignment of overlapping sequence elements essential for gene expression and reverse transcription: (**A**) promoters, enhancers (EN), and polyadenylation (PolyA) signal; (**B**) protein open reading frames; (**C**) direct repeats (DR) and encapsidation signal (ε).

semiconservative replication in the nucleus, as the intracellular HBV DNA pool can be supplemented only by reverse transcription in the cytoplasm, as described below. In contrast to serum HBV DNA, which has a half-life of just 1–3 d, cccDNA is a remarkably stable species in hepatocyte nuclei. It is resistant to direct elimination by antiviral agents, and is lost only upon destruction of the host cell. The half-life of infected hepatocytes is quite long, 10–100 d or more, depending on the extent of liver injury. Accordingly, antiviral therapy with reverse transcriptase inhibitors requires an extended course of treatment to achieve complete clearance, especially in mild disease with a relatively low rate of hepatocyte turnover.

Transcription

In contrast to other DNA viruses, HBV appears not to utilize post-transcriptional alternative mRNA splicing to maximize its coding capacity. Instead, HBV makes exquisitely economic use of its genome at the transcriptional level by embedding regulatory elements—even overlapping open reading frames (ORFs)—within concise protein coding sequences (Fig. 2). Despite its small size, the HBV cccDNA genome is sufficient to direct the synthesis of four classes of RNA transcripts by host RNA polymerase II. A pair of ~3.5 kb RNAs, differentially-regulated by the core promoter, function as templates for HBV DNA synthesis, and serve as mRNAs for pre-core, core, and polymerase proteins. The 2.4 kb and 2.1 kb pre-S/S mRNAs encode three envelope proteins, designated S(mall), M(iddle), and L(arge). A 0.7 kb transcript directs synthesis of the HBV X protein (HBxAg).

Transcription of each HBV RNA initiates from one or more unique promoters, which are regulated by two shared enhancer elements, EN I and II. Activity of liver-enriched transcription factors (TFs) at these sites is thought to contribute to tissue specificity of HBV infection, as the observed multifactorial cis-regulation of viral promoters takes place only in well-differentiated liver cells *(4)*. All transcripts terminate at a common polyadenylation signal, which is located in the core ORF. This signal is read-through during transcription of the pregenomic RNA, generating a terminally redundant greater-than-genome-length transcript. Hepatitis delta RNA selectively inhibits transcription of pregenomic HBV RNA in vitro, and this effect likely contributes to the frequently-observed pre-core antigen seroconversion in carriers superinfected with HDV.

Translation

Efficient use of coding sequences, the hallmark of HBV biology, is also apparent during translation. The envelope components, S, M, and L, are generated by usage of three different in-phase start codons. Translation of the pre-core/core ORF originates from one of two in-frame start codons; initiation from the upstream site generates the pre-core polypeptide, which is post-translationally modified to form the hepatitis B e-antigen (*see* discussion of HBeAg function below). Translation of the polymerase gene initiates from an out-of-frame start codon located in the C-terminal coding region of the core ORF. The inefficiency of this unconventional and, as yet, poorly-understood process, yields a core:polymerase molar ratio of ~250:1. Interaction between the HBV polymerase and the 5'-end of its own mRNA is sufficient to block further translation, and to precipitate the events of genomic replication.

Encapsidation and Reverse Transcription

HBV RNA packaging and reverse transcription have been well characterized *(5)*. The N-terminal domain of the polymerase protein binds to pregenomic mRNA at a stem-loop secondary structure designated "epsilon". This event is facilitated by host-cell chaperones, such as p23 and heat shock protein (Hsp)70; inhibitors of Hsp90 have been shown to block HBV RNA packaging and subsequent DNA synthesis. Formation of the polymerase–RNA complex triggers assembly of the viral nucleocapsid. The capsid is composed of 120 disulfide-linked core dimers, which collectively bind RNA via a C-terminal domain of the core polypeptide.

Reverse transcription occurs within the nucleocapsid, which contains small pores to allow influx of deoxynucleotides and other small molecules. Initiation of reverse transcription is accomplished by a protein-priming mechanism, utilizing an amino-terminal tyrosine residue of the polymerase and the epsilon structure as a replication origin. The C-terminal catalytic domains of the HBV polymerase protein exhibit reverse transcriptase, DNA-dependent DNA polymerase, and RNase H activities. In the presence of requisite host-cell chaperones and possibly other cofactors, the polymerase carries out synthesis of viral pdsDNA and nearly complete degradation of the pregenomic RNA template. Phosphorylated metabolites of the antiviral compounds lamivudine, famciclovir, lobucavir, and adefovir dipivoxil inhibit this step of HBV replication by competing with deoxynucleotide triphosphates for incorporation into HBV DNA, thereby causing premature termination of nascent polynucleotide chains.

One notable feature of the HBV-polymerization process is its discontinuous nature. pdsDNA synthesis requires dissociation of the polymerase and nascent DNA from the RNA template, and annealing to a homologous direct repeat sequence on the 3'-end of the pregenome. Polymerization from primers which fail to undergo template switching ("*in situ* priming") results in the formation of double-stranded linear (dslDNA) genomes. Although illegitimate recombination events can convert dslDNA into cccDNA, they may also cause integration of HBV sequences into host DNA.

Integration

The integration of HBV DNA is apparently a common event. Even in the majority of patients who develop spontaneous or treatment-induced HBeAg seroconversion and normalization of aminotransferase (ALT) levels and histology, HBV DNA sequences can be detected by PCR-based diagnostic tests. HBV dslDNA is likely the predominant integrating species, although the gap structure in pdsDNA may facilitate integration of this form as well. Commonly, the core and polymerase genes are disrupted by integration, whereas the X and envelope ORFs remain intact. Transcription from integrated DNA accounts for hepatitis B surface antigen (HBsAg) secretion observed in the absence of viral replication.

Integrated HBV DNA is found in the majority of HBsAg-positive hepatocellular carcinomas (HCCs). As with other viruses, insertional mutagenesis may cause activation of a proto-oncogene or inactivation of a tumor suppressor gene in cis. In woodchuck hepatitis virus, there is evidence of specific activation of the myc family of genes by this mechanism. In isolated cases of human HCC, HBV insertion has been observed near cyclin A, retinoic acid receptor β, and p53 loci. However, the HBV-integration site is conspicuously random, and integration of full-length HBV genomes does not commonly lead to transformation of cultured cells.

X Protein and Hepatocarcinogenesis

The oncogenic potential of HBV integration likely derives from activation of host gene transcription in trans, rather than in cis *(6)*. Truncated forms of the HBV pre-S/S envelope proteins may be formed as a result of integration. These exhibit potent transactivation in vitro, and can stimulate the c-myc promoter, as seen in woodchuck hepatitis virus-related HCC. Integrated HBV DNA isolated from tumor nodules preferentially encompasses the X protein ORF. X is required for infection in vivo, but is dispensable for viral replication in transfection-based cell culture models. The X protein regulates transcription from viral and host RNA polymerase I, II, and III promoters in vitro *(7)*. Although X has been shown to dimerize—a feature common to DNA-binding TFs—it likely acts as a coactivator. X associates with a myriad of host cell proteins, including transcriptional regulators. It influences other TFs without binding them directly, and so is thought to act by more global mechanisms, such as interaction with general transcription factors (TFIIB, RNA polymerase subunit 5).

Among the multitude of cis-acting genetic elements responsive to X activity is HBV enhancer I: thus X may regulate its own synthesis. X-responsive host genes include many involved in acute inflammatory and immune responses (e.g., major histocompatibility complex (MHC), tumor necrosis factor (TNF)-α1, interleukin-6), signal transduction, cell proliferation, and apoptosis. HBxAg sensitizes cells to TNFα, and is suspected to influence other apoptotic pathways. Overall, the transcriptional regulatory effects of X may contribute to viral persistence, increased cell turnover, and HBV-related hepatocarcinogenesis.

Distinct from its transactivation function, HBxAg may disrupt DNA repair and normal cell-growth regulation by direct interaction with host regulatory proteins. X associates with a cellular factor called UV-damaged DNA binding protein, and downregulates nucleotide excision repair pathways. Sequestration by X protein also inhibits p53 nuclear translocation and tumor suppressor activities, disrupting transcription-coupled repair mechanisms. Consequently, X may sensitize cells to genotoxic stimuli and promote integration events and overall genetic instability common in HCC. Interestingly, HBxAg has been reported to exhibit endogenous adenosine monophosphate (AMP) kinase/ATPase activities, and to colocalize with proteasome subunits, which may be mechanistically relevant to its observed effects on growth regulators. Stimulation of the Ras-Raf-mitogen-activated protein kinase pathway, and activation of protein kinase C, c-Src, and c-Fyn have been reported in cell-culture models of X expression. The retinoblastoma (Rb) tumor suppressor is inactivated by hyperphosphorylation in the presence of HBxAg.

In vitro and transgenic studies indicate that X promotes cell transformation and carcinogenesis, but only upon overexpression to levels well beyond those typical of infected cells. Integration of X may lead to such overexpression, as subcellular localization studies indicate that expression of X from integrated templates leads to its accumulation and redistribution. Notably, an X-responsive bZip-family TF was found to be overexpressed in HCCs. However, cell transformation has been observed with expression of the X gene product N-terminal domain, which lacks the transactivation function altogether. Indeed, most of the proposed actions of X have not been demonstrated in the context of HCC-derived cells; it is possible that HBV-associated carcinogenesis is solely due to induction of chronic hepatocellular necrosis and regeneration. Given that HBV-related HCC is closely associated with cirrhosis, and that the peak incidence occurs 30–50 years after HBV infection, it is likely that the contribution of X expression alone is limited, relative to other factors, such as the extent of immune-mediated pathogenesis.

Virion Production

Newly synthesized pdsDNA may be imported into the nucleus, resulting in replenishment of the cccDNA pool, or secreted from the cell in virions. Completion of pdsDNA synthesis in some way facilitates nucleocapsid translocation into the endoplasmic reticulum (ER) and entry into the secretory pathway. The mechanism of this coupled maturation process is unknown, but may involve a conformational shift in the nucleocapsid exterior. Other factors, such as core protein phosphorylation state, or regulation by HBeAg, may influence the relative rate of cccDNA accumulation and virion production. Secretion is also dependent on the concentration of L envelope protein, as the pre-S1 domain mediates association of the envelope with core particles. Through budding, the nucleocapsid acquires a coating of the S, M, and L transmembrane proteins. Transport of virions through the Golgi apparatus results in the maturation of envelope proteins into N-glycosylated disulfide-linked multimers.

HBV is continuously released into the bloodstream, with a daily production of up to 10^{11} enveloped virions. Envelopes lacking enclosed nucleocapsids can be secreted at more than a 100-fold excess over virions, resulting in very high serum concentrations of "surface antigen particles." Extrahepatic symptoms may result from deposition of antigen-antibody complexes formed when these particles are neutralized by anti-HBsAg antibodies.

Immune System Evasion

Infection of a high percentage of hepatocytes is observed even in acute, resolved cases, suggesting a delayed immune response to HBV antigens. Patients recovering from acute HBV infection exhibit humoral response to pre-S and S antigens, as well as vigorous, polyclonal cytotoxic T lymphocyte (CTL) activity against multiple epitopes of HBV envelope, core, and polymerase proteins. However, given the large quantity of hepatocytes infected, and the rapid rate of clearance following transient infection, it has been proposed that HBV nucleic acids can be eliminated from infected hepatocytes by means other than direct CTL killing and replacement by noninfected cells. cccDNA may be lost from cell nuclei during mitosis. Additionally, the activation of an intracellular antiviral response by cytokines, such as TNF-α, interleukin-12 and interferons (IFNs) alpha and gamma, is known to induce noncytocidal loss of viral RNA and proteins. At high doses, TNF and interferons downregulate the core promoter.

Immunotolerance of HBV antigens may play a central role in viral persistence. Most infections in immunocompromised adults, and ~90% of perinatal infections, progress to chronicity. These patients exhibit generally less severe liver disease than immunocompetent adults, despite higher viral load. The CTL and CD4+ T cell response in chronically infected patients is weak and restricted to relatively few epitopes. Hepatitis B e-antigen is not essential for infection in vivo, but appears to play an immunosuppressive role contributing to the maintenance of high level viremia. HBeAg bears an N-terminal signal peptide, and is actively secreted. It has been proposed to cross-react with antibodies to core, or antagonize the inflammatory Th1 response, thereby suppressing the host's ability to generate a sufficient CTL attack on infected hepatocytes. HBeAg may cross the placenta to establish T-cell tolerance to HBV e- and core antigens, setting the stage for perinatally acquired chronic infection. Consistent with these proposed interactions, clearance of HBeAg during primary and chronic infections is frequently associated with ALT flare-ups. HBV mutant strains defective for e-antigen expression generally induce more severe immune-mediated liver injury than wild type, and are more likely to be cleared during the acute phase of infection.

Viral Mutation

The genetic stability of HBV is evidenced by the fact that each of the major genotypes exhibits only a few of the possible HBsAg subtypes. The development of effective anti-HBV vaccines has been greatly facilitated by the high degree of sequence conservation in neutralization epitopes (e.g., the "a" determinant, amino acids 99–169) of the HBV envelope proteins. Even the most divergent genotype, F, retains approx 85% genomic sequence identity with the other genotypes. Despite a prodigious daily virion production, and a polymerase misincorporation rate of 10^{-4} per base per replication cycle, the observed HBV mutation rate is less than 2×10^{-4} base substitutions per year. This frequency is 1–2 orders of magnitude lower than that for other viruses lacking polymerase-associated proofreading.

The remarkably low tolerance for mutation is most likely a consequence of the overlapping nature of the HBV genome, which dictates that a single point mutation can affect multiple coding sequences and/or regulatory elements. Nonetheless, mutations in each of the four HBV genes have been clinically isolated, and these variants frequently arise in response to immune system selection and antiviral therapy *(8)*. In several cases, the emergence of a particular mutant is known to be contingent upon nearby wild type sequences; therefore, HBV genotyping is valuable for the prediction and assessment of the clinical implications of viral mutation.

Immune–Escape Mutants

The emergence of HBV mutants has been implicated in vaccine failure and immune system evasion. The common G-to-A transition at nucleotide 1896 causes premature translation termination of the pre-core ORF and prevents synthesis of HBeAg. Notably, this mutation is found in association with T1858, a sequence characteristic of HBV genotypes B–E, possibly because this pairing maintains stability of the pregenomic RNA encapsidation signal. The relative rarity of this mutation in genotype A may contribute to the observed low perinatal transmissibility of HBV from healthy HBsAg carrier mothers in Northwestern Europe, where genotype A predominates.

Pre-core mutants may replicate more efficiently than wild type, but are most likely selected due to their ability to escape anti-HBe surveillance. Their pathogenic significance is unclear, as mixed viremia brings about a complex set of dynamic interactions with the host immune response *(8)*. Recently, mutations in the core promoter and enhancer II, which alter the binding sites for host TFs, have been identified in patient isolates. In addition to their possible impact on the overlapping X protein coding sequence, these have been found to reduce HBeAg expression, and influence viral pathogenicity in a manner similar to pre-core mutations.

Envelope gene mutations are detected in roughly half of all individuals who develop post-vaccination HBV infection, and are particularly prevalent in infants born to carrier mothers. The most common of these so-called "vaccine-escape" mutants is G145R in the "a" determinant of HBsAg. Mutations within this locus have also been found in orthotopic liver transplant recipients who developed reinfection despite human immunoglobulin prophylaxis. The presence of escape variants correlated with a high incidence of graft failure, nearly double the percentage observed for patients lacking variants. The S140 residue, unique to HBV E and F genotypes, may predispose patients to a vaccine escape mutation at an adjacent locus, as K141E has been observed only in West Africa, where genotype E predominates.

Pre-S1/S2 deletions and start codon mutants have been detected in patients with chronic and fulminant hepatitis, perhaps arising in response to strong humoral and T cell activity against this highly-immunogenic region. Selection of emergent mutations in CTL epitopes of the envelope and core genes has been observed, though escape is incomplete due to the multispecific nature of the CTL response. Some of these mutant-derived core sequences act as antagonists of CTL response against the wild type epitope, and may contribute to viral persistence.

Polymerase Mutants

HBV integration typically yields replication-deficient integrated genomes. Therefore, inhibition of reverse transcriptase for a sufficiently long duration should permit eventual immune-mediated clearance of the pre-existing cccDNA pool. However, long term monotherapy with lamivudine or other polymerase inhibitors is often unsuccessful due to breakthrough infection by drug-resistant polymerase gene mutants after approx one year of therapy *(9)*. Polymerase mutants are absent from untreated patients, and exhibit generally lower virulence than wild-type, due to lower catalytic activity, or possible missense disruption of the overlapping *S* gene. Clinical manifestations of breakthrough infection are variable: most patients sustain lower-than-pretreatment serum DNA and ALT levels, but in rare occasions, emergence is accompanied by ALT flares and hepatic decompensation. Upon therapy withdrawal, the re-emergence of wild-type HBV typically yields further bouts of hepatitis.

Several mutations which confer resistance to lamivudine have been shown to cause substitutions within or adjacent to the "YMDD" motif at the catalytic site of the polymerase. A protein structure-based model by which these mutated residues block drug action has been proposed *(10)*. Famciclovir-associated polymerase gene mutations, commonly affecting upstream domains of the protein, have been identified in immunocompromised patients. Upstream mutations are more likely to affect immune epitopes on HBsAg, although the effect on antigenicity has yet to be determined. Unfortunately, the two most common famciclovir-resistance mutations, L528M and V521L, are also observed with lamivudine treatment, suggesting that patients who develop lamivudine-resistant mutants may not respond favorably to famciclovir treatment, and vice-versa. Phase III clinical trials for lobucavir and adefovir treatment will permit the identification of mutants associated with these agents. Recent in vitro and in vivo studies indicate that YMDD gene variants resistant to lamivudine remain sensitive to adefovir, suggesting that the antiviral effects of these drugs will be additive. The identification of such mutually exclusive resistance profiles may be useful in the design of effective sequential or combination therapy regimes.

HEPATITIS C VIRUS

The most remarkable feature of hepatitis C virus is its ability to establish chronic infection, which occurs in 55–85% of patients *(11)*. In contrast to HBV, HCV exhibits extreme variability in nucleotide sequence. At least 11 different genotypes, exhibiting diverse clinical outcomes, have been identified. For a genotype 1a strain, the complete ~9600 nucleotide (nt) RNA genome has been verified by in vivo chimpanzee transfection, using transcripts derived from consensus cDNA clones. During the course of an infection, HCV mutations accrue at the rate of $1-2 \times 10^{-3}$ per base per year. Variants reflecting slight modifications to the coding sequence, so-called "quasispecies", are commonly found to co-exist simultaneously within a patient, and any given serum-derived HCV inoculum contains a population of closely related viruses. The observed "hypervariability" in HCV-envelope proteins is one explanation for the exceptional ability of HCV inocula to reinfect the same host following seroconversion and resolution of acute infection. The absence of protective immunity against HCV continues to thwart vaccine development, and the emergence of drug-resistant strains will likely pose a future obstacle to long-term efficacy of inhibitors designed to target the enzymes responsible for viral replication.

Replication Cycle

Chimpanzee infection studies revealed the principal etiologic agent of non-A, non-B hepatitis to be an enveloped, positive-sense RNA virus,

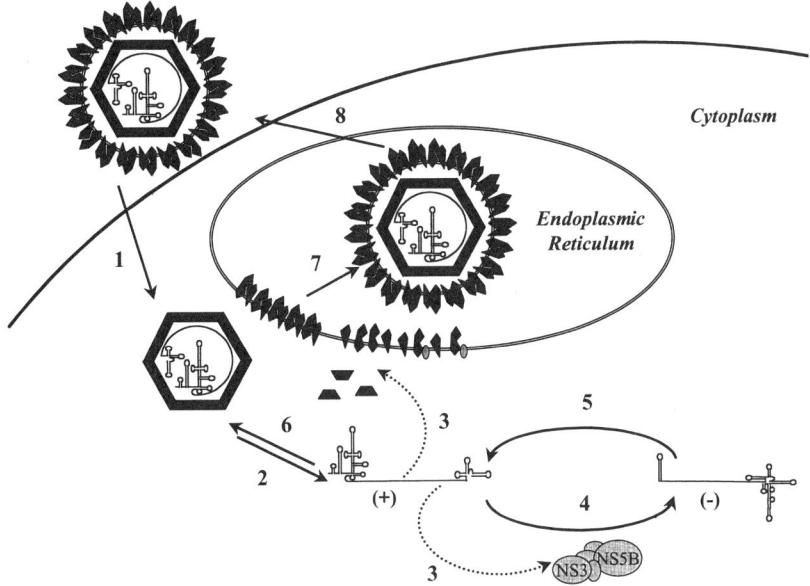

Fig. 3. HCV Replication Cycle. The events of hepatocellular HCV infection are indicated: (**1**) endocytosis, (**2**) uncoating, (**3**) translation and polyprotein processing, (**4**) negative strand synthesis and (**5**) positive strand synthesis by viral nonstructural (NS) proteins, (**6**) encapsidation, (**7**) budding, (**8**) secretion.

and HCV has since been characterized extensively in vitro *(12,13)*. The 5'-untranslated region (UTR) of virion RNA directs the cap-independent translation of a polyprotein, which is cleaved into structural (C, E1, E2, p7) and nonstructural (NS2, 3, 4A, 4B, 5A, 5B) viral proteins *(14)*. Replication of the viral RNA is carried out by an HCV-encoded RNA-dependent RNA polymerase, through a full-length negative strand RNA intermediate (Fig. 3). Nascent positive strand RNAs can be utilized for translation, subsequent rounds of RNA replication, or packaging into virions. Although development of hepatitis in immunocompromised individuals suggests that HCV proteins may be directly cytopathic, the replication process is generally noncytolytic. In most cases, chronic infection continues for many years without evidence of hepatocyte injury.

Many details of the viral replication cycle, including the mechanisms of viral entry, RNA replication, packaging, and budding, remain obscure due to the lack of a complete cell culture replication system or a convenient animal model. Although HCV infection in several human lymphoblastoid and hepatocyte-derived cell lines has been reported, these systems exhibit low titer and poor reproducibility. Only recently has the cultivation of RNA replicons encompassing the HCV UTRs and nonstructural region permitted high level RNA replication and analysis of interferon-mediated inhibition *(15–17)*.

Viral Entry

Recent studies have identified viral and host cell components involved in HCV cell entry. The HCV envelope integral membrane proteins are glycosylated noncovalent heterodimers of two polypeptides, E1 and E2. The latter of these is apparently responsible for viral attachment, as E2-specific antisera can prevent HCV binding to cultured cells. Circulating HCV virions have been shown to associate with β-lipoproteins. The capsid protein, core, colocalizes with apolipoprotein AII and intracellular lipid droplets; this interaction may contribute to hepatic steatosis observed in core-transgenic mice. Notably, the expression of LDL receptor in some cell types was shown to induce HCV binding, which does not otherwise occur. The endocytosis of HCV particles appears to be mediated by LDL receptor, but may be assisted by other interactions. E2 was shown to bind a human cell-surface membrane protein, CD81. This interaction may contribute to entry of HCV virions into hepatocytes, although expression of CD81 not restricted to the liver.

HCV replication has been reported to occur in extrahepatic sites, most notably peripheral blood mononuclear cells (PBMCs) from chronically infected patients. High HCV RNA titers are observed in lymph nodes, and approx 50% of patients develop circulating HCV-associated cryoglobulins. An association with lymphoproliferative disorders such as non-Hodgkin's lymphoma has been reported. Lymphotropic variants of HCV have been isolated from passage in cell culture and chimpanzee PBMCs. Comparison of HCV RNA sequences isolated from viruses propagated in lymphocyte vs. hepatocyte cell lines revealed that the majority of amino acid positions which putatively influence cell tropism are located in E2.

Events following HCV-cell attachment remain to be elucidated. The E2 glycoprotein is insufficient for membrane fusion, and a hydrophobic region of the E1 glycoprotein has been proposed to mediate fusion of the viral envelope to the cell membrane. Upon cell entry, core associates with 60S ribosomal subunits, which may contribute to uncoating of RNA and initiation of HCV translation.

Translation

There is no evidence that HCV positive-strand RNA bears the 5'-methylguanidine cap and 3'-polyadenylate tail typical of eukaryotic messenger RNAs, but it is nonetheless sufficient to direct translation of the ~3000 amino acid-long HCV open reading frame. The 5'-UTR sequence folds into a complex secondary and tertiary RNA structure. Notably, it is one of the few regions of the genome exhibiting little sequence variation among all HCV genotypes. The ~300 nt region upstream of the initiator codon functions as an internal ribosome entry site (IRES). It directly recruits 40S ribosomal subunits to the start codon, and can do so even in the absence of any canonical eukaryotic initiation factors. The unique internal entry, and factor-independence of HCV ribosome binding stand in marked contrast to cap-dependent translation initiation of host cell genes, making the IRES a potential target for specific inhibition.

Sequences adjacent to the minimal IRES element are thought to influence its activity either by preventing disruption of RNA secondary structure, or possibly by recruiting host cell factors. Various host RNA-binding proteins have been isolated via their direct interaction with the HCV UTRs, although in many cases their identity and contribution to translation initiation remain obscure. Disruption of these interactions might destabilize the IRES structure or diminish ribosome entry, and could be explored as a treatment strategy. Indeed, the inhibition of translation, and/or the direct cleavage of positive strand RNA, may be essential components of an effective antiviral therapeutic regime. Because HCV translation does not require the preexistence of virally encoded factors, any remaining RNA is sufficient to initiate new rounds of replication, even if all HCV enzymes are simultaneously inhibited.

Protein Processing

Proteolytic processing of the HCV polyprotein is co- and post-translational, and mediated by both host and viral proteases (Fig. 4). The host signal peptidase, resident in the ER lumen, is responsible for cleavage between the HCV structural proteins, and separation at the p7/NS2 junction. The E1 and E2 proteins are translocated into the lumen of the ER, with the C-terminal domains remaining embedded the membrane.

Enzymatically-active viral proteases are essential for productive infection in the chimpanzee model *(18)*. Autocatalytic cleavage at the NS2/3 site is carried out by the flanking protein domains, initially believed to function as a metalloprotease, but whose structural motifs are more indicative of a zinc-stabilized cysteine protease. All other principal cleavage sites within the HCV nonstructural region are hydrolyzed by a serine protease embodied in the N-terminal domain of the NS3 protein. (There is some evidence for further processing within the NS3 region by a cellular protease, which may contribute to proposed nonenzymatic functions of

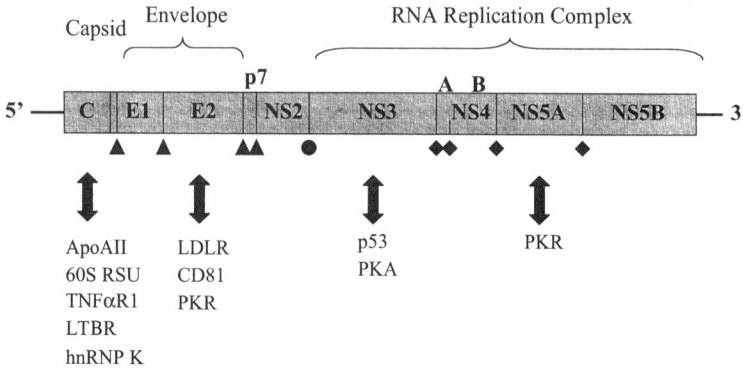

Fig. 4. HCV Polyprotein Processing and Host Factor Binding. Cleavage sites processed by host signal peptidase (△), NS2/3 protease (○), and NS3/4A protease (◇) are indicated. Putative interactions between the processed polypeptides and host cell factors are listed. (Abbreviations: ApoAII, apolipoprotein AII; RSU, ribosomal subunit; TNαR1, tumor necrosis factor-alpha receptor-1; LTBR, lymphotoxin-beta receptor; hnRNP, heterogeneous nuclear ribonucleoprotein; LDLR, low density lipoprotein receptor; PKR, double-stranded RNA-activated protein kinase; PKA, cyclic AMP-dependent protein kinase.)

various NS3 domains, discussed below.) Importantly, the stability and full activity of the NS3 protease requires association with the NS4A polypeptide, and the enzyme active site may be subject to steric inhibition by the C-terminus of the NS3 protein. These properties, in addition to the known substrate specificity and crystal structure of the NS3/4A complex, will be important considerations for the design of HCV protease inhibitors.

Immune System Evasion

Once synthesized, the various HCV proteins are subject to host-mediated proteolytic degradation and presentation on the cell surface as foreign antigens. Epitopes from all HCV proteins can be presented by multiple MHC Class I and II haplotypes, and are susceptible to recognition by immunoglobulins and T cell receptors *(19)*. In acute and IFN-resolved cases, humoral, CD4+ T cell, and CD8+ CTL responses are directed against all viral antigens, and are especially vigorous against epitopes on core and NS3. In comparison to HBV, viral antigen expression is relatively low in hepatitis C, but unlike some other viruses, HCV does not appear to actively subvert antigen processing and/or presentation. To the contrary, the expression of molecules which mediate antigen recognition, such as MHC, intracellular adhesion molecules, TNF-α, and Fas antigen, is upregulated in HCV-infected cells. In chronic infection, the HCV-specific CTL response is effective enough to maintain some control over viral load, but the majority of patients develop only a modest humoral response, and are unable to establish a robust CTL activity sufficient to achieve clearance.

How HCV is able to persist in the face of an active, concerted immune response is unclear. The lack of a virus-associated reverse transcriptase activity precludes integration into the host genome. Given the quasispecies nature of HCV infection, it is likely that "escape mutations" arise from nucleotide misincorporation by NS5B RNA-dependent RNA polymerase activity. It has long been presumed that sequence heterogeneity in immunodominant epitopes allows immune-mediated selection of resistant quasispecies. There is some evidence that selection of humoral escape variants can occur during the course of HCV infection in humans and chimpanzees. The principal neutralization epitope, hypervariable region-1 (HVR1, a 27–30 residue amino acid sequence located in the E2 N-terminus) exhibits extreme variation among known isolates. Quasispecies with mutated HVR1 have been shown to arise in response to antibody selection against the parent sequence. It is also possible that mutations modify a dominant CTL epitope, as has been observed in chimpanzee acute infection. Mutation may even convert viral polypeptides to potent antagonists of CTL directed against the wild type sequence. This scenario has been observed with an NS3 epitope.

Further analysis suggests that the immune escape strategy is a secondary effect. The CTL response in chronic infection is typically polyclonal and multispecific. It is unlikely that escape variants arise continuously and simultaneously for all determinants. Recent chimpanzee transfection studies demonstrate that persistent infection is possible in the absence of inoculum sequence diversity, without mutation of any previously identified immune epitopes, even for deletion mutants lacking HVR1 altogether *(20)*. While immune escape may provide one avenue for maintenance of high levels of viremia in a pre-existing infection, it does not appear to be necessary for the establishment of chronicity.

The failure to clear HCV infection could conceivably result from a quantitative overwhelming of the T-cell response. The kinetics of viral replication may yield an insurmountably high ratio of infected hepatocytes to effector T cells. High viral load may also induce peripheral tolerance or T-cell "anergy", wherein HCV-specific CTL, activated in secondary lymphoid organs, are subsequently inactivated in the liver, because the viral antigen is presented in the absence of requisite costimulatory signals. HCV may exacerbate this scenario from within the host cell by debilitating the host cell response to cytotoxic mediators or other cytokines.

Inhibition of the Intracellular Antiviral Response

Several HCV-encoded proteins actively subvert the intracellular antiviral response. NS5A and E2 are known to inhibit the double-stranded RNA-activated protein kinase (PKR), an effector of the IFN-α pathway. Activation of PKR by double-stranded RNA substrates, such as viral RNA replication intermediates, causes phosphorylation of eukaryotic initiation factor 2, thereby shutting down translation of any host genes which might aid in viral replication. Binding by NS5A is thought to block dimerization of PKR, preventing its activation. The sequence of a relatively conserved 40 amino acid region within the putative PKR-binding domain of NS5A (the "interferon sensitivity-determining region," ISDR) was previously shown to correlate with resistance to interferon treatment for Japanese patients infected with certain HCV genotypes. However, the correlation is weak or nonexistent when the analysis is extended to other geographic regions or genotypes, and the selection of resistant ISDR sequences during the course of interferon treatment does not appear to be common. The NS5A protein may disrupt the interferon response in other ways, as the C-terminal region exhibits transcriptional activation properties and bears a nuclear localization signal. Although these functions are not evident in the full-length protein, liberation of the C-terminus by proteolytic processing raises the possibility that NS5A might influence expression of other host genes involved in the antiviral immune response.

HCV-core protein is known to inhibit apoptosis in various cell types. Although results from some experimental systems suggest that core actually sensitizes cells to TNF- or Fas-mediated apoptosis, it is possible that this viral protein modulates intracellular signal transduction pathways so as to abrogate cell death signals. The interaction of core protein with the lymphotoxin-Beta receptor and TNF receptor-1, and concomitant effects on intracellular signaling, have been demonstrated in vitro. It has been proposed that in this way, HCV disrupts host nuclear factor-κB-mediated signaling, so as to confer a survival advantage to infected hepatocytes, or to prevent activation of B cells.

The NS3 protein may disrupt signal transduction pathways governing cell death and proliferation. The helicase domain includes a short amino acid sequence similar to autophosphorylation and inhibitor regulatory sites of cyclic AMP-dependent protein kinase (PKA). Polypeptides bearing this NS3 sequence bind to the PKA catalytic subunit, inhibiting its nuclear translocation and phosphorylation of host cell substrates. The NS3 protease domain suppresses actinomycin D-induced apoptosis in some cell types, apparently by sequestering or decreasing the expression of p53.

HCV Proteins and Hepatocarcinogenesis

The anti-apoptotic effects of viral proteins, in addition to increased cellular turnover resulting from chronic inflammation, may contribute to the development of HCV-associated HCC *(21)*. The prevalent HCC incidence in HCV carriers, estimated at 20%, suggests an important role for the virus in hepatocarcinogenesis. HCV proteins are almost invariably expressed in these tumors, and some chronically infected patients develop HCC even in the absence of cirrhosis.

Although the C-terminal hydrophobic region of full-length HCV core renders the polypeptide membrane-associated and localized to cytoplasmic membranes, the N terminus bears a nuclear localization signal. Some in vitro expression studies suggest that core, and particularly its C-terminally truncated forms, can be phosphorylated by protein kinases A and C, and translocated to the nucleus. Core may exhibit transcriptional regulatory activity on cellular promoters, so as to induce host cell proliferation. Accordingly, core has been shown to activate the c-myc promoter, and to suppress transcription of c-fos, p53, Rb, and β-IFN. Additionally, it may interact with heterogeneous nuclear ribonucleoprotein K, so as to derepress the human thymidine kinase gene promoter.

In coexpression studies with H-ras oncogene, core contributed to the tumorigenic transformation of primary rodent fibroblast cells. HCC development reportedly occurs in transgenic mice expressing core, and C-terminal mutations in the core coding sequence have been observed in HCV RNA isolated from human HCC tissue. The serine protease domain of NS3 has also been reported to transform murine cells, and to induce HCC in transgenics. In addition to the possible direct oncogenic effects of these proteins, neoplastic transformation likely arises as an inevitable consequence of chronic liver cell proliferation, a condition which may be deliberately induced by HCV in order to maximize viral replication.

RNA Replication

The RNA polymerase activity responsible for HCV RNA synthesis is encoded in the NS5B region. This viral protein is sufficient for synthesis of full length HCV RNA in vitro, although many host proteins are known to bind HCV 3'-terminal sequences, and may influence template specificity in vivo. The HCV 3'-UTR contains a polypyrimidine (U/UC) sequence of variable length, and terminates in a highly conserved 98 nt sequence, the "X region." X is nearly identical in every isolate analyzed thus far, consistent with its essential role in replication. Deletion of X, or of the polypyrimidine sequence immediately upstream, renders RNA noninfectious in the chimpanzee model. Although the negative strand 3'-terminus lacks a large polypyrimidine tract, the terminal 239 nt have been shown to function in vitro as a template for NS5B RDRP activity.

In vitro NS5B assays indicate that HCV RNA synthesis is initiated by a primer-independent *de novo* mechanism. Notably, the 3'-terminal 45 nt of the positive strand fold into a thermodynamically-stable stem-loop structure, which may require unwinding by an RNA helicase in order for the polymerase to gain access. Accordingly, NS3, found to colocalize with NS5B, bears an NTPase/helicase activity in its C terminal domain. NS3 helicase binds HCV UTR sequences, unwinds RNA duplexes in a 3' to 5' direction, and is essential for infection in the chimpanzee model *(18)*. The helicase is thought to dissociate nascent complementary strands from the HCV RNA template, although NS3 activity has not yet been demonstrated in the context of viral RNA synthesis.

The C-terminal hydrophobic sequence of NS5B is necessary for its localization into membrane-associated complexes in the perinuclear region, the proposed site of HCV replication. These complexes are thought to form by noncovalent protein-protein linkage of all HCV NS proteins, with the exception of NS2, in association with one or more host-encoded factors. These protein aggregates are tethered to ER membranes by the NS4A peptide. Dissociation of replication complexes, or disruption of their anchorage to membranes, present possible means to inhibit RNA replication. Also, the recently solved crystal structures of NS5B and the NS3 helicase domain will facilitate the rational design of inhibitors.

HCV RNA replication appears to be influenced in subtle ways by the NS5A protein. Two forms of NS5A, differing in the extent of serine phosphorylation, are generally present within infected cells. This phosphorylation may serve to regulate NS5A subcellular localization and putative transcriptional regulatory activity. However, the utility of NS5A hyperphosphorylation, and the identity of the kinase responsible for it, remain to be determined. Interestingly, mutation of serine phosphorylation sites, or deletion of the ISDR, greatly enhances replication of subgenomic HCV replicons in cell culture *(16)*.

Like the HBV polymerase, HCV NS5B lacks proofreading activity and exhibits a high rate of nucleotide misincorporation. To some degree, HCV may avoid replicating lethally mutated genomes by utilizing only the genomic RNA template from which NS5B is translated. Still, it is thought that the majority of serum HCV RNA is replication-defective, bearing one or more mutations prohibitive of viral replication. Because its coding sequence is non-overlapping, HCV presumably exhibits a higher tolerance for mutation than HBV. Therefore, HCV escape variants may present an even greater obstacle for therapy than the HBV mutants. The oral nucleoside analogue, ribavirin, has shown promise as an inhibitor of HCV replication, but its effects on HCV RNA levels are generally transient.

Assembly and Secretion

The details of HCV virion assembly are very poorly understood at present, but the recent development of cell-culture-based systems for the production of virus-like particles may soon shed light on the relevant mechanisms. Although core protein oligomerization and specific interaction with E1 have been demonstrated, core exhibits only non-specific RNA binding. Core may preferentially bind positive strand RNA, but no discrete encapsidation signal is apparent. By analogy to HBV pregenomic RNA, which binds to both of its gene products to facilitate packaging and replication, the HCV positive strand may bind core and NS5B cotranslationally. Binding to core might suppress IRES activity, leading to a transition from replication to assembly. Another event which may contribute to virion formation is the C-terminal proteolytic processing of the core and E2 proteins. At the time of translation, the cleavage between E2 proper and p7 is incomplete, giving rise to two forms of the envelope protein. An as yet unidentified protease, possibly signal peptide peptidase, is believed to trim the E1 signal sequence from the core C-terminus posttranslationally.

The E2 C-terminal domain acts as an ER retention signal; the glycoproteins are not translocated through the Golgi apparatus to the cell surface unless incorporated into virion envelopes. Therefore, cytoplasmic HCV core-encapsidated RNA particles are thought to bud through the ER membrane, rather than the cell membrane. In so doing, they acquire a coating of E1-E2 heterodimers. The complete virions progress through the Golgi apparatus, and are released into the extracellular space by exocytosis. Interestingly, transgenic mice expressing HCV E1 and E2 exhibit salivary and lachrymal exocrinopathy resembling Sjogren's syndrome, suggesting that these proteins may disrupt cellular exocytosis, and contribute to pathogenesis of this disorder in chronically infected patients.

It is estimated that a typical infected liver releases $\sim 10^{12}$ HCV virions per day. Assuming 10% of hepatocytes are infected, this amounts to 50 particles per cell per day. Hepatocytes generally maintain a low level of intracellular RNA; approx 3×10^{11} RNA molecules are produced daily. Thus, as with HBV, there is evidence that a substantial portion of released particles are replication-defective virions, or naked core structures. With a virion half-life of just 4–7 h, most patients have an understandably low serum titer.

CONCLUSION: FUTURE TREATMENT STRATEGIES

It is apparent from the above discussion that, given the compactness of HBV and HCV genomes, conserved sites exhibiting multiple essential functions can be readily identified. It may be possible to design single inhibitors, or therapeutic regimes, which target these important viral functions simultaneously. Our expanding knowledge of hepatitis virus molecular biology has provided a wealth of novel strategies to achieve maximal genomic coding capacity, persistence of infection, and immune system evasion. Application of these concepts may be useful for the design of gene therapy constructs, perhaps even hepatotropic vectors based on HBV- or HCV-derived replicons.

ACKNOWLEDGMENT

The support of the grant NIDDK-42182 from NIH, the Herman Lopata Chair in Hepatitis Research, and the secretarial assistance of Mrs. Martha Schwartz is gratefully acknowledged.

REFERENCES

1. Seeger C, Mason WC. Hepatitis B virus biology. Microbiol Mol Biol Rev 2000; 64: 51–68.
2. Magnius LO, Norder H. Subtypes, genotypes and molecular epidemiology of the hepatitis B virus as reflected by sequence variability of the S-gene. Intervirology 1995; 38: 24–34.
3. Lok AS. Hepatitis B infection: pathogenesis and management. J Hepatol 2000; 32 (1 Suppl): 89-97.
4. Kramvis A, Kew MC. The core promoter of hepatitis B virus. J Viral Hepat 1999; 6: 415–427.
5. Nassal M. Hepatitis B virus replication: novel roles for virus-host interactions. Intervirology 1999; 42: 100–116.
6. Feitelson MA. Hepatitis B virus in hepatocarcinogenesis. J Cell Physiol 1999; 181: 188–202.
7. Murakami S. Hepatitis B virus X protein: structure, function and biology. Intervirology 1999; 42: 81–99.
8. Brunetto MR, Rodriguez UA, Bonino F. Hepatitis B virus mutants. Intervirology 1999; 42: 69–80.
9. Hussain M, Lok ASF. Mutations in the hepatitis B virus polymerase gene associated with antiviral treatment for hepatitis B. J Viral Hepat 1999; 6: 183–194.
10. Doo E, Liang TJ. Molecular anatomy and pathophysiologic implications of drug resistance in hepatitis B virus infection. Gastroenterology 2001; 120: 1000–1008.
11. Liang TJ, Rehermann B, Seeff LB, Hoofnagle JH. Pathogenesis, natural history, treatment, and prevention of hepatitis C. Ann Int Med 2000; 132: 296–305.
12. Hagedorn CH, Rice CM, editors. The hepatitis C viruses (Current Topics Microbiol Immunol, Vol. 242). Springer-Verlag, New York, NY.

13. Bartenschlager R, Lohmann V. Replication of hepatitis C virus. J Gen Virol 2000; 81: 1631–1648.
14. Suzuki R, Suzuki T, Ishii K, Matsuura Y, Miyamura T. Processing and functions of hepatitis C virus proteins. Intervirology 1999; 42: 145–152.
15. Lohmann V, Korner F, Dobierzewska A, Bartenschlager R. Mutations in hepatitis C virus RNAs conferring cell culture adaptation. J Virol 2001; 75: 1437–1449.
16. Blight KJ, Kolykhalov AA, Rice CM. Efficient initiation of HCV RNA replication in cell culture. Science 2000; 290: 1972–1975.
17. Frese M, Pietschmann T, Moradpour D, Haller O, Bartenschlager R. Interferon-α inhibits hepatitis C virus subgenomic RNA replication by an MxA-independent pathway. J Gen Virol 2001; 82: 723–733.
18. Kolykhalov AA, Mihalik K, Feinstone SM, Rice CM. Hepatitis C virus-encoded enzymatic activities and conserved RNA elements in the 3' nontranslated region are essential for virus replication in vivo. J Virol 2000; 74: 2046–2051.
19. Cerny A, Chisari FV. Pathogenesis of chronic hepatitis C: immunological features of hepatic injury and viral persistence. Hepatology 1999; 30: 595–601.
20. Forns X, Thimme R, Govindarajan S, Emerson SU, Purcell RH, Chisari FV, Bukh J. Hepatitis C virus lacking the hypervariable region 1 of the second envelope protein is infectious and causes acute resolving or persistent infection in chimpanzees. Proc Natl Acad Sci USA 2000; 97: 13,318–13,323.
21. Colombo M. Hepatitis C virus and hepatocellular carcinoma. Semin Liver Disease 1999; 19: 263–267.

2 Epidemiology of Hepatitis B and Hepatitis C

Robert L. Carithers, Jr., MD

CONTENTS

INTRODUCTION
PREVALENCE OF HEPATITIS B AND HEPATITIS C
RISK OF CHRONIC INFECTION AND SEQUELAE OF DISEASE
MODES OF TRANSMISSION
SPECIAL PATIENT POPULATIONS
SUMMARY
REFERENCES

INTRODUCTION

There are striking epidemiological and clinical parallels between hepatitis B and hepatitis C virus infections. Each virus can be transmitted by bloodborne routes, such as transfusions or injection drug use. Acute infections often are asymptomatic, but can result in persistent viremia and chronic liver injury. Finally, chronic infection with either virus may cause minimal symptoms for decades, but ultimately can progress to cirrhosis and hepatocellular carcinoma (HCC).

There also are distinctive differences between hepatitis B and hepatitis C. The risk of developing chronic hepatitis B is closely correlated with the patient's age at the time of infection. Most infants and children exposed to hepatitis B develop chronic infection, but adults typically have self-limited infection. By contrast, the risk of developing chronic hepatitis C (CHC) is high, irrespective of the age at which initial infection occurs. There also are marked differences in the risk of sexual and maternal–fetal transmission of the two viruses. Highly effective methods are available for preventing infection with hepatitis B. By contrast,

From: *Clinical Gastroenterology: Diagnosis and Therapeutics*
Edited by: R. S. Koff and G. Y. Wu © Humana Press Inc., Totowa, NJ

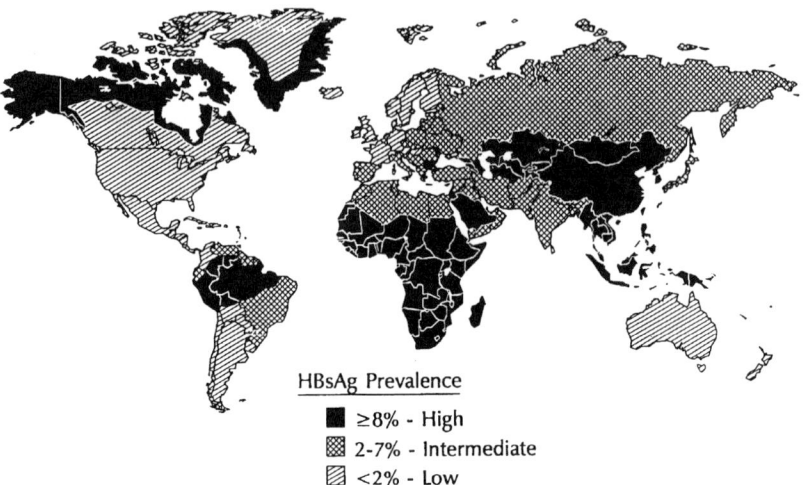

Fig. 1. Geographical distribution of hepatitis B. Reproduced with permission from ref. *1a*.

no effective means of active or passive prevention of HCV infection are currently available.

A clear understanding of similarities and differences in the transmission, natural history, and methods for preventing the spread of these important hepatitis viruses is essential to optimal care and education of patients and their families.

PREVALENCE OF HEPATITIS B AND HEPATITIS C

More than 300 million individuals throughout the world have chronic HBV infection *(1)*. The prevalence of hepatitis B varies widely from one geographic region to another (Fig. 1). In many parts of Asia and Africa, as many as 10% of the population have active infection with hepatitis B. By contrast, the prevalence of chronic hepatitis B in the United States is only 0.4%, with an estimated 1 million hepatitis B virus (HBV) carriers. Although the global impact of hepatitis C has yet to be conclusively determined, similar variations in infection rates occur from one geographical region to another. Chronic infection rates as high as 10–15% have been reported in some African and Middle Eastern countries *(2)*. In the United States, approx 1.8% of the population, or 3.9 million individuals, have antibodies to hepatitis C. Approximately 75% of these individuals have circulating HCV RNA, indicating active infection *(3)*.

Within the United States, the prevalence of both hepatitis B and hepatitis C is higher among African Americans and Hispanics (Fig. 2) *(3,4)*. In addition, chronic hepatitis B is particularly common among Alaskan

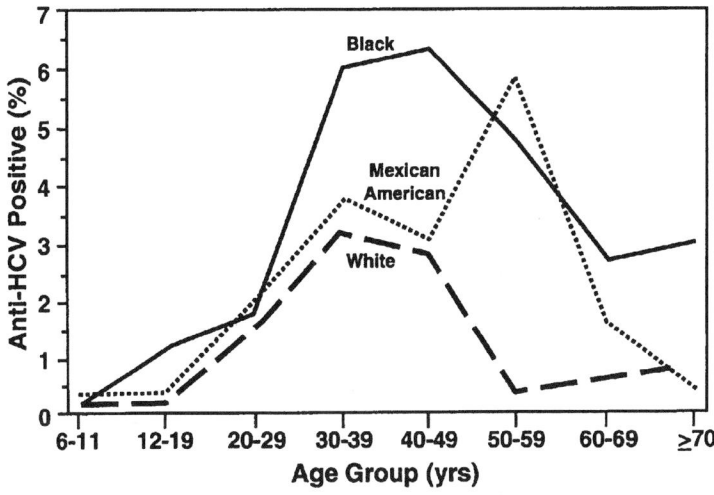

Fig. 2. Prevalence of HVC infection by age and race/ethnicity: United States 1988–1994. Reproduced with permission from ref. *13*.

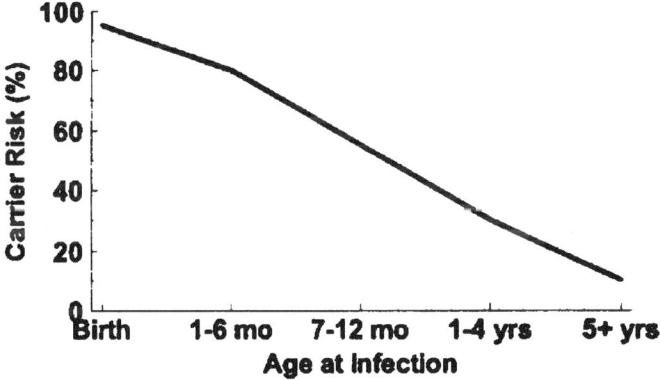

Fig. 3. Risk of developing chronic hepatitis B by age at infection. Reproduced by permission of Hepatitis Branch Centers of Disease Control, Atlanta, GA.

Eskimos, Pacific Islanders, and immigrants from countries where hepatitis B is endemic *(5)*. Hepatitis B and hepatitis C infections also are more frequent among individuals from low socioeconomic groups.

RISK OF CHRONIC INFECTION AND SEQUELAE OF DISEASE

Both the severity of acute hepatitis and the risk of developing chronic hepatitis B are related to the age at which the infection is acquired (Fig. 3). Infants and children typically have asymptomatic acute hepatitis, but have an inordinately high risk of developing chronic hepatitis B and suffering the sequelae of cirrhosis and HCC later in life. Over 90% of infants who acquire hepatitis B at birth develop chronic infection. Children exposed to the virus within the first 5 yr of life have a 25–50% risk of developing chronic infection. By contrast, acute hepatitis B can be severe in older individuals, but no more than 5% of adolescents and adults develop chronic infection *(6)*.

Both the severity of acute hepatitis and the risk of developing CHC are more uniform among various age groups. Most patients have anicteric hepatitis, with few symptoms. Approximately 85% of adults with acute hepatitis C develop chronic viremia, and 70% have biochemical or histological evidence of chronic liver disease *(7)*. Infection among adults over the age of 40 yr is associated with more rapidly progressive chronic disease *(8)*. By contrast, children infected within the first decade of life have only a 50% chance of developing CHC, and often have mild liver disease *(9,10)*.

Acute infection during infancy or childhood with either hepatitis B or hepatitis C usually is characterized by a mild, often asymptomatic illness, with a high rate of progression to chronic infection. Among adults, hepatitis B infection may result in severe illness, including fulminant hepatic failure; however, the risk of chronic infection is low. By contrast, adults who acquire hepatitis C often have a relatively asymptomatic acute illness, but a high risk of developing chronic infection. Few, if any, patients with acute hepatitis C develop fulminant hepatic failure. As a consequence, the morbidity and mortality of acute hepatitis B is considerably higher than hepatitis C. The long-term sequelae of hepatitis B and hepatitis C are similar in countries in which hepatitis B is endemic, because of the high rate of chronic hepatitis B virus infection among infants and children. By contrast, in countries such as the United States, where most HBV and HCV infections are acquired later in life, the overall impact of chronic hepatitis C virus infections is far greater than that of chronic hepatitis B.

MODES OF TRANSMISSION

In contrast to hepatitis A and E, in which most infections occur from oral ingestion of the virus, or from contact with infected individuals, hepatitis B and hepatitis C are transmitted primarily by parenteral routes.

Blood and Tissue Transmission

Both hepatitis B and hepatitis C can be very efficiently transmitted by blood transfusions, transplantation of infected organs, or injection drug use. In addition, administration of contaminated vaccines and use of non-

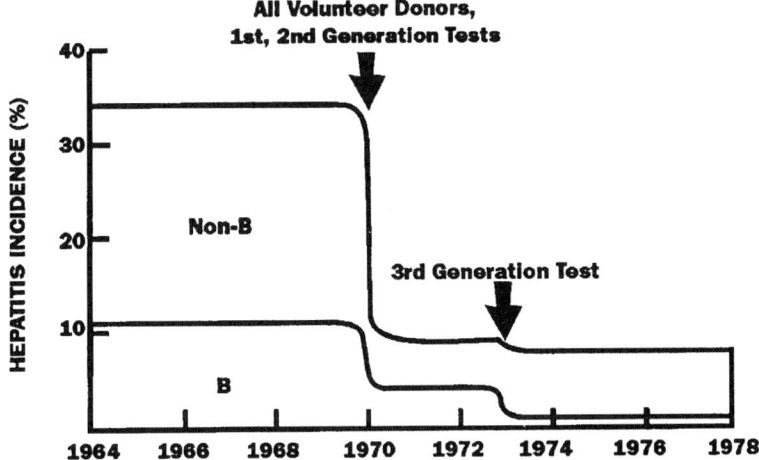

Fig. 4. Incidence of posttransfusion HBV infection. Reproduced with permission from ref. *11*.

disposable instruments have resulted in inadvertent transmission of both viruses. Other potential modes of transmission include tattooing, body piercing, acupuncture, and sharing razors and toothbrushes.

BLOOD TRANSFUSIONS

Jaundice and liver injury occurred in a disturbing number of individuals following the increased use of blood transfusions during and after World War II. These clinical observations offered strong evidence for an infectious cause of transfusion-associated jaundice, and stimulated research to identify the agents responsible. Shortly after the discovery of the virus in 1967, hepatitis B was identified as a major cause of posttransfusion hepatitis, accounting for approx 25% of cases. Exclusion of paid blood donors, and screening with increasingly accurate diagnostic tests for hepatitis B rapidly eliminated this virus as an important cause of posttransfusion hepatitis by the early 1970s (Fig. 4) *(11)*. Approximately 80 cases of transfusion-associated hepatitis B now are reported annually in the United States *(12)*.

From the 1970s until the early 1990s, hepatitis C accounted for over 90% of all cases of posttransfusion hepatitis. The highest risk was among individuals who received multiple transfusions or pooled products such as clotting factor concentrates. In the 1970s, 40% of all new cases of hepatitis C were acquired from blood transfusions *(13)*. However, following discovery of the HCV in 1988, sensitive and specific diagnostic tests to detect HCV infection became available. Widespread application of these tests in blood banks led to a precipitous drop in posttransfusion hepatitis C. Since 1992, the risk of acquiring hepatitis C from blood products is estimated to be only 0.001% per unit transfused *(14)*. However, it is recommended that individuals exposed to potentially infective blood products before 1992 undergo testing for hepatitis C *(15)*.

Currently, the risk of posttransfusion hepatitis B or hepatitis C is quite low *(14)*. Since 1992, no cases of posttransfusion hepatitis C have been reported in the United States *(11)*. However, there is a window between HBV or HCV infection and the development of circulating antigens or antibodies. Since potential donors in this window period might not be detected by the currently employed screening tests, blood banks are currently exploring the feasibility of evaluating potential donors using polymerase chain reaction-based techniques for detecting HBV DNA and HCV RNA in donor mini-pools *(14,16)*.

TRANSPLANTATION

Hepatitis B and hepatitis C can be transmitted during bone marrow or solid organ transplantation and occasionally even by transplantation of corneas and bone *(17,18)*. All organ donors currently undergo serologic testing for hepatitis B surface antigen (HBsAg), hepatitis B cone antibody (anti-HBc), and anti-HCV. HBsAg-positive donors usually are excluded, because of the high risk of viremia and transmission of hepatitis B to the recipient. Organs from HBsAg-negative donors with serologic evidence of past HBV infection (anti-HBc or anti-HBc and anti-HBs) can usually be used safely for kidney, pancreas, heart, and lung transplants *(19)*. However, organs from such donors not infrequently transmit HBV to liver transplant recipients *(20)*.

Approximately 4.2% of U.S. organ donors have positive tests for anti-HCV, which is over twice the prevalence in the general population *(21)*. Slightly more than one-half of these potential donors have circulating HCV RNA, indicating active HCV infection. Use of organs from HCV RNA-positive donors almost invariably results in HCV transmission to the transplant recipient *(22)*. Unfortunately, there is no rapid screening test available to quickly evaluate the presence of HCV RNA among anti-HCV-positive donors. As a result, there is considerable controversy on the use of organs from these donors. The safest approach is to exclude all anti-HCV-positive donors; however, in some parts of the country, this would result in loss of up to 10% of all potential organ donations. Given the drastic shortage of donor organs, organ procurement agencies and transplant programs are exploring a variety of options, including using anti-HCV-positive organs only in life-threatening situations or only in anti-HCV-positive recipients. The safety of these approaches has yet to be determined *(22)*.

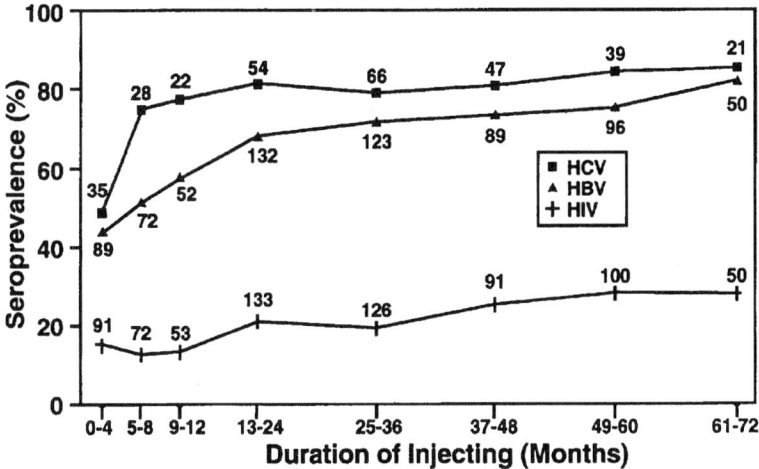

Fig. 5. Prevalence of HCV, HBV, and HIV infection with increasing duration of injection drug use. Modified with permission from ref. 23.

INJECTION DRUG USE

Injection drug use is an important means of transmitting both hepatitis B and hepatitis C. Many injection drug uses have serologic evidence of infection with both viruses. Within the first year, 50% of drug users acquire hepatitis B (Fig. 5) (23). The risk of hepatitis C is even higher, with 80% of young drug abusers infected within the first year (23). Injection drug use now is responsible for 60% of new cases of hepatitis C in the United States (15). Intranasal cocaine use also has been suggested as a possible cause of HCV infection (24). The vast majority of young people who acquire hepatitis C from injection drug use develop chronic infection. By contrast, the risk of developing chronic hepatitis B virus infection from injection drug use is less than 10%.

NOSOCOMIAL TRANSMISSION

Hepatitis B and hepatitis C also have been transmitted via various medical interventions. Nearly 350,000 U.S. soldiers acquired hepatitis B during World War II from a yellow fever vaccine contaminated with the virus. Transmission of hepatitis C appears to have occurred in many countries from folk treatments in which nonsterilized instruments are used (25). In Egypt, which has the highest prevalence of hepatitis C of any country, the virus appears to have been transmitted via injection therapy for schistosomiasis, in which nondisposable needles and syringes were used (2). Isolated outbreaks of hepatitis C also have resulted from iv immunoglobulin preparations contaminated with the virus (26). Iatrogenic transmission of hepatitis B and hepatitis C remains a concern in many countries *(27)*.

OTHER POTENTIAL MODES OF BLOODBORNE TRANSMISSION

Tattooing and body piercing using nonsterile instruments are other potential means of transmitting both hepatitis B and hepatitis C. Although well-documented in other countries, these modes of transmission appear to be uncommon in the United States. However, more study is needed, especially when these procedures are performed under substandard conditions, such as in prisons.

Maternal–Fetal Transmission

Maternal–fetal transmission of hepatitis B is virtually universal when the mother has active infection at the time of delivery. In countries where hepatitis B is endemic, maternal–fetal transmission is the primary mode of infection, and is responsible for 40–50% of cases of chronic hepatitis B. On a global basis, this is the most important mode of HBV transmission. In the United States, an estimated 20,000 infants are exposed to HBV at birth each year. Maternal transmission usually occurs at delivery, as the newborn is exposed to maternal blood and secretions during passage through the birth canal. Infected infants typically show serological evidence of asymptomatic HBV infection 2–6 mo after birth. Over 90% of these children develop chronic infection and face inordinate risks of developing liver failure and HCC later in life. For example, young men who acquire hepatitis B at birth have a relative risk of developing HCC 100× higher than age-matched controls *(28)*.

Maternal–fetal transmission of hepatitis C occurs much less frequently. Approximately 3–6% of infants born to mothers with CHC acquire the infection during the perinatal period. Women with higher levels of circulating virus and co-infection with HIV appear more likely to transmit infection to their newborn infants *(29)*. Current studies suggest that liver injury in these infected infants is very mild. Since the risk of perinatal transmission is small, and the morbidity of liver disease among infected children appears to be low, women with CHC do not need to avoid pregnancy *(13)*. However, children born to mothers with CHC should be tested for HCV, and, if chronic infection is documented, long-term follow-up with periodic liver function tests is warranted.

There is no convincing evidence that either hepatitis B or hepatitis C is transmitted by breastfeeding *(30,31)*. Therefore, there is no scientific basis for mothers with chronic hepatitis B or hepatitis C to avoid breastfeeding unless their nipples are cracked or bleeding *(13)*.

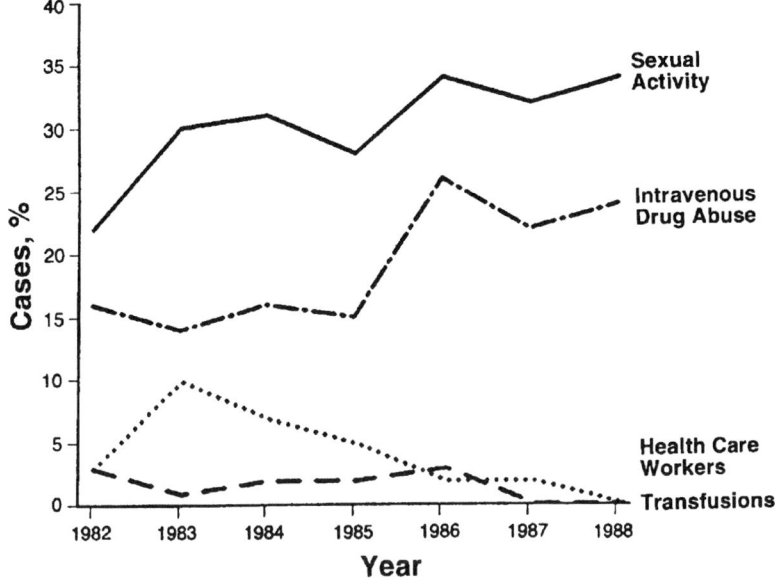

Fig. 6. Selected risk factors for acquiring hepatitis B in females. Centers of Disease Control Sentinel County Studies: 1982–1988. Modified with permission from ref. *4*.

Household Contacts

Hepatitis B infection can be acquired from household contacts. This is particularly true among children in countries where the prevalence of HBV is high. Contacts with serologic evidence of active chronic infection (HBsAg or HBV DNA) are the most prone to transmit HBV to other family members. By contrast, acquisition of HCV infection from household contacts appears to be uncommon.

Sexual Transmission

In the United States, almost two-thirds of reported cases of hepatitis B occur in young people between 15 and 29 yr of age *(4)*. Sexual transmission is the most common mode of transmission, accounting for almost one-third of the cases (Fig. 6) *(4)*. Men who have sex with men have a particularly high risk of harboring HBV infection.

The risk of sexual transmission of hepatitis C is a highly controversial and unresolved issue. The prevalence of hepatitis C is 2–3× higher among individuals with multiple sexual partners than in the general population. However, the risk of HCV infection is far lower than for hepatitis B, HIV, or other sexually transmitted diseases. In 15–20% of newly diagnosed cases of hepatitis C, sexual activity is the only risk factor that can be identified *(32)*. By contrast, the prevalence of HCV infection among long-term sexual partners of patients with CHC is no higher than the general population *(15)*. Thus, although sexual transmission of hepatitis C may occur, it seems to be very inefficient *(15)*.

Unknown Source of Infection

Even in the most carefully performed epidemiological studies, no specific risk factor can be found in approx 25% of patients with HBV infection and 10% of patients with HCV infection *(13)*. These findings leave considerable gaps in understanding of the epidemiology of these viral infections. Undoubtedly, some of these patients have risk factors, such as injection drug use, which they refuse to share with health care professionals. However, some patients appear to have no clear-cut risk factors for acquiring either hepatitis B or hepatitis C. One can only speculate as to the source of these infections.

SPECIAL PATIENT POPULATIONS

Hepatitis B and hepatitis C infections are particularly common in certain populations. The highest rates of infection are seen among patients who received multiple transfusions or blood products prepared from pooled donors, such as clotting factor concentrates. Chronic infection among transplant recipients also is common. Prisoners and other institutionalized individuals also have inordinate risks for these infections. In some, but not all, studies, retired military personnel, especially those who served in Vietnam, also have a high frequency of infection with hepatitis B or hepatitis C.

Hemophilia Patients

Before 1990, hemophilia patients, who received factor concentrates produced from pooled plasma, faced inordinately high risks of acquiring hepatitis B and HCV infections. Over one-half of these patients have evidence of exposure to hepatitis B; however, the carrier rate for chronic hepatitis B is <10% *(33)*. By contrast, between 75 and 90% of hemophilia patients who received factor concentrates during the 1970s and 1980s developed CHC. Although the full impact of these infections is not known, the risk of HCC is markedly increased among hemophilia patients, compared to the general population *(34–37)*.

Hepatitis infections among hemophilia patients have been virtually eliminated by adoption of virucidal methods of treating factor concentrates, screening plasma donors for HCV RNA by polymerase chain reaction techniques, and development of recombinant coagulation factors. No cases of hepatitis C from the use of factor concentrates have been reported since 1994 *(38)*.

Transplant Recipients

Hepatitis B and hepatitis C infections are common among transplant recipients. Although many patients are asymptomatic, with clinical and histological features of mild disease, infection with either of these viruses can be life-threatening.

Hepatitis B can be a lethal infection in immunosuppressed patients. Some patients have active HBV infection prior to transplantation. Other patients, with inactive disease and serologic features suggesting recovery from a prior infection (anti-HBc and anti-HBs), experience reactivation of disease with cancer chemotherapy or high-dose immunosuppression *(39)*. Patients also can acquire hepatitis B at the time of transplantation.

Many liver transplant recipients with active HBV infection in the past developed rapidly progressive, fatal disease following the operation. Reactivation of previously inactive disease, which is seen most commonly in marrow recipients who receive chemotherapy and immunosuppression, also can result in fulminant hepatic failure *(40)*. A variety of innovative strategies have been employed to overcome these challenges *(41)*. With specialized care, the outcome of patients with HBV infection has dramatically improved following transplantation.

Although less overt, CHC infection also can significantly affect long-term survival of transplant recipients. Cirrhosis secondary to hepatitis C has emerged as one of the leading causes of death in long-term survivors of bone marrow and kidney transplants *(42,43)*.

Injection Drug Users

Preventing transmission of hepatitis B and hepatitis C among young drug abusers is a critically important, but difficult, task. Most young people are unaware of the risk of acquiring these infections from drug use. Furthermore, very few young drug abusers have been vaccinated against hepatitis B, despite having contact with medical care providers *(44)*. Preventing hepatitis C transmission among young drug abusers is an even more difficult task. Needle exchange programs have been shown in some studies to reduce the risk of infection *(45)*. Such programs, in combination with drug treatment programs and intensive community-based education programs, will remain the mainstays of HCV prevention, until a vaccine is developed.

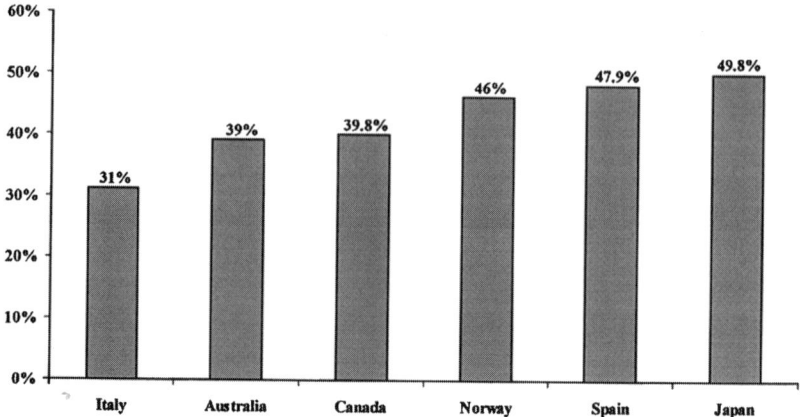

Fig. 7. Worldwide prevalence of hepatitis C in correctional populations. Reproduced with permission from ref. 46.

Prisoners

The prevalence of hepatitis C among prisoners ranges from 30 to 50% (Fig. 7) *(46)*. The overwhelming risk factor in this population is injection drug use, either before or during incarceration. Another potentially high risk means of exposure is tattooing with nonsterile instruments *(46)*. The overall impact of hepatitis B and hepatitis C on the correctional populations of the world remains to be determined.

Military Veterans

Chronic hepatitis infections also are common among military veterans. Although the risk of chronic hepatitis B is less than 5%, chronic hepatitis C virus infection has been reported in 7–36% of patients who use Veterans Administration hospitals in the United States *(47)*. The highest prevalence is among men 40–50 yr of age. Over 80% of these infections appear to have been acquired from iv drug use *(47)*. The long-term sequelae of these infections have yet to be determined.

Dialysis Patients

Numerous outbreaks of hepatitis B occurred among dialysis patients and staff in the 1970s. The patients often had asymptomatic chronic disease. In contrast, nurses and physicians often developed overt and serious acute illness. Aggressive infection control practices have dramatically reduced the incidence and prevalence of hepatitis B within dialysis units. For example, in 1976, the prevalence of HBsAg among dialysis patients was 7.8%, compared to 0.1% in 1993 *(48)*. However, occasional outbreaks of hepatitis B in dialysis units continue to occur, when rigorous infection control precautions are not maintained *(49)*.

Approximately 10–20% of hemodialysis patients have serologic evidence of HCV infection *(50,51)*. These patients are usually asymptomatic, and often have normal aminotransferase values. Most of these patients probably acquired hepatitis C from previous blood transfusions, although there have been isolated reports of HCV transmission within dialysis units. The incidence of new HCV infections in dialysis units has declined appreciably in recent years, largely as the result of improved safety of the blood supply and reduction in the number of transfusions administered.

Health Care Workers

Hepatitis B is the most commonly transmitted bloodborne virus in the health care setting *(52)*. The highest risk is among health care providers who have daily exposure to blood and tissues (dentists, surgeons, pathologists, and laboratory technicians). Widespread hepatitis B vaccination among health care providers has significantly reduced this risk over the past two decades.

The prevalence of HCV among health care workers is 10× lower than that of HBV *(15)*. In fact, the risk of HCV is no higher among health care providers than the general population of the United States *(15)*. Seroconversion rates after needlestick exposure to patients with active hepatitis C infections range from 0- to 7%. There is no effective means of preventing transmission in this setting *(15)*.

The transmission of either hepatitis B or hepatitis C from health care providers to patients is extremely rare. Most cases have been associated with breaks in sterile technique. However, isolated episodes of transmission from infected surgeons to patients have been reported for both hepatitis B and hepatitis C, despite adequate sterile precautions *(53,54)*.

SUMMARY

There are two global epidemiological patterns of HBV transmission. In populations in which the prevalence of hepatitis B is high, most new infections occur at birth or within the first 5 yr of life from maternal–fetal or horizontal transmission of the virus within families. Most of the infected infants and children develop chronic hepatitis B infection and face high risks of morbidity and mortality from chronic hepatitis and HCC later in life. By contrast, among populations in which the prevalence of hepatitis B is low, most new infections occur among adolescents and young adults from sexual transmission or injection drug use. The risk of chronic infection in this setting is generally less than 5%, and the long-term sequelae of chronic disease are much lower. Vaccination is effective in preventing transmission of hepatitis B at each of these settings. As a result, hepatitis B could potentially be eliminated as a global health problem within the next 30–50 yr.

The highest risk for acquisition of hepatitis C is among adolescents and young adults. The high rate of chronic infection exposes these young people to excessive risk of cirrhosis and HCC later in life. Unfortunately, no effective means of preventing transmission of hepatitis C are currently available. Nevertheless, the rate of new infections in the United States has declined sharply in recent years. This encouraging trend offers hope that aggressive educational programs may be effective in reducing transmission of this important pathogen.

REFERENCES

1. Maynard JE. Hepatitis B: global importance and need for control. Vaccine 1990; 8(Suppl): S18–S20.
1a. Mahoney FJ. Update on diagnosis, management, and prevention of hepatitis B virus infection. Clin Microbiol Rev 1999; 12: 351–366.
2. Frank C, Mohamed MK, Strickland GT, et al. Role of parenteral antischistosomal therapy in the spread of hepatitis C virus in Egypt. Lancet 2000; 355: 887–891.
3. Alter MJ, Kruszon-Moran D, Nainan OV, et al. Prevalence of hepatitis C virus infection in the United States, 1988 through 1994. N Engl J Med 1999; 341: 556–562.
4. Alter MJ, Hadler SC, Margolis HS, et al. Changing epidemiology of hepatitis B in the United States: need for alternative vaccination strategies. JAMA 1990; 263: 1218–1222.
5. Margolis HS, Alter MJ, Hadler SC. Hepatitis B: evolving epidemiology and implications for control. Semin Liver Dis 1991; 11: 84–92.
6. Lee WM. Hepatitis B virus infection. N Engl J Med 1997; 337: 1733–1745.
7. Alter MJ, Margolis HS, Krawczynski K, et al. Natural history of community-acquired hepatitis C in the United States. The Sentinel Counties Chronic Non-A, Non-B Hepatitis Study Team. N Engl J Med 1992; 327: 1899–1905.
8. Poynard T, Bedossa P, Opolon P. Natural history of liver fibrosis progression in patients with chronic hepatitis C. Lancet 1997; 349: 825–832.
9. Vogt M, Lang T, Frosner G, et al. Prevalence and clinical outcome of hepatitis C infection in children who underwent cardiac surgery before the implementation of blood-donor screening. N Engl J Med 1999; 341: 866–870.
10. Jonas MM. Hepatitis C infection in children. N Engl J Med 1999; 341: 912–913.
11. Alter H. Discovery of non-A, non-B hepatitis and identification of its etiology. Am J Med 1999; 107: 16S–20S.
12. Dodd RY. Risk of transfusion-transmitted infection. N Engl J Med 1992; 327: 419–421.
13. Williams I. Epidemiology of hepatitis C in the United States. Am J Med 1999; 107: 2S–9S.
14. Schreiber GB, Busch MP, Kleinman SH, Korelitz JJ. Risk of transfusion-transmitted viral infections. N Engl J Med 1996; 334: 1685–1690.

15. Centers for Disease Control and Prevention. Recommendations for prevention and control of hepatitis C virus (HCV) infection and HCV-related chronic disease. MMWR 1998; 47: 1–39.
16. Roth WK, Weber M, Seifried E. Feasibility and efficacy of routine PCR screening of blood donations for hepatitis C virus, hepatitis B virus, and HIV-1 in a bloodbank setting. Lancet 1999; 353: 359–363.
17. Hoft RH, Pflugfelder SC, Forster RK, et al. Clinical evidence for hepatitis B transmission resulting from corneal transplantation. Cornea 1997; 16: 132–137.
18. Conrad EU, Gretch DR, Obermeyer KR, et al. Transmission of the hepatitis-C virus by tissue transplantation. J Bone Joint Surg Am 1995; 77: 214–224.
19. Turner DP, Zuckerman M, Alexander GJ, et al. Risk of inappropriate exclusion of donor organs by introduction of hepatitis B core antibody testing. Transplantation 1997; 63: 775–777.
20. Dickson RC, Everhart JE, Lake JR, et al. Transmission of hepatitis B by transplantation of livers from donors positive for antibody to hepatitis B core antigen. The National Institute of Diabetes and Digestive and Kidney Diseases Liver Transplantation Database. Gastroenterology 1997; 113: 1668–1674.
21. Pereira BJ, Wright TL, Schmid CH, et al. Screening and confirmatory testing of cadaver organ donors for hepatitis C virus infection: a U.S. National Collaborative Study. Kidney Int 1994; 46: 886–892.
22. Terrault NA, Wright TL, Pereira BJG. Hepatitis C infection in the transplant recipient. Infect Dis Clin North Am 1995; 9: 943–964.
23. Garfein RS, Vlahov D, Galai N, et al. Viral infections in short-term injection drug users: the prevalence of the hepatitis C, hepatitis B, human immunodeficiency, and human T-lymphotropic viruses. Am J Public Health 1996; 86: 655–661.
24. Conry-Cantilena C, VanRaden M, Gibble J, et al. Routes of infection, viremia, and liver disease in blood donors found to have hepatitis C virus infection. N Engl J Med 1996; 334: 1691–1696.
25. Kiyosawa K, Tanaka E, Sodeyama T, et al. Transmission of hepatitis C in an isolated area in Japan: community-acquired infection. The South Kiso Hepatitis Study Group. Gastroenterology 1994; 106: 1596–1602.
26. Bresee JS, Mast EE, Coleman FJ, et al. Hepatitis C virus infection associated with administration of intravenous immune globulin: a cohort study. JAMA 1996; 276: 1563–1567.
27. Mast EE, Alter MJ, Margolis HS. Strategies to prevent and control hepatitis B and C virus infections: a global perspective. Vaccine 1999; 17: 1730–1733.
28. Beasley RP. Hepatitis B virus. Major etiology of hepatocellular carcinoma. Cancer 1988; 61: 1942–1956.
29. Ohto H, Terazawa S, Sasaki N, et al. Transmission of hepatitis C virus from mothers to infants. The Vertical Transmission of Hepatitis C Virus Collaborative Study Group. N Engl J Med 1994; 330: 744–750.
30. Beasley RP, Stevens CE, Shiao IS, Meng HC. Evidence against breast-feeding as a mechanism for vertical transmission of hepatitis B. Lancet 1975; 2: 740–741.
31. Mast EE, Alter MJ. Hepatitis C. Semin Pediatr Infect Dis 1997; 8: 17–22.
32. Alter MJ. Epidemiology of hepatitis C. Hepatology 1997; 26: 62S–65S.
33. Kumar A, Kulkarni R, Murray DL, Gera R, Scott-Emuakpor AB, Bosma K, et al. Serologic markers of viral hepatitis A, B, C, and D in patients with hemophilia. J Med Virol 1993; 41: 205–209.
34. Colombo M, Mannucci PM, Brettler DB, et al. Hepatocellular carcinoma in hemophilia. Am J Hematol 1991; 37: 243–246.

35. Rabkin CS, Hilgartner MW, Hedberg KW, et al. Incidence of lymphomas and other cancer in HIV-infected and HIV uninfected patients with hemophilia. JAMA 1992; 267: 1090–1094.
36. Darby SC, Ewart DW, Giangrande PL, et al. Mortality from liver cancer and liver disease in hemophilic men and boys in UK given blood products contaminated with hepatitis C. Lancet 1997; 350: 1425–1431.
37. Tradati F, Colombo M, Mannucci PM, et al. Prospective multicenter study of hepatocellular carcinoma in Italian hemophiliacs with chronic hepatitis C. Blood 1998; 91: 1173–1177.
38. Mannucci PM, Tuddenham EGD. Hemophilias: progress and problems. Semin Hematol 1999; 36(Suppl 7): 104–117.
39. Davis GL, Hoofnagle JH. Reactivation of chronic hepatitis B virus infection. Gastroenterology 1987; 92: 2028–2030.
40. Webster A, Brenner MK, Prentice HG, Riffiths PD. Fatal hepatitis B reactivation after autologous bone marrow transplantation. Bone Marrow Transplant 1989; 4: 207–208.
41. Davis CL, Gretch DR, Carithers RL, Jr. Hepatitis B and transplantation. Infect Dis Clin North Am 1995; 9: 925–941.
42. Mathurin P, Mouquet C, Poynard T, et al. Impact of hepatitis B and C virus on kidney transplantation outcome. Hepatology 1999; 29: 257–263.
43. Strasser SI, Sullivan KM, Myerson D, et al. Cirrhosis of the liver in long-term marrow transplant survivors. Blood 1999; 93: 3259–3266.
44. Seal KH, Edlin BR. Risk of hepatitis B infection among young injection drug users in San Francisco: opportunities for intervention. West J Med 2000; 172: 16–20.
45. Hagan H, Des Jarlais DC, Friedman SR, et al. Reduced risk of hepatitis B and C among participants in a syringe exchange program. Am J Public Health 1995; 85: 1531–1537.
46. Reindollar RW. Hepatitis C and the correctional population. Am J Med 1999; 107: 100S–103S.
47. Cheung RC. Epidemiology of hepatitis C virus infection in American veterans. Am J Gastroenterol 2000; 95: 740–747.
48. Tokars JI, Alter MJ, Favero MS, et al. National surveillance of dialysis associated diseases in the United States, 1993. ASAIO J 1996; 42: 219–229.
49. Favero MS, Alter MJ. Reemergence of hepatitis B virus infection in hemodialysis centers. Semin Dial 1996; 9: 373–374.
50. Chan TM, Lok ASF, Cheng IKP, Chan RT. Prevalence of hepatitis C virus infection in hemodialysis patients: a longitudinal study comparing the results of RNA and antibody assays. Hepatology 1993; 17: 5–8.
51. Seelig R, Renz M, Bottner C, Seelig HP. Hepatitis C virus infection in dialysis units; prevalence of HCV RNA and antibodies to HCV. Ann Med 1994; 26: 45–52.
52. Gerberding JL. Infected health care provider. N Engl J Med 1996; 334: 594–595.
53. Harpaz R, Von Seidlein L, Averhoff FM, et al. Transmission of hepatitis B virus to multiple patients from a surgeon without evidence of inadequate infection control. N Engl J Med 1996; 334: 549–554.
54. Esteban JI, Gomez J, Martell M, et al. Transmission of hepatitis C virus by a cardiac surgeon. N Engl J Med 1996; 334: 555–560.

3 Natural History of Hepatitis B Virus Infection

*David G. Forcione, MD,
Raymond T. Chung, MD,
and Jules L. Dienstag, MD*

CONTENTS

INTRODUCTION
ACUTE HBV INFECTION
CHRONIC HEPATITIS B VIRUS INFECTION
IMPACT OF IMMUNOPATHOGENETIC MECHANISMS
  OF HEPATITIS INJURY ON OUTCOME OF HEPATITIS B
EXTRAHEPATIC MANIFESTATIONS IN CHRONIC HEPATITIS B
  VIRUS INFECTION
PROGNOSIS AND SURVIVAL IN CHRONIC HEPATITIS B
HCC AND CHRONIC HEPATITIS B VIRUS INFECTION
INFECTION WITH HBV MUTANTS
VACCINATION IN HBV INFECTION
ANTIVIRAL THERAPY FOR CHRONIC HEPATITIS B VIRUS
  INFECTION
ROLE OF LIVER TRANSPLANT IN HEPATITIS B
FUTURE CONSIDERATIONS
REFERENCES

INTRODUCTION

Hepatitis B virus (HBV) infects over 350 million persons, and represents one of the world's leading public health problems. Although viral hepatitis has been known to mankind since the days of Hippocrates, it has only been in the last half century that the complex interactions between

From: *Clinical Gastroenterology: Diagnosis and Therapeutics*
Edited by: R. S. Koff and G. Y. Wu © Humana Press Inc., Totowa, NJ

HBV and its human host have been unraveled. Understanding of the natural history of HBV infection has evolved significantly since Blumberg's discovery of the Australia antigen (hepatitis B surface antigen [HBsAg]) in 1965. This landmark finding has been followed by a research explosion that has produced new insights into molecular virology and pathogenesis, a wide array of diagnostic assays, a safe and effective vaccine, and the introduction of effective treatment strategies designed to reduce the rate of complications.

Hepatitis B is associated with a wide spectrum of human disease, from acute, self-limited hepatitis to fulminant liver failure, and, in some, chronic hepatitis that may lead to cirrhosis, progressive hepatic failure, and neoplasia. Clinical observation and laboratory investigation have established that the natural history of HBV infection is determined by a dynamic interplay between virus, host immune response factors, and environmental cofactors.

ACUTE HBV INFECTION

Acute infection with HBV can occur through several different modes of transmission, with clear geographic variation. In many areas, especially those with a high prevalence of infection (East Asia, China, sub-Saharan Africa), perinatal transmission accounts for the majority of cases; however, in low-prevalence areas, such as Western Europe and the United States, sexual activity and percutaneous exposures appear to be the most common forms of transmission. Therefore, in high-prevalence areas, most HBV infections occur during infancy; in low-prevalence areas, most HBV infections occur during adulthood. In turn, age at time of infection is an important variable in outcome.

The clinical spectrum of acute hepatitis B infection in adults varies from a subclinical variant (approx two-thirds) to symptomatic hepatitis (approx one-third), and rarely fulminant liver failure requiring urgent liver transplantation (<1%). The vigor of the host cellular response probably determines which of the three patterns an infected individual will follow. In the great majority of acute HBV infections, the cellular immune response to viral peptides presented at the hepatocyte cell surface leads to effective immunologic clearance of virus-infected cells.

In the extreme case of fulminant hepatitis, an intense cytolytic T-lymphocyte response has been postulated to occur, resulting in massive hepatocyte necrosis and acute liver failure. Support for this concept comes from the finding that, in most of these cases, there are low to occasionally undetectable levels of viremia as determined by HBV DNA assays. A picture of fulminant or subfulminant liver failure may also be seen in

Table 1
Chronic Infection Rates by Age

Age at Acquisition	Infected
<1 yr old	>90%
1–6 yr old	20–50%
Adulthood	<5%

patients with chronic hepatitis B virus infection who are tapered off immunosuppressive agents, particularly corticosteroids, which enhance viral replication. In these cases, immune reconstitution, with withdrawal of immunosuppression in the face of enhanced replication, can lead to an overwhelming necroinflammatory response. In some populations (particularly Israel and Japan), fulminant HBV has been linked to the presence of specific mutants, especially the pre-core mutant, in which HBeAg, encoded by the C gene, is not expressed because of the formation of a premature stop codon. However, pre-core mutants can also be found in less severe episodes of hepatitis.

The rate of progression from acute infection to chronic infection is most closely linked to age at the time of infection, and, by inference, to the maturity of the immune response. Chronic infection occurs in <5% of patients who are infected in adulthood, but rises to 20–50% between the ages of 1 and 6 yr of age, and to 90%, if the infection is acquired during the perinatal period (1–3) (see Table 1). The low frequency of chronicity among adult-exposed cases was highlighted in an analysis of 330,000 U.S. soldiers in World War II, who were exposed to a contaminated lot of yellow fever vaccine. Thirty thousand developed clinical hepatitis, and, of nearly 600 veterans who were followed for 40 yr, fewer than 1% were still HBsAg-positive (4). Similarly, the frequency of chronic infection among healthy Greek military recruits with acute hepatitis B was 0.2% (5).

One group of investigators (6) demonstrated a protective effect of the human lymphocyte antigen (HLA) class II allele, DRB1*1302, in a Gambian population composed of both children and adults. Additional associations with specific polymorphic alleles linked to immune response are likely to be identified in the future; however, a comprehensive understanding of the determinants of a successful host response remains elusive. Although host immune factors appear critical in determining the outcome of acute HBV infection, viral factors appear to contribute little to outcome. The weight of evidence suggests that no one viral serotype is inherently more virulent or more likely to produce chronicity. Still,

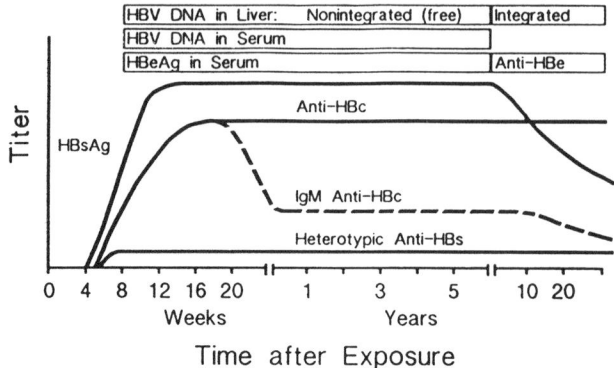

Fig. 1. Natural history of chronic hepatitis B virus infection (from AGA Teaching Collection).

preliminary information suggests potential differences in outcome, chronicity, and carcinogenicity among the six recognized HBV genotypes.

CHRONIC HEPATITIS B VIRUS INFECTION

Chronic hepatitis B infection becomes established following failure to clear HBsAg after 6 mo of infection (*see* Fig. 1). As noted, the development of chronicity is dependent on the failure of the immune system to effect clearance of virus-infected hepatocytes. chronic hepatitis B virus infection may be divided into two phases: highly replicative and relatively nonreplicative.

Perinatally acquired HBV infection appears to be associated with immunologic tolerance to the virus (postulated to be the result of *in utero* exposure to HBeAg, which functions as a tolerogen) (*see* Fig. 2a). This results in high levels of viral replication, without a robust immune response, and, therefore, minimal evidence of hepatic injury by histologic, biochemical, or clinical criteria. This phase may last decades, with low rates of spontaneous HBeAg seroconversion; studies have shown that, at 20 yr, fewer than 20% have seroconverted *(7,8)*. Episodes of seroconversion are often heralded by flares of alanine aminotransferase (ALT) levels, and have been molecularly linked to overexpression and relocation of hepatitis B core antigen from the nucleus to the cytoplasm. In general, these episodes are asymptomatic, but have been reported, uncommonly *(9)*, to result in acute decompensation and liver failure. The observation that men are more apt to experience exacerbations *(10)* has been pro-

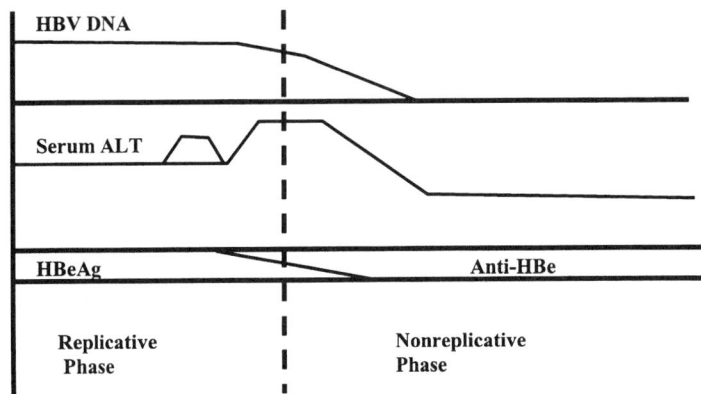

A Adult-acquired HBV infection

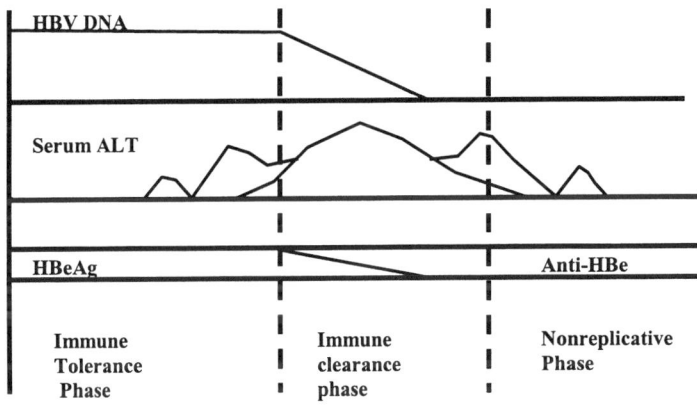

B Perinatally-acquired HBV infection.

Fig. 2. Natural history of HBV infection among HBeAg (+) and HBeAg (–) patients. (**A**) Adult-acquired HBV infection. (**B**) Perinatally acquired HBV infection. Adapted from *44–46*.

posed as one explanation for the higher frequency of acute liver failure and hepatocellular carcinoma (HCC) in men.

In adolescents and adults who acquire HBV, the replicative phase is characterized by a dynamic balance between high levels of HBV replication and expression and a vigorous immune response, which results in hepatic injury (*see* Fig. 2B). As a result, acute, clinically apparent hepatitis B in a healthy adult culminates, as a rule, in self-limited infection; chronicity is rare *(11)*.

The relatively nonreplicative phase characterizes the patient who has seroconverted to being anti-HBe-reactive. In nonreplicative HBV infection, low levels of HBV DNA are still detectable by ultrasensitive polymerase chain reaction assays. In general, HBeAg- to-anti-HBe seroconversion is accompanied by a marked reduction in infectivity, and, in liver injury, i.e., a change from chronic hepatitis to a carrier state, with limited or no hepatic inflammation. Overall, the estimated annual rate of spontaneous seroconversion is 7–20%. The rate of spontaneous HBeAg loss is approx 1–2%/yr. Indeed, highly replicative disease (HBeAg-reactive) is associated with an increased risk for cirrhosis, HCC, and mortality *(12–14)*.

There is one condition in which replicative infection may be associated with the HBeAg-negative, anti-HBe-reactive profile. Some such individuals harbor the previously mentioned pre-core or core-promoter mutants, and are thereby unable to generate detectable HBeAg, but can still have highly replicative HBV infection, and progressive liver disease.

IMPACT OF IMMUNOPATHOGENETIC MECHANISMS OF HEPATITIS INJURY ON OUTCOME OF HEPATITIS B

As noted, the most important determinants of chronicity are the age at acquisition of infection and the vigor of the host immune response. Further evidence for the importance of the immune system in control of HBV disease comes from observations demonstrating high levels of replicative HBV disease in HIV-co-infected persons. The host immune response to HBV is accountable for the massive necrosis found in patients with fulminant hepatitis, and for the development of chronic hepatitis. Even successful seroconversion may not reflect true viral eradication; in patients who clear HBeAg successfully, and in whom liver injury and chronic sequelae never materialize, traces of HBV DNA can be identified in liver years later, by polymerase chain reaction, raising the question of whether there is ever complete viral clearance following natural infection *(15)*.

Clearly, a better understanding of the intricate immune response mechanisms activated in HBV infection will permit identification of those individuals at greatest risk for chronicity. What is known is that recovery from acute HBV infection requires competent humoral and cellular responses. Neutralizing antibodies to the products of the pre-*S* and *S* genes are protective against subsequent re-infection. Perhaps the most effective and potent means of immune response is derived from the HLA class I-restricted $CD8^+$ T-lymphocytes. Adequate polyclonal T-lymphocyte activation results in effective recovery for individuals who have self-limited viral hepatitis. Such T-lymphocyte populations remain present for many years after the initial infection, and, in all likelihood, maintain surveillance over low levels of HBV that persist in hepatocytes and other sites.

In patients with chronic hepatitis B, $CD8^+$ and $CD4^+$ T-lymphocyte responses appear to be weaker and less likely to be polyclonal. Furthermore, in such patients viral antigen presentation on hepatocyte membranes is reduced, and a larger proportion of hepatocytes is infected. In patients who acquire HBV perinatally, immune tolerance occurs to the virus, despite high levels of virus, resulting in an enfeebled immune response and a milieu for chronicity. Chronicity in this setting does not appear to result from an HBV-specific T-cell clonal depletion; its mechanism has not been defined. Low-level transplacental passage of HBeAg has been postulated by some to induce tolerance by exhausting the fetal immune system, thus rendering the virus less susceptible to normal clearance mechanisms *(16)*.

In addition to direct T-cell-mediated lysis of infected hepatocytes, cytokine-mediated mechanisms probably play a role in viral clearance. For example, higher interleukin-12 levels, a T-helper 1 cytokine, have been associated with a higher likelihood of HBeAg seroconversion *(17)*. The preponderance of evidence argues against a substantial, direct cytopathic effect of HBV, although, under specific clinical conditions, high levels of HBV may be cytotoxic. One such example is fibrosing cholestatic hepatitis, a clinicopathologic entity seen in liver transplant recipients with recurrent HBV infection. Developing in up to 20% of patients with recurrent allograft HBV infection, fibrosing cholestatic hepatitis is associated with a paucity of inflammation, but severe ballooning degeneration in association with drastically elevated viral protein expression (especially HBcAg) *(18)*.

The same immune mechanisms responsible for limiting viral replication are also likely to be important mediators of malignant transformation associated with chronic hepatitis B virus infection. Such immune responses trigger inflammatory changes in the hepatic parenchyma, which, after long-standing disease, create a milieu suitable for local free-radical insult to genomic DNA, thus predisposing to oncogenicity. Supportive data for this hypothesis derive from mouse models in which S antigen overexpression itself is associated with an increased risk of neoplasia. Less information exists to support the mechanism of proto-oncogene activation via HBV DNA genomic integration, although the occasional occurrence of HCC in the noncirrhotic HBV carrier suggests that this event may be an important mechanism. Some experimental evidence exists for a potential role for the HBV X protein as a potent oncogene tranactivator.

EXTRAHEPATIC MANIFESTATION IN CHRONIC HEPATITIS B VIRUS INFECTION

Although HBV is hepatotropic, viral proteins and HBV DNA sequences have been found in other tissues, including peripheral blood lymphocytes. Nonetheless, other organs are rarely targets for HBV-associated injury. The exceptions are extrahepatic disorders attributable to circulating immune complexes. The two most common manifestations, which affect a small proportion of patients with chronic hepatitis B, are immune-mediated glomerulonephritis and vasculitis. Hepatitis B-associated glomerulopathy affects more children than adults, and generally causes a membranous or membranoproliferative appearance on electron microscopy. Clinically, most patients have mild liver disease, but have nephrotic-range proteinuria, and, in up to 30% of patients, end-stage renal disease may ensue *(19)*. A similar association between chronic hepatitis B and generalized vasculitis, i.e., polyarteritis nodosa, has been established *(20)*. Although therapeutic options exist for these disorders, glomerulonephritis and polyarteritis nodosa may increase the morbidity and mortality of chronic hepatitis B. In this cohort, factors associated with progression to cirrhosis included advanced age at initial presentation, a history of hepatic decompensation, repeated episodes of acute exacerbation, severe acute exacerbation without HBeAg seroconversion, and HBV reactivation.

PROGNOSIS AND SURVIVAL IN CHRONIC HEPATITIS B

Outcomes for patients chronically infected with HBV vary widely. Although the factors determining survival have not been completely elucidated, early age of acquisition and long duration of HBeAg positivity (i.e., of high virus replication and associated liver injury) are considered important factors. In one study, the 5-yr survival rate, among 98 patients who were HBsAg-reactive, and who had compensated end-stage liver disease, was 97% for those who were HBeAg-negative, compared to 72% for those were HBeAg-reactive, which was consistent with a twofold mortality benefit for the HBeAg-negative group *(21)*. This has been confirmed in a larger study, as well *(22)*. In an Asian cohort, the 5-yr rate of progression to cirrhosis was 2.4%/yr for HBeAg-reactive vs 1.3%/yr for anti-HBe-reactive patients *(23)*. There are a number of other factors that affect prognosis and survival. Alcoholics with chronic hepatitis B virus infection have been shown to have higher rates of cirrhosis and HCC, compared to nonalcoholics with HBV *(24)*. The risk of HCC was about 6× higher among HBsAg-positive alcoholics, compared to nonalcoholics *(25)*. Other factors include older age, markers of portal hypertension (hypersplenism with thrombocytopenia), markers of synthetic dysfunction (low albumin), elevated prothrombin time, and markers of excretory dysfunction (jaundice) *(25)*.

Co-infection with other hepatotropic viruses has also been evaluated in terms of prognosis and survival. Approximately 15% of chronically HBV-infected patients are also infected with hepatitis C virus (HCV). Those who are acutely co-infected tend to have reduced HBV replication, suggesting that viral interference occurs. Nonetheless, there have been case series suggesting an increased risk of acute liver failure in the setting of acute co-infection *(26)*. In the setting of chronic hepatitis B, studies have shown that co-infection accelerates progression to cirrhosis and HCC. Similarly, acute co-infection and super-infection with hepatitis D virus has been associated with a worse outcome, increasing the likelihood of acute liver failure and more progressive chronic hepatitis *(27)*. The data for hepatitis A virus super-infection are less clear. A prospective study of 163 patients with chronic hepatitis B virus infection, over 7 yr documented 10 cases of hepatitis A super-infection. Of the 10, only 1 experienced worsening of hepatitis *(28)*. These data contrast with those in studies demonstrating a worse outcome in hosts with chronic hepatitis C virus infection who are superinfected with hepatitis A virus.

Limited data have been collected on long-term survival and morbidity of chronic hepatitis B. One of the earliest studies of natural history was conducted by Weissberg et al. *(29)*, who found that 5-yr survival varied as a function of the histologic severity of liver disease. Among patients with mild chronic hepatitis B, the 5-yr survival was 97%; among those with moderate-to-severe chronic hepatitis, the 5-yr survival was 86%; and among those with chronic hepatitis B in whom cirrhosis was present, the 5-yr survival fell to 55%. At 15 yr, in the same cohort, survival in the three groups was 77, 66, and 40%, respectively.

The milder the disease at baseline, the less progressive it appears to be. For example, in 68 Italian asymptomatic HBsAg-positive blood donors with normal ALT levels, only 3% had a worsening of histology over a 130-mo mean follow-up period, during which no HCC cases of mortality occurred *(30)*. Similarly, of 317 blood donors in Montreal who had HBsAg, only three died of HBV-related complications at 16 yr follow-up *(31)*. However, the overall 5-yr survival data for those patients with chronic hepatitis infection (particularly those who acquire HBV peri-

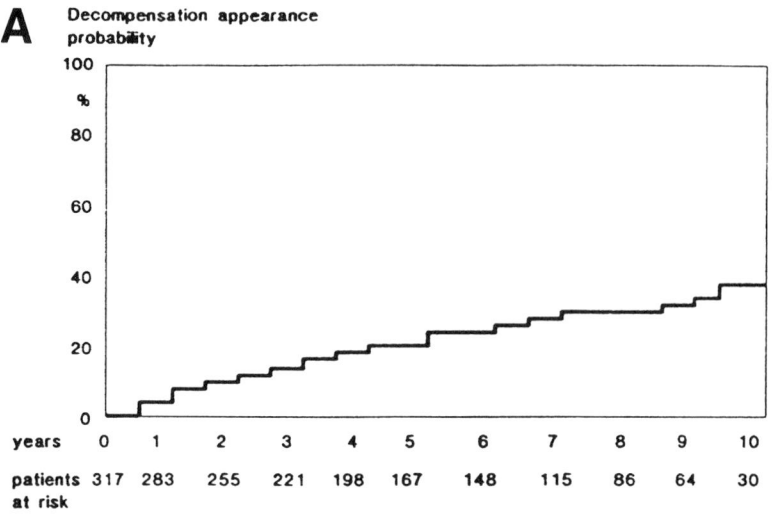

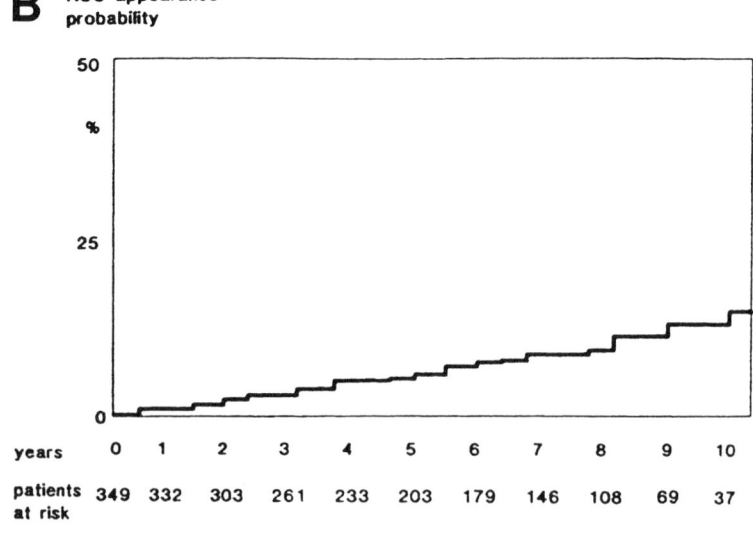

Fig. 3. Progression of HBV infection: (**A**) Progression to decompensated cirrhosis (%); (**B**) probability of HCC appearance (%). From *(33)*.

natally), are not as sanguine. Fattovich et al. *(32)* have reported natural history data in such patients. At 5 yr, up to 20% progress from chronic hepatitis to cirrhosis, approx 23% from compensated cirrhosis to hepatic decompensation, and up to 15% from cirrhosis to HCC *(32,33)* (*see* Fig. 3A–D). Cumulative data suggest that the overall 5-yr survival is approx

Chapter 3 / Natural History of HBV   51

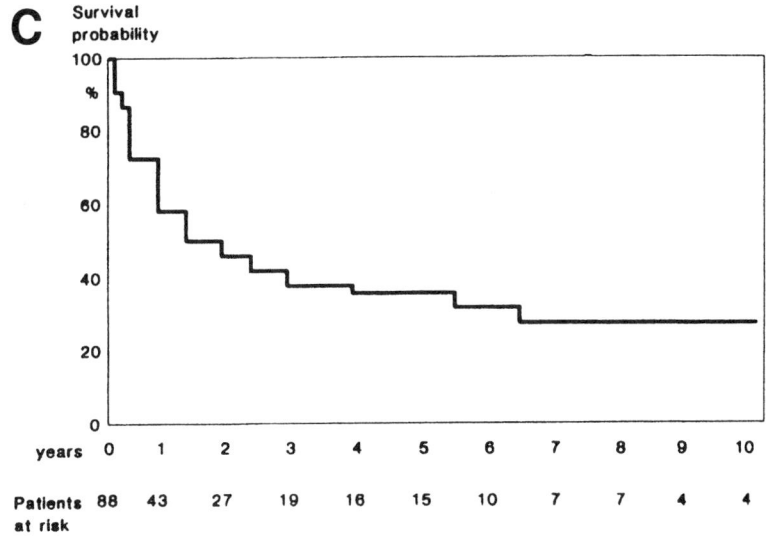

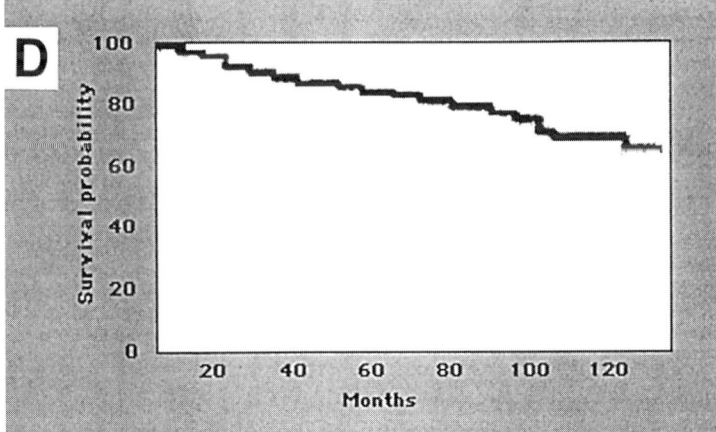

Fig. 3. (**C**) survival probability in decompensated HBV cirrhosis (%). From *(33)*.
(**D**) survival probability in compensated HBV cirrhosis (%). Adapted from *(22)*.

71% among all patients with chronic hepatitis B virus, but only 14% in those with decompensated cirrhosis *(33)*. In fact, of all prognostic variables for progression, sustained, high-level virus replication appears to stand out, as cited above. For example, among 44 patients with histologically mild hepatitis B, followed for a mean of 4 yr, histologic progression did not occur in any patient who had undetectable serum HBV DNA at baseline; progression was confined essentially to those who had detectable HBV DNA at baseline, and who failed to clear viremia, and this group experienced histologic deterioration in more than 50% of cases.

HCC AND CHRONIC HEPATITIS B VIRUS INFECTION

Epidemiologic studies have demonstrated an increased incidence of HCC among patients with chronic hepatitis B virus infection. Although the mechanisms by which malignant transformation occur are unknown, in all likelihood, the chronic inflammatory state established results in oxidative stress and increased cellular turnover, thereby increasing the risk of genetic mutations. Duration of infection appears to be the most important predictor of the risk for HCC, with most instances of HCC occurring some 25–30 yr after infection. Fattovich et al. *(33)* demonstrated that at 10 yr, approx 20% of patients with HBV-related cirrhosis will have progressed to HCC. Furthermore, host genetics and geography also influence the risk of HCC. The relative risk for HCC is 148:1 in Alaska, compared to 30:1–98:1 in Asia *(34)*. Also, animal data support a role for the *X* gene, which encodes a transcriptional activator, as a potent co-factor in the process of malignant transformation.

INFECTION WITH HBV MUTANTS

Recent advances in molecular biology have allowed for the reclassification of the HBVs from the traditional four main serotypes into six genotypes: A–F. In addition, there has been an increasing awareness and characterization of HBV mutants. Because of its much more compact genomic structure, HBV mutants are much less frequent than the quasispecies seen in HCV. HBV variants, predominantly found in the S and C genes, are thought to confer replication and host–immune response evasion advantage over wild-type strains.

A G→A change at the 1896 nucleotide position of the C gene results in the most common form of the pre-core mutation. This mutation results in the formation of a stop codon and premature termination of HBeAg. Although now thought to be an increasingly prevalent variant, the pre-core mutant was initially described among Greek patients who were serologically positive for anti-HBe, but who also had high levels of circulating HBV DNA, indicating ongoing replication. The prevalence of this mutant appears to be higher in HBV genotypes B–E. Pre-core-mutant HBV has also been linked to outbreaks of acute liver failure in Japan and Israel. This link has not been confirmed in other studies; further, this mutant has also been found in asymptomatic carriers. The survival advantage that the pre-core mutant provides is not clear, although some investigators have demonstrated a replication advantage on the basis of genomic stability. Although the clinical significance of the pre-core mutant remains to be fully defined, many observations support an association between such cases and more progressive chronic hepatitis B.

Perhaps of more concern, from the perspective of global vaccination programs, has been the description of so-called "vaccine escape" mutants. Such S gene variants were initially reported in children of HBV-carrier mothers who acquired HBV infection, despite adequate vaccination. These surface antigen mutants are felt to emerge as a result of selective pressure associated with immunization. The most common of such variants involves the substitution of an arginine for glycine at amino acid position 145. This change results in an important conformational change in a key determinant to which the common vaccine-induced antibodies bind. Thus, immunized individuals exposed to this mutant will not generate neutralizing antibody. A study of 345 infants in Singapore, born to mothers positive for HBsAg and HBeAg, who had received perinatal hepatitis B immunoglobulins and standard hepatitis B vaccination, revealed 41 cases of breakthrough infection, despite adequate titers of anti-HBs *(35)*. In the United States, one study showed a frequency of breakthrough infection of 8.6%, again with the 145 amino acid variant predominating *(36)*. This variant has also been described among liver transplant patients who acquired recurrent infection, despite the use of prophylactic HBI. Although concern has been voiced over the impact of vaccination programs on selection of such escape mutants, these fears have not been realized.

VACCINATION IN HBV INFECTION

Approximately 25 yr after Blumberg's landmark discovery of the Australia antigen, the first vaccine targeting HBV became commercially available. Early on, these vaccines were plasma-derived HBsAg subunits. As the molecular understanding of the HBV genome advanced, however, the original vaccine was replaced by a recombinant-DNA-derived surface antigen subunit. Hepatitis B vaccine has been used widely over the past two decades, and is now recommended for neonates of HBsAg-positive mothers, all children and adolescents through age 18 yr, adults with multiple sexual partners, injection drug users, homosexual and bisexual men, patients on chronic hemodialysis, and health care workers.

Hepatitis B vaccination, once universally deployed, is predicted to eliminate new cases of HBV infection within two generations. Already, vaccination has had an impact on the natural history of hepatitis B. For example, the effective implementation of a universal vaccination program in Taiwan has resulted in a 785% reduction in the HBV carrier rate prevalence among young children over a 10-yr period *(37)*. This change has resulted in a near-halving of the incidence of HCC *(39)*.

ANTIVIRAL THERAPY FOR CHRONIC HEPATITIS B VIRUS INFECTION

The goal for treatment of chronic hepatitis B virus infection is control of viral replication, which would reduce infectivity, prevent progression to cirrhosis and/or HCC, and thereby prolong survival. In the United States, there are only two agents that are currently FDA-approved interferon α (IFN-α) and lamivudine.

IFN-α was first tested against HBV in the 1970s, and was proven effective during a series of trials in the 1980s. A 1993 meta-analysis of the randomized clinical trials of IFN-α therapy vs placebo, for 6 mo, showed that it is effective in inducing the loss of HBeAg (33 vs 12%), HBV DNA (37 vs 17%), and HBsAg (7.8 vs 1.8%) *(39)*.

Data are beginning to accumulate to demonstrate the impact of IFN therapy on the natural history of chronic hepatitis B. Among patients who have lost HBeAg and HBV DNA by hybridization assays during IFN treatment, the life-table loss rate of HBsAg and frequency of sustained-normal ALT approaches 80% *(40)*. Among patients who lose HBeAg during therapy, long-term observation and comparison to untreated controls has documented an improvement in clinical outcome (reduced fatality, prolonged survival, prolonged survival without complications of liver disease, even reduced frequency of HCC) *(41,42)* (*see* Fig. 4). Thus, data are beginning to accumulate to support the beneficial impact of successful antiviral therapy on the long-term natural history of chronic hepatitis B. An analysis of all available studies suggests that treatment of chronic hepatitis B virus infection with IFN-α is associated with a 13% reduction in cirrhosis, 9% reduction in decompensation cirrhosis, and 4% reduction in the development in HCC.

Although lamivudine is promising in early trials as an effective nucleoside analog, sufficient time has not elapsed to address the impact of this therapy on the natural history of chronic hepatitis B. Still, studies of the natural history of hepatitis B, and observations after IFN treatment, suggest that any approach that reduces HBV replication will have a beneficial outcome on the con-sequences of HBV infection.

The benefit and safety profile of lamivudine has permitted expansion of the potential target pool for treatment of chronic hepatitis B to patients with decompensation disease. In studies of lamivudine for patients with class B and C cirrhosis, who are awaiting liver transplant, a substantial

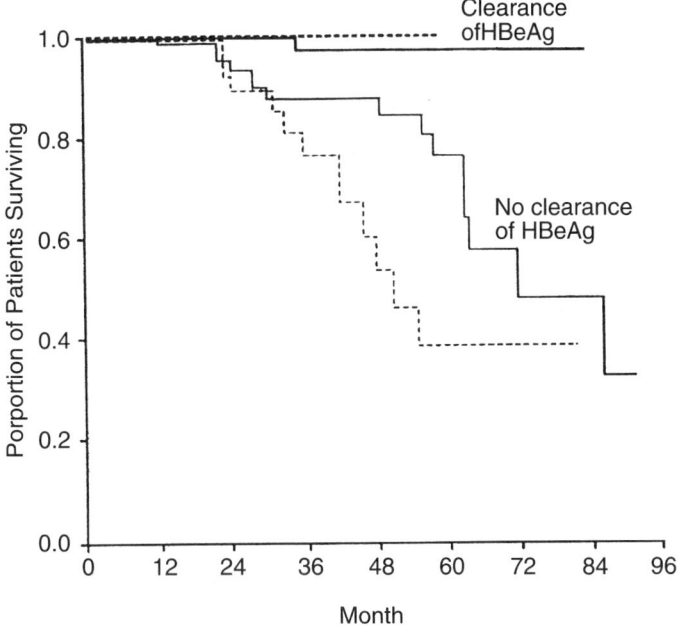

Fig. 4. Natural history of among HBeAg (+) and HBeAg (–) patients. From *(41)*.

proportion have improved clinically, and in a small proportion, liver transplant has been delayed, occasionally indefinitely *(43)*.

ROLE OF LIVER TRANSPLANT IN HEPATITIS B

Despite advances in the understanding of the immunopathogenesis of HBV, and development of new treatment strategies, there are approx 4500 deaths/yr in the United States, attributable to HBV infection. As mentioned, there is only a 14% 5-yr survival among patients with decompensation HBV cirrhosis.

Although full consideration of liver transplant for hepatitis B is beyond the scope of this chapter, the availability of liver transplant has the potential to reduce the impact of progressive hepatitis on mortality. Among patients who would otherwise succumb to end-stage cirrhosis or fulminant hepatitis resulting from HBV infection, liver transplant can lead to long-term survival: 80% at 1 yr, and 65% at 5 yr, comparable to survival figures for liver transplant in nonviral liver disease. Such excellent outcomes, however, would not be possible without effective antiviral strategies to prevent recurrent infection in the allograft.

A number of strategies have been developed to reduce the re-infection rate. At present, the most effective strategy appears to be immunoprophylaxis with hepatitis B immunoglobulins. In theory, providing patients with high levels of anti-HBs antibodies will neutralize circulating virions and decrease graft re-infection. Despite the high cost of therapy ($15,000–$30,000/yr), and the possible emergence of "escape mutants," long-term therapy with hepatitis B immunoglobulins remains the standard of care to decrease the incidence of recurrent HBV infection in the transplanted patient.

Current studies are ongoing to evaluate the benefit of combination therapy of nucleoside analogs together with hepatitis B immunoglobulins.

FUTURE CONSIDERATIONS

Since Blumberg's discovery of the Australia antigen, progress in understanding HBV and the natural hepatitis B has been substantial. Effective and safe vaccination is now available to prevent new infections, and, for those infected, increasingly effective antiviral thers are available. Both of these interventions have already affected the natural history of hepatitis B.

Future success in the struggle against hepatitis B infection will depend on universal application of vaccination programs, and the development of more effective multidrug combination thers aimed at multiple targets within the virion. With such advances, global eradication of hepatitis B within several decades is a realistic goal.

REFERENCES

1. Beasley RP, Hwang LY, Liu CC, et al. Incidence of hepatitis B virus infections in preschool children in Taiwan. J Infect Dis 1982; 146: 198–204.
2. Coursaget P, Yyonnet B, Chotaro J, et al. Age- and sex-related study of hepatitis B virus chronic carrier state in infants from an endemic area (Senegal). J Med Virol 1987; 22: 1–5.
3. Stevens CE, Beasley RV, Tsui J, et al. Vertical transmission of hepatitis B antigen in Taiwan. N Engl J Med 1975; 292: 771–774.
4. Sawyer WA, Meyer KF, Eaton MD, Bauer JH, Putnam P, Schwentker FF. Jaundice in Army personnel in the western region of the United States and its relation to vaccination against yellow fever. Am J Hygiene 1944; 39: 337–430.
5. Tassopoulos NC, Papnevangelou W, Sjogren MH, et al. Natural history of acute hepatitis B surface antigen-positive hepatitis in Greek adults. Gastroenterology 1987; 92: 1844–1850.
6. Thursz MR, Kwiatkowski D, Allsopp CE, et al. Association between an MHC class II allele and clearance of hepatitis B virus in the Gambia. N Engl J Med 1995; 332: 1065–1069.
7. Lok AS, Lai CL, Wu PC, et al. Spontaneous hepatitis B e antigen to antibody seroconversion and reversion in Chinese patients with chronic hepatitis B virus infection. Gastroenterology 1987; 92: 1839–1843.

8. Chang MH, Hsu HY, Hsu HC, et al. Significance of spontaneous hepatitis B e antigen seroconversion in childhood: with special emphasis on the clearance of hepatitis B e antigen before 3 years of age. Hepatology 1995; 22: 1387–1392.
9. Sheen IS, Liau YF, Tai DI, et al. Hepatic decompensation associated with hepatitis B e antigen clearance in chronic type B hepatitis. Gastroenterology 1985; 89: 732–735.
10. Lok AS, Lai CL. alpha-Fetoprotein monitoring in Chinese patients with chronic hepatitis B virus infection: role in the early detection of hepatocellular carcinoma. Hepatology 1989; 9: 110–115.
11. Liaw YF, Chu CM, Lin DY, et al. Age-specific prevalence and significance of hepatitis B e antigen and antibody in chronic hepatitis B virus infection in Taiwan: a comparison among asymptomatic carriers, chronic hepatitis, liver cirrhosis, and hepatocellular carcinoma. J Med Virol 1984; 13: 385–391.
12. Alward WL, McMahon BJ, Hall DB, et al. Long-term serological course of asymptomatic hepatitis B virus carriers and the development of primary hepatocellular carcinoma. J Infect Dis 1985; 151: 604–609.
13. Liaw YF, Sheen IS, Chen TJ, et al. Incidence, determinants and significance of delayed clearance of serum HBsAg in chronic hepatitis B virus infection: a prospective study. Hepatology 1991; 13: 627–631.
14. Chung HT, Lai CL, Lok AS. Pathogenic role of hepatitis B virus in hepatitis B surface antigen-negative decompensated cirrhosis. Hepatology 1995; 22: 25–29.
15. Lok AS, Chung HT, Liu VW, et al. Long-term follow-up of chronic hepatitis B patients treated with interferon alfa. Gastroenterology 1993; 105: 1833–1838.
16. Hsu HY, Chang MH, Hsieh KH, et al. Cellular immune response to HBcAg in mother-to-infant transmission of hepatitis B virus. Hepatology 1992; 15: 770–776.
17. Guidotti LG, Chisari FV. To kill or to cure: options in host defense against viral infection. Curr Opin Immunol 1996; 8: 478–483.
18. Davies SE, Portmann BC, O'Grady JG, et al. Hepatic histological findings after transplantation for chronic hepatitis B virus infection, including a unique pattern of fibrosing cholestatic hepatitis. Hepatology 1991; 13: 150–157.
19. Lai KN, Lai FM, Chan KW, et al. Clinico-pathologic features of hepatitis B virus-associated glomerulonephritis. Q J Med 1987; 63: 323–333.
20. Agnello V, Chung RT, Kaplan LM. A role for hepatitis C virus infection in type II cryoglobulinemia. N Engl J Med 1992; 327: 1490–1495.
21. de Jongh FE, Janssen HL, deMan HK, et al. Survival and prognostic indicators in hepatitis B surface antigen-positive cirrhosis of the liver. Gastroenterology 1992; 103: 1630–1635.
22. Realdi G, Fattovich G, Haoziyannis S, et al. Survival and prognostic factors in 366 patients with compensated cirrhosis type B: a multicenter study. The Investigators of the European Concerted Action on Viral Hepatitis (EUROHEP). J Hepatol 1994; 21: 656–666.
23. Ohnishi K, Iida S, Iwama S, et al. Effect of chronic habitual alcohol intake on the development of liver cirrhosis and hepatocellular carcinoma: relation to hepatitis B surface antigen carriage. Cancer 1982; 49: 672–677.
24. Liaw YF, Tai DI, Chu CM, et al. Development of cirrhosis in patients with chronic type B hepatitis: a prospective study. Hepatology 1988; 8: 493–496.
25. Laskus T, Raokowski M, Lupa E, et al. Prevalence of markers of hepatitis viruses in out-patient alcoholics. J Hepatol 1992; 15: 174–178.
26. Feray C, Gigou M, Samuel D, et al. Hepatitis C virus RNA and hepatitis B virus DNA in serum and liver of patients with fulminant hepatitis. Gastroenterology 1993; 104: 549–555.

27. Smedile A, Farci V, Veume G, et al. Influence of delta infection on severity of hepatitis B. Lancet 1982; 2: 945–947.
28. Vento S, Garofano T, Renzini G, et al. Fulminant hepatitis associated with hepatitis A virus superinfection in patients with chronic hepatitis C. N Engl J Med 1998; 338: 286–290.
29. Weissberg JI, Andres LL, Smith CI, et al. Survival in chronic hepatitis B. An analysis of 379 patients. Ann Intern Med 1984; 101: 613–616.
30. de Franchis R, Meucci G, Vecchi M, et al. The natural history of asymptomatic hepatitis B surface antigen carriers. Ann Intern Med 1993; 118: 191–194.
31. Villeneuve JP, et al. A long-term follow-up study of asymptomatic hepatitis B surface antigen-positive carriers in Montreal. Gastroenterology 1994; 106: 1000–1005.
32. Fattovich G, Brollo L, Giustina G, et al. Natural history and prognostic factors for chronic hepatitis type B. Gut 1991; 32: 294–298.
33. Fattovich G, Giustina G, Schalm SW, et al. Occurrence of hepatocellular carcinoma and decompensation in western European patients with cirrhosis type B. The EUROHEP Study Group on Hepatitis B Virus and Cirrhosis. Hepatology 1995; 21: 77–82.
34. McMahon BJ, Alberts SK, Wainwright RB, et al. Hepatitis B-related sequelae. Prospective study in 1400 hepatitis B surface antigen-positive Alaska native carriers. Arch Intern Med 1990; 150: 1051–1054.
35. Oon CJ, Lim GK, Ye Z, et al. Molecular epidemiology of hepatitis B virus vaccine variants in Singapore. Vaccine 1995; 13: 699–702.
36. Nainan OV. HBV antibody resistant mutants among mothers and infants with chronic HBV infection. In: *Viral Hepatitis and Liver Disease* (Rizzetto M, Purcell RH, Gerin JL, Verme G, eds.). Edizioni Minervi, Medica. Turin, Italy, 1997, pp. 132–134.
37. Chen HL, Chang MH, Ni YH, et al. Seroepidemiology of hepatitis B virus infection in children: ten years of mass vaccination in Taiwan. JAMA 1996; 276: 906–908.
38. Chang MH, Chen W, Lai MS, et al. Universal hepatitis B vaccination in Taiwan and the incidence of hepatocellular carcinoma in children. Taiwan Childhood Hepatoma Study Group. N Engl J Med 1997; 336: 1855–1859.
39. Wong DK, Cheung AM, O'Rourke K, et al. Effect of alpha-interferon treatment in patients with hepatitis B e antigen-positive chronic hepatitis B. A meta-analysis. Ann Intern Med 1993; 119: 312–323.
40. Lau DT, et al. Long-term follow-up of patients with chronic hepatitis B treated with interferon alfa. Gastroenterology 1997; 113: 1660–1667.
41. Niederau C, Heintges T, Lange S, et al. Long-term follow-up of HBeAg-positive patients treated with interferon alfa for chronic hepatitis B. N Engl J Med 1996; 334: 1422–1427.
42. Lin SM, Sheen IS, Chien KN, et al. Long-term beneficial effect of interferon therapy in patients with chronic hepatitis B virus infection. Hepatology 1999; 29: 971–975.
43. Villeneuve JP, Conoreay LD, Willems B, et al. Lamivudine treatment for decompensated cirrhosis resulting from chronic hepatitis B. Hepatology 2000; 31: 207–210.
44. Realdi G, Alberti A, Rugge M, et al. Seroconversion from hepatitis B e antigen to anti-HBe in chronic hepatitis B virus infection. Gastroenterology 1980; 79: 195–199.
45. Hoofnagle JH, Dusheiko GM, Seeff LB, et al. Seroconversion from hepatitis B e antigen to antibody in chronic type B hepatitis. Ann Intern Med 1981; 94: 744–748.
46. Lok AS. Natural history and control of perinatally acquired hepatitis B virus infection. Dig Dis 1992; 10: 46–52.

4 Natural History of Hepatitis C

Gregory T. Everson, MD

CONTENTS

INTRODUCTION
PREVALENCE, RISK FACTORS, AND INCIDENCE
ACUTE HEPATITIS C
FULMINANT HEPATITIS C
CHRONIC INFECTION AND SEQUELAE
CHRONIC INFECTION WITH NORMAL ALT ("CARRIER")
DISEASE PROGRESSION IN PATIENTS WITH CHRONIC
   HEPATITIS C
RISK FACTORS FOR DISEASE PROGRESSION
RISK OF DECOMPENSATION IN CHILD'S A CIRRHOSIS
OUTCOME AFTER DECOMPENSATION IN CIRRHOTIC
   PATIENTS
RISK OF HCC
SUMMARY
REFERENCES

INTRODUCTION

The natural history of infection with hepatitis C is incompletely understood, because the exact date of acquisition of infection is often unknown, many patients with hepatitis C escape detection, and current, widely used treatments may affect outcome. Seeff *(1)* proposed that the most accurate study to evaluate the natural history of hepatitis C should have five basic components. First, the date of onset of acute hepatitis C should be documented to properly determine duration of disease. Second, the study should include the full spectrum of acute disease, to avoid bias toward ascertainment of only the more severe forms of the disease. Third, the

From: *Clinical Gastroenterology: Diagnosis and Therapeutics*
Edited by: R. S. Koff and G. Y. Wu © Humana Press Inc., Totowa, NJ

study should encompass the whole disease process, with complete follow-up to resolution of disease or clinical end points, regardless of the duration of disease must be examined. Fourth, the outcome of disease must be examined in the absence of treatment that could modify the course of the disease. Fifth, properly matched controls, followed with the same clinical intensity as patients with hepatitis C should be included. Another consideration is that studies of natural history should examine cohorts that are representative of the overall population with the infection. Unfortunately, no single study meets all of these criteria. Nonetheless, there are numerous studies of natural history and disease progression that shed light on the nature of this indolent, but highly significant chronic liver disease.

PREVALENCE, RISK FACTORS, AND INCIDENCE

Prevalence

Current estimates of the prevalence of hepatitis C in the United States are based on data from the third study of the National Center for Health Statistics (NHANES III), Centers for Disease Control and Prevention (CDC) (2). Serum samples from 21,241 persons, age ≥6 yr, who participated in the study between 1988 and 1994, were analyzed for both antibody to hepatitis C and HCV RNA. The results indicate that the prevalence of seropositivity to hepatitis C virus antibody in the general population of the United States is 1.8%, representing approx 3,900,000 citizens. 74% of patients positive for hepatitis C virus antibody were also positive for HCV RNA, indicating that 2,700,000 U.S. citizens are currently chronically infected with hepatitis C. The number of patients with CHC dwarfs the number infected with either HBV (~1.25 million) or HIV (~0.9 million).

Despite these impressive statistics, the United States is considered a low-prevalence population (3). Surveillance studies from across the world indicate relatively low prevalence (<2.5%) in North America, Europe, Russia, and Japan, and high prevalence (>2.5%) in South America, Africa, and Southeast Asia, including China. In some countries, prevalence exceeds 10% (Bolivia, Egypt, and Mongolia).

Risk Factors

Risk factors for acquisition of hepatitis C (Table 1) primarily involve activities that increase likelihood of exposure to contaminated blood or blood products (4–7). A major risk factor is any current or past experimentation with intravenous drugs. Today, intravenous drug users represent the majority of cases of acute hepatitis C in the United States. Prior

Table 1
Current Risk Factors for Acquisition of Hepatitis C in United States

Definite
   Intravenous drug abuse
   Receipt of blood transfusion or solid organ transplant prior to 1992
   Receipt of clotting factor concentrates prior to 1987
   Receipt of contaminated units of immunoglobulin preparations
   Hemodialysis
   High-risk sexual behavior
   Vertical transmission to neonate from infected mother
   Inadequate sterilization of needles or medical devices
   Hepatitis B or HIV infection
   Alcohol abuse and alcoholic liver disease
   Accidental needlestick
Possible
   Nasal cocaine
   Tattoos
   Body piercing
   Acupuncture
   Use of shared sharps or toothbrushes
   Health care worker
   Prior surgery when there was risk for transfusion
   Prior dental procedures
Surrogates
   Use of cocaine
   Use of marijuana
   Divorced or separated
   Income below poverty level
   12 yr or fewer education
Not a Risk Factor
   Infant breastfeeding from infected mother
   Race or ethnicity

to 1990 and the availability of tests to detect hepatitis C, transfusion of contaminated blood accounted for a substantial proportion of cases; the risk per unit transfused was 0.45%/U. However, risk decreased dramatically with testing of donors for hepatitis C virus antibody. Current, third-generation tests for hepatitis C virus antibody are so sensitive and specific that risk of acquisition of hepatitis C through transfusion has dramatically diminished, to nearly zero (.001%/U).

The NHANES III study suggested that CHC was more prevalent in users of marijuana and cocaine, and that risk increased with increasing use of either illicit substance *(2)*. Other risk factors included high-risk sexual activity* and co-infection with hepatitis B. Prevalence was also greater in patients who were divorced or separated, had incomes below poverty level, or who had 12 yr or fewer of education. Although prevalence of hepatitis C was greatest in middle-aged, African American males, neither race nor ethnicity were independently associated with infection. Likewise, the prevalence of hepatitis C was not associated with employment in the health care profession, surgery that might have included blood transfusion (hysterectomy), or higher frequency of dental visits.

A large case-control study of U.S. blood donors indicated that injection drug users, sex with an injection drug user, and past history of blood tranfusion are the three greatest risk factors for hepatitis C *(8)*. Weaker associations were found with incarceration, religious scarification, body piercing, being pierced with a bloody object, and immunoglobulin injection. In that study, drug inhalation and high number of lifetime sex partners were not independently associated with hepatitis C. These results suggest that use of intranasal cocaine may not be a mode of transmission, but simply a surrogate for other high-risk behaviors, such as illicit injection drug use. In addition, sexual activity is only weakly associated with transmission of hepatitis C.

Hepatitis C may be transmitted from mother to infant at time of delivery. The risk in otherwise healthy mother–infant pairs is approx 6%, but risk increases dramatically, to approx 20%, if mothers are co-infected with HIV *(9)*. A recent Italian study examined vertical transmission in 15,250 pregnant women *(10)*. Three-hundred-seventy women were seropositive to hepatitis C virus antibody, and 72% of these were positive for HCV RNA. The risk of development of CHC in the offspring of viremic mothers was 5.1%. Pregnancy did not affect level of viremia, but tended to ameliorate ongoing liver injury in the mothers; 56.4% of mothers had elevated alanine aminotransferase (ALT) in the first month of pregnancy, but only 7.4% had abnormal ALT in the last trimester. After delivery, 54.5% of mothers had elevated ALT. Those authors also observed that infants of mothers seropositive for HIV, but, when treated with highly active antiretroviral therapy, did not have an increased risk for acquisition of HCV. Limited data from that and other studies suggest that hepatitis C is not transmitted from mother to infant during breastfeeding.

---

*High-risk sexual activity is defined as early age at first sexual intercourse, having more than 10 sexual partners, and infection with herpes simplex virus type 2. Nonuse of condoms, vigorous sexual practices that traumatize the mucosal lining, and male homosexual activity may also increase likelihood of transmission. In heterosexuals with high-risk sexual behavior, male-to-female transmission may be more common than female-to-male transmission.

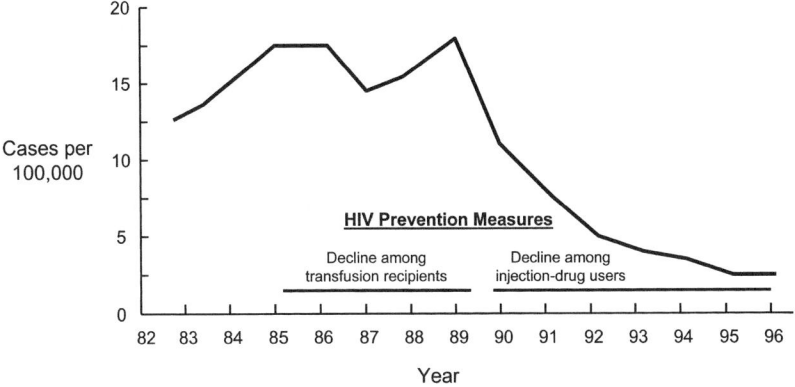

Fig. 1. The estimated incidence of hepatitis C in the United States between the years 1982 and 1996. The decline in incidence coincided with both the institution of effective screening of blood donors and measures to prevent spread of HIV. (Adapted with permission from ref. *14*.)

Risk may also be increased by certain medical or cultural practices. Surveillance of 3999 residents of a village in the Nile delta indicated 24.3% seropositivity to hepatitis C virus antibody. A major correlate of the high rate of seropositivity was prior exposure to antischistosomal injection therapy *(11,12)*. In Japan, community-acquired infection has been traced to folk remedies, including acupuncture and cutting of the skin with unsterilized knives *(13)*. Suspected, but unproven, risk factors for transmission of hepatitis C include tattooing, body piercing, and shared use of sharps (razor blades).

Incidence

The current incidence of hepatitis C in the United States is on the decline, because of effective means of screening for HCV in the blood donor population, and changes in behavior of injection drug users related to awareness of AIDS and hepatitis *(14)*. The CDC estimates that there were approx 180,000 new infections/yr in the mid 1980s, but that the incidence had dropped to 28,000 cases/yr by 1995 (Fig. 1). Currently, it is estimated that there are 30,000–40,000 new infections annually. Given the relatively slow progression in liver disease of 20–30 yr, large numbers of patients who were infected in the 1970s and 1980s are just now beginning to report to physicians with advanced liver disease and hepatocellular carcinoma (HCC). Worldwide incidence of hepatitis C is unknown, but the World Health Organization estimates that about 3% of the world population is chronically infected with hepatitis C; these 170 million individuals are at risk for cirrhosis and liver cancer *(15)*.

ACUTE HEPATITIS

Approximately 10–20% of cases of acute viral hepatitis (AVH) in the United States are due to hepatitis C *(16)*. There is a mean incubation period of 7 wk between the exposure to hepatitis C and development of clinical liver disease. Serum concentrations of ALT may be minimally elevated, but as many as 80% experience peak ALT, elevated >10-fold above the normal range. Clinical illness lasts for 2–12 wk, and spontaneously resolves. Fulminant hepatic failure (FHF) is uncommon *(17)*.

FULMINANT HEPATITIS

In a recent survey of FHF in the United States, no cases could be attributed to hepatitis C *(18)*. Likewise, in the two series from Europe of acute exposure to anti-D immunoglobulin *(19,20)*, there were no cases of fulminant hepatitis caused by hepatitis C. In contrast, reports from Asia indicate that hepatitis C may account for as many as one-half of their cases of FHF resulting from non-A, non-B causes *(21,22)*. One study from California *(23)* of Hispanic patients of low socioeconomic status, indicated that 60% had seropositivity for hepatitis C. Farci et al. *(24)* described a case of a 68-yr-old man who died of fulminant posttransfusion hepatitis (PTH). Serial performance of clinical, virologic, and histologic tests firmly established hepatitis C as the etiology. The latter authors reviewed their past experience with PTH and concluded that this was the sole patient who developed fulminant hepatitis. Thus, although it can be a consequence of acute hepatitis C, it must be a rare event, probably occurring with a frequency of less than 1/1000.

CHRONIC INFECTION AND SEQUELAE

Most patients with CHC cannot recall a previous illness consistent with acute hepatitis, and only one-third experience clinical jaundice or symptoms *(25)*. For this reason, patient recall of past events is not likely to yield a clear picture of the spectrum of acute hepatitis C. Accurate assessment of the natural history of acute hepatitis C can only be gained by studying a population of patients with a known time-point of exposure to the virus, such as occurs with acquisition of hepatitis C by transfusion or by widespread use of a contaminated blood product.

The prolonged time-course of disease progression after acute hepatitis C was suggested by two older studies. Kiyosawa *(26)* studied 231 patients with transfusion-related hepatitis C. 96 had chronic hepatitis without cirrhosis, 81 had cirrhosis, and 54 had HCC. The time of acquisition of infection was presumed to be the time of transfusion. Using

Table 2
Clinical Outcomes After Infection with HCV

A. Rates of progression to cirrhosis and HCC

	Cirrhosis (yr)	HCC (yr)
Kiyosawa (26)	21.2	29
Tong (27)	20.6	28

B. Risk of developing cirrhosis, HCC, or death related to liver disease

Patient group (ref)	Yr Obs	Cirrhosis %	HCC %	Death %
CHC (27,46,48)	4–11	30–50	11–19	15.3
PTH (28–32)	7–14	8–24	0.7–1.3	1.6–6
NHLBI (33,43)	18–20	15–20	—	3.2
Military recruits (35)	45	18.2	—	9.1
Irish women (19)	17	2	0	0
German women (20)	20	0.4	0	0.2
Aust CA study (34)	25	8	0	1

See text for discussion of the individual studies. CHC, retrospective studies of patients referred to liver centers for chronic hepatitis C; PTH, prospective studies patients who experienced posttransfusion hepatitis; NHLBI, National Heart, Lung, and Blood Institute study; Military recruits, 45-yr follow-up of 11 military recruits who were both HCV-antibody- and HCV RNA-positive; Irish and German women, followed after acquisition of HCV via anti-D immunoglobulin; Aust CA Study, study of a cohort of patients diagnosed with community-acquired (CA) acute hepatitis C between 1971 and 1975.

these assumptions, they estimated that development of cirrhosis required 21.2 yr, and development of HCC required 29 yr of chronic infection. Tong (27) used similar analyses to determine that the time to development of cirrhosis and HCC were 21 and 28 yr, respectively. In five separate, but small, prospective studies (Table 2) of transfusion-associated hepatitis C (or non-A, non-B), 8–24% of patients had developed cirrhosis within 8–14 yr of acquisition of infection, 0–1.3% had developed HCC, and 1.6–6.0% had experienced liver-related death (28–32). These data suggested that hepatitis C is a serious progressive disease, with potentially fatal complications occurring within 15 yr of infection.

A study by the U.S. National Heart, Lung, and Blood Institute suggested a more benign outcome from infection with hepatitis C. Persons were evaluated who had experienced transfusion-associated non-A, non-B hepatitis between the years 1968 and 1980 (33). Outcome in 568 cases of transfusion-associated hepatitis was compared to outcome in 984 controls, who had not developed chronic hepatitis. Overall mortality at

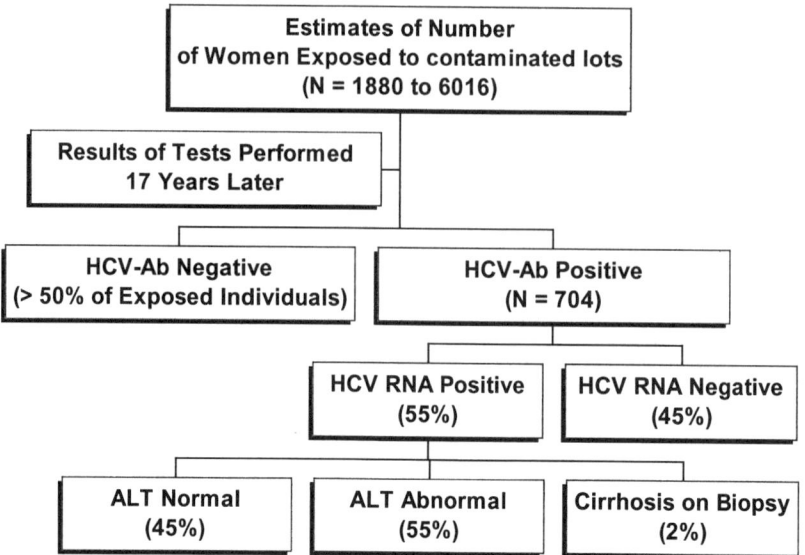

Fig. 2. Algorithm depicting the outcome of Irish women who acquired hepatitis C via contaminated anti-D immunoglobulin, given to them to prevent Rh isoimmunization. Many of the exposed patients failed to seroconvert. The clinical course in those who seroconverted was relatively benign.

20 yr posttransfusion was high in both groups (51%), related to their underlying medical condition, such as advanced cardiovascular disease. Liver-related mortality was significantly higher in the patients with CHC (3.2%), compared to controls (1.5%, $P = .033$). In addition, there was histologic or radiologic evidence of cirrhosis in 15–20% of these patients after 18–20 yr of follow-up. However, the incidence of serious complications of liver disease, or mortality from liver disease, was low. 71% of patients who experienced liver-related morbidity or mortality were noted to be heavy drinkers, and had been hospitalized for alcohol-related medical problems.

The Irish women's study also confirmed a low rate of serious complications after infection with hepatitis C *(19)* (Fig. 2). Between 1977 and 1978, batches of anti-D immunoglobulin used to prevent Rh isoimmunization in Irish women, were contaminated with hepatitis C from a single infected donor. In a nationwide screening campaign aimed at recipients of anti-D immunoglobulin, 704 women were identified as positive for hepatitis C virus antibody. However, more than half of the recipients of contaminated lots tested negative. 390 of the 704 women with hepatitis C virus antibody were also positive for HCV RNA, and were referred for clinical evaluation and treatment. Of these, 376 underwent further study.

At the time of evaluation, in 1994, the women had been infected with hepatitis C for 17 yr. 81% reported symptoms, mostly fatigue (66%), arthralgia or myalgia (38%), or anxiety or depression (16%). ALT was elevated in 55%. The concentration of ALT was greater than 100 IU/L in only 8%. Liver biopsies were performed in 96.5% of patients, and 98% of the biopsies demonstrated at least some degree of inflammation. Inflammation was mild in 41%, moderate in 52%, and severe in 4%. 51% of biopsies demonstrated an increase in fibrosis, but only 2% had cirrhosis. 15% demonstrated either portal–portal or portal–central bridging fibrosis.

Several findings of this study were noteworthy. First, nearly half (45%) of the women exposed to hepatitis C infection had cleared the infection, and were no longer viremic. Second, nearly half of the women with viremia had normal ALT (45%). Third, in most cases, liver inflammation was mild-to-moderate (93%), and fibrosis limited (83%). Fourth, over a 17-yr period, only 2% of women infected with hepatitis C developed cirrhosis, and there were no reported liver-related deaths or deaths caused by HCC. This female cohort was otherwise relatively healthy, and only 5% reported significant alcohol consumption. Few had other risk factors for hepatitis C, such as blood transfusion (17%) or injection drug use (1%).

A study from East Germany reported an even more benign course of hepatitis C in another cohort of women infected with hepatitis C via contaminated anti-D immunoglobulin *(20)*. A cohort of 1018 were studied at nine centers with 20 yr of retrospective data available for analysis. Within 6 mo of exposure to anti-D immunoglobulin, 90% developed acute hepatitis, and 10% had no evidence of infection or hepatitis. There were no cases of FHF. Of those with acute hepatitis, 22% had icteric disease, 27% were anicteric but symptomatic, and 39% were both anicteric and asymptomatic. The median ALT elevation in icteric cases was higher than anicteric cases (765 vs 348 [symptomatic] and 390 [asymptomatic] IU/L). In addition, ALT elevations were similar in symptomatic and asymptomatic anicteric cases. Although 85% remained positive for hepatitis C virus antibody in 20-yr follow-up, only 55% remained positive for HCV RNA (Fig. 3). Patients who had experienced icteric illness during acute hepatitis were more likely than anicteric patients to clear hepatitis C and remain negative for HCV RNA.

Long-term prognosis was excellent. After 20 yr of follow-up, there were only four cases of overt cirrhosis (0.4% incidence). One cirrhotic, who was also alcoholic, died, and another noncirrhotic patient died of

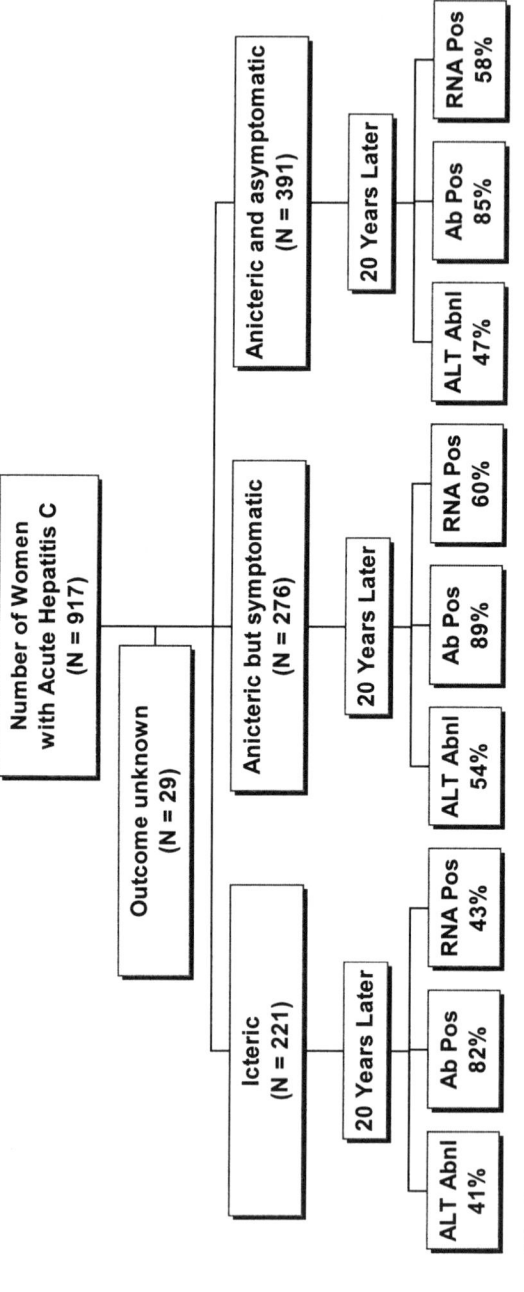

Fig. 3. Algorithm depicting the outcome of German women who acquired hepatitis C via contaminated anti-D immunoglobulin, given to them to prevent Rh isoimmunization. 90% had acute hepatitis, but nearly 40% were asymptomatic. Icteric AH was more likely to lead to HCV RNA clearance than anicteric hepatitis.

superimposed fulminant hepatitis B. Liver biopsies in 241 women, who were HCV RNA-positive, revealed mild-to-moderate inflammation in 96%, and lack of significant fibrosis (only 3% had focal bridging fibrosis) or cirrhosis (0%). The four patients with overt clinical features of cirrhosis did not undergo biopsy.

These patients were relatively healthy: only 4% were obese, 1% had diabetes mellitus, none were co-infected with hepatitis B, and only 2% had significant alcohol intake. The one drawback of this study was the inability to obtain liver histology on a greater proportion of infected patients. Nonetheless, the results are consistent with the findings in the Irish women's study.

A criticism of the latter two studies is that the populations studied are not representative of the usual population of patients with hepatitis C, or the cohort of patients with community-acquired infection. Rodger et al. *(34)* evaluated a cohort of patients admitted to an infectious disease hospital in Melbourne, Australia, between 1971 and 1975, with a diagnosis of AVH, and for whom stored serum were available. The majority were male (65%) and injection drug users (87%). Tattooing and unprotected sex were more frequent in hepatitis C virus antibody-positive patients. 16% ($N = 238$) tested positive for hepatitis C virus antibody on admission. Outcome in 98 of these patients, followed for 25 yr, was compared to 201 controls from the same cohort, who tested negative for hepatitis C virus antibody. At the 25-yr mark, 54% of hepatitis C virus antibody-positive patients were HCV RNA-positive; the rest were negative. 69% of HCV RNA-positive patients had elevated liver enzymes, but only 8% had progressed to cirrhosis, and none developed hepatoma. Chronic excessive consumption of alcohol (>50 g/d) was a risk factor for progression to cirrhosis. Excess mortality in the HCV-positive group was not caused by liver disease, suggesting that, even in a male injection drug user population, the course may be relatively benign and prolonged, with slow progression of fibrosis.

All of the above studies have examined outcomes over a period of <25 yr follow-up. However, one study carefully examined outcome in 17 patients followed over a period of 45 yr. The results again emphasize the potentially benign course of hepatitis C. Seeff et al. *(35)* examined serum samples from 8568 military recruits, obtained between 1948 and 1954, for the presence of hepatitis C virus antibody *(35)*. 17 recruits were positive to hepatitis C virus antibody by both enzyme-linked immunosorbent assay and recombinant immunoblot assay; 11/17 were positive for HCV RNA. There was one death attributed to liver disease, and one case of chronic liver disease in these 11 patients (18.2%). 9/11 (82%), failed to experience liver-related morbidity or mortality in this 45-yr follow-up study. None of the 17 patients with positive hepatitis C virus antibody reported alcohol or iv drug abuse. However, extrapolation of these results to the total population of patients with hepatitis C is not possible, because of two drawbacks: the small number of patients and the high mortality rate from causes other than liver disease (29%).

CHRONIC INFECTION WITH NORMAL ALT ("CARRIER")

Patients with hepatitis C, who have a persistently normal ALT, represent a unique subgroup of patients. One early study indicated that 26% of patients with positive hepatitis C virus antibody had normal ALT *(36)*. But, as noted previously, this is likely an underestimate of the true proportion of patients with positive hepatitis C virus antibody who are ALT-normal. In the two studies of women who acquired hepatitis C after administration of anti-D immunoglobulin, nearly two-thirds of those who were antibody-positive had normal ALT *(19,20)*. Approximately one-half were positive for HCV RNA, and one-half were negative for HCV RNA. Women are more likely than men to have normal ALT, but normal ALT is not related to viral load, genotype, or degree of quasispecies. Other factors, such as human lymphocyte antigen (HLA) type, cell-mediated immune response, hepatic iron (Fe) concentration, and obesity may be important. Long-term follow-up, with repeat testing of HCV RNA, is required to determine whether patients with normal ALT and negative HCV RNA are truly free of viral infection, and represent recovery from the acute infection. In the author's experience, the vast majority of these patients remain negative for HCV RNA. However, an occasional, rare patient will exhibit intermittent positive HCV RNA, usually in low titer (<10,000 vEq/mL).

Although the bulk of the literature indicates that viremic patients with normal ALT typically exhibit a benign, nonprogressive clinical course, some centers have suggested that this group of patients is still at risk for progressive liver disease *(37)*. In addition, the National Institutes of Health consensus conference suggested that liver biopsy is required in these patients, to define activity and stage disease *(38)*. Also, patients with persistently normal ALT, but who have ALTs in the upper half of the normal range, are the subgroup at particular risk to have more aggressive grades of inflammation or grades of fibrosis. Heavy alcohol consumption is a risk factor for active disease and disease progression in this population.

Despite the concern regarding the potential for significant liver disease, four recent studies *(39–42)* attest to the relatively benign nature of

CHC in patients with persistently normal ALT. Mathurin et al. *(39)* performed a case-control study of 102 patients with positive hepatitis C virus antibody and normal ALT and 102 patients with positive hepatitis C virus antibody and abnormal ALT. HCV RNA was positive in 66 and 97%, respectively. Histology grade (0.6 vs 1.38; $P < .0001$) and stage of fibrosis (.95 vs 1.8; $P < .001$) were much lower in the normal ALT group. Patients with normal ALT, who were positive for HCV RNA, had histology scores as low as those with negative HCV RNA. In addition, patients with normal ALT had much slower rates of disease progression than the patients with abnormal ALT, regardless of HCV RNA status (fibrosis progression of .05 vs .13 (F-METAVIR) U/yr. The only patients with normal ALT who developed severe fibrosis or cirrhosis were those with a history of heavy alcohol consumption.

Jamal et al. *(41)* performed a case-control study of 75 patients with normal ALT and 200 with abnormal ALT, all of whom were positive for HCV RNA. They also observed lesser grades of inflammation and lower stages of fibrosis in the normal ALT group. Levels of HCV RNA were lower, and disease progression, measured by fibrosis score divided by estimated years of disease, was significantly slower in patients with normal ALT (.08 vs .15 F-ISHAK U/yr). One study of serial liver biopsies *(42)* demonstrated no change in either histologic inflammatory grade or fibrosis stage, over a period of 5 yr.

These data indicate that patients with normal ALT, who are HCV RNA negative, may be free of hepatitis C, and are not at risk for disease progression. Those who have a normal ALT, but are positive for HCV RNA, are likely to have limited liver disease and slow rates of disease progression.

One is left to conclude that the natural history of hepatitis C has not yet been fully defined *(43)*. Current data suggest that the course of CHC is variable, and that some patients appear to demonstrate little evidence of disease progression; others are at risk for development of cirrhosis and its complications. Serious sequelae may emerge in a subgroup after a prolonged period of infection, usually beyond two decades.

DISEASE PROGRESSION IN CHRONIC HEPATITIS

The major determinant of clinically significant liver disease in patients with CHC is the progressive accumulation of hepatic fibrosis *(27,33,44–53)*. The rate of progression in fibrosis is highly variable, generally requiring 20–40 yr from initiation of infection to result in death from cirrhosis *(1,19,20,25–33,35,43)*. Yano et al. have suggested that the degree of necrosis, inflammation, and fibrosis on liver biopsy predicts risk of pro-gression to cirrhosis (Fig. 4) *(48)*. Studies examining progression of fibrosis,

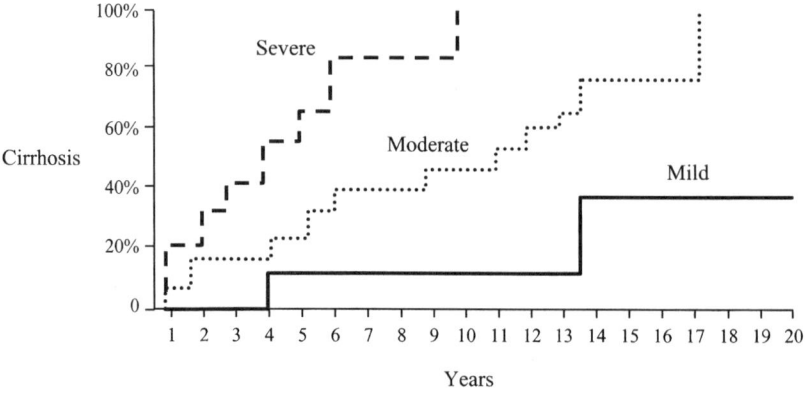

Fig. 4. Graph showing that patients with more severe inflammation and necrosis on baseline liver biopsy were at greatest risk to develop cirrhosis in long-term follow-up. (Adapted with permission from ref. *48*.)

from serial liver biopsies in a population of HCV patients with chronic hepatitis and variable degrees of fibrosis, have demonstrated an average rate of increase in METAVIR fibrosis score of 0.133 U/yr *(47,54)*.

In the study by Poynard *(47)*, in which risk factors for progression of hepatitis C were studied in 2235 patients, disease progression ranged within a spectrum from rapid to indolent. Only three factors were associated with disease progression: age >40 yr at time of infection, ethanol >50 g/d, and male gender. There was no correlation with viral level or genotype. Some patients rapidly progressed from infection to cirrhosis in less that 10 yr. Others, called "slow fibrosers," who often had normal ALT, progressed to cirrhosis only after 30 yr or more of disease.

If one assumes linear progression in disease, the annual rate of fibrosis can be calculated for a given patient simply by dividing the METAVIR fibrosis score on liver biopsy (F-METAVIR), by the estimated number of years that the patients has had disease. The projected length of time required to develop cirrhosis (F-METAVIR stage 4) is calculated by dividing 4 by the fibrosis progression per year. For example, a patient with CHC has an F-METAVIR stage 2, and presumably acquired hepatitis C by blood transfusion 20 yr ago. He asks, "When am I going to get cirrhosis?" Using the above method, one might answer, 4 / (2/20) = 40 yr from time of infection to time of cirrhosis, or 20 yr from now. A word of caution: hepatitis C may not follow a linear course. This simple prognostic tool has not been validated, and certainly does not account for changes in rates of disease progression. When counseling patients, give guidelines, rather than absolute projections, and insist that patients continue to be followed for changes in their course.

Table 3
Factors Associated with Disease Progression in Patients with CHC

Host
    Age >50 yr
    Race other than African American
    Male gender
    Fe overload
    Steatosis
    Possibly differences in immunologic response
Viral
    Possibly size of initial inoculum
    Possibly genotype 1, particularly 1B
    Possibly quasispecies
Extraneous
    Alcohol
    Co-infection with HBV
    Co-infection with HIV
    Possibly smoking
    Possibly other environmental factors
    Possibly geographic location

RISK FACTORS FOR DISEASE PROGRESSION

Patients with abnormal ALT are at greatest risk of disease progression, and most of the information regarding evolution of fibrosis in patients with hepatitis C is obtained in patients with biopsy evidence of active chronic hepatitis and abnormal ALT. Because disease progression is so highly variable, it is likely that a number of factors affect disease progression (Table 3). These risk factors are categorized as primarily host, viral, or extraneous.

A word of caution regarding the interpretation of risk factors as potentially contributing to disease pathogenesis. Risk factors are usually defined by their statistical association with the prevalence of a given disease. Ideally, risk factors should be identified in the context of randomized, controlled studies, in which the outcome of the disease in question can be assessed in the presence or absence of the risk factor. Authors often infer a direct role of risk factors in disease pathogenesis, but only rarely is experimental support provided.

Host Factors

AGE AND DURATION OF INFECTION

Separating the role of age, *per se*, from length or duration of infection is often difficult, when examining relationships to disease progression. One study *(55)*, of 838 patients referred to an outpatient hepatology clinic for management of CHC, examined patients for factors associated with disease progression. Most of the patients had established liver disease, 16.8% had cirrhosis on entry, and 7.4% died during a mean follow-up of 26.9 mo. Death resulting from complications of liver disease, including liver failure and HCC, occurred only in cirrhotics and accounted for half of the total deaths. Risk of death was increased in patients with cirrhosis, long duration of disease, alcohol consumption, injection drug use, and older age. Acquisition of infection at a young age was associated with higher risk of dying from liver disease. Risk of death was decreased by use of interferon.

The Niederau study *(55)* also suggested that young age at acquisition of infection was associated with higher risk of liver disease. In contrast, other studies *(47)* have suggested that the rate of disease progression is more rapid, the older the age at the time of infection. This discrepancy may result from the unique characteristics of the study populations, and simply reflect the most important variable, duration of disease, which can be related to age.

Prevalence studies, which examine a cross-section of a population at a given point in time, indicate that more severe histology changes are found in older patients with high levels of HCV RNA, genotype 1 or 1B, and more extensive quasispecies diversity *(56–61)*. Cohorts followed for a short period of time after acute infection tend to be younger and have relatively benign outcomes; but cohorts followed later, after development of established hepatitis, tend to be older, and to have higher risk of morbidity and mortality related to liver disease *(62)*.

Mode of Transmission

Several pieces of evidence suggest that transfusion-acquired hepatitis C is more rapidly progressive than community-acquired hepatitis C. First, posttransfusion acute hepatitis C is histologically worse that sporadic acute hepatitis C *(63)*. Second, histology tends to be worse in patients with CHC acquired by transfusion *(64,65)*. Third, the link of PTH to more aggressive disease was convincingly demonstrated in a large sample of 6664 patients, studied at 30 French health centers *(66)*. The cases were representative of patients with established disease, who would be referred to a treatment center. The average length of time between estimated time of exposure and referral was 11 yr, and most patients exhibited biochemical evidence of hepatitis for 2 yr prior to establishment of the diagnosis of hepatitis C.

As expected from the above discussion, these cases represented later-stage disease with 20% of patients who underwent liver biopsy demonstrating cirrhosis. Cirrhosis was more common in patients who acquired hepatitis C via blood transfusion, had longer duration of disease, were heavy users of alcohol, and had co-infection with hepatitis B. HCC was only observed in patients with cirrhosis. Fourth, Gordon et al. studied 627 patients at one U.S. medical center, and confirmed the link of PTH to more aggressive disease. Logistic regression analysis revealed that the risk of liver failure was predicted primarily by acquisition of infection through transfusion *(67)*. Those authors also found that serum albumin, prothrombin time, and platelet count predicted risk of future hepatic decompensation, and that the risk of developing HCC in cirrhotics was 1.2%/yr. The finding that acquisition by transfusion predicted subsequent late clinical events suggests that the load of the initial viral inoculum may modify either the innate cytotoxicity of the virus or the immunological response of the host.

GENDER

Male sex may be another risk factor for more rapid progression of fibrosis *(47,54)*. Or, conversely, female sex may be protective. In the studies of women who acquired hepatitis C after anti-D immunoglobulin, rates of development of cirrhosis, after approx 20 yr of infection, were 0.4–4% *(19,20)*. In contrast, a group of predominantly male injection drug users experienced an 8% risk of cirrhosis after 25 yr *(34)*. Patients in the latter study, however, also had other risk factors for disease progression, such as heavy alcohol consumption. One report of a small number of patients *(35)* suggested that the risk of cirrhosis in males, without other risk factors for disease progression, followed for 45 yr, was 18.2%. It is intriguing to speculate that disease expression might be modified by gender, because several investigations have demonstrated significant differences in effects of male and female steroid hormones on hepatic metabolism and protein synthesis.

RACE

Existing data, although inconclusive, suggest that African Americans may have slower rates of disease progression than their white counterparts. Also, results from therapeutic trials suggest that the ability of African Americans to clear hepatitis C, when treated with current antiviral regimens, is limited. Additional studies are needed to determine if these observations are true, or simply reflect other confounding variables, such as duration of disease, mode of acquisition, viral factors, or other extraneous risk factors.

PEDIATRIC POPULATIONS

Hepatitis C is acquired by infants and young children via transfusion of blood or blood products, by vertical transmission from an infected mother at the time of delivery, or by horizontal transmission from infected siblings or playmates. In general, pediatric cases of CHC are mild, with little evidence of disease progression for at least two decades. A minority will develop fibrosis that progresses with age and duration of disease *(68,69)*. Vogt et al. *(70)* examined the outcome of hepatitis C in children who had undergone cardiac surgery prior to 1991, at a mean age of 2.8 yr. They identified 67 cases that were hepatitis C virus antibody-positive, out of a cohort of 458 children. The mean follow-up after the first operation was 19.8 yr. 37/67 who had positive hepatitis C virus antibody also tested positive for HCV RNA; infection had supposedly cleared in the other 30. Only 1/37 had abnormal liver enzymes, but this patient also had congestive hepatopathy from right heart failure. 17 had liver biopsies, 14 were essentially normal, but 3 did show evidence for progressive liver damage. 2/3 had congestive heart failure, and the third was co-infected with hepatitis B. Thus, for at least 20 yr, children infected with hepatitis C have an excellent prognosis, with little evidence of either chronic hepatitis or disease progression. Long-term follow-up for 30–50 yr will be required to determine whether the disease remains quiescent, or becomes progressive with risk of fibrosis, cirrhosis, or liver cancer *(71)*.

SEVERITY OF HEPATIC INFLAMMATION

Other factors that predict more rapid progression of disease are high-grade inflammation or fibrosis on initial liver biopsy *(47)*. Two studies indicate that patients with severe grades of inflammation or more extensive fibrosis are more likely to progress to either cirrhosis or decompensation within a follow-up period of 10 yr *(48,49)*.

IMMUNOLOGIC RESPONSE

Hepatitis C persists as a chronic infection, despite a diversified host humoral and cellular immune response. Host defense mechanisms against viral pathogens include antibody formation, natural killer cells, interferon production, and CD4 and CD8 T-cell responses *(72)*. Viruses persist by interfering with one or several of the mechanisms of viral clearance. One mechanism by which hepatitis C avoids immunologic clearance is the development of a limited and inadequate T-cell response, because of minimal expression of viral proteins at the cell surface, a single viral peptide–HLA complex *(73)*. Although several immunologic mechanisms have been proposed, and are currently under investigation, there is no unifying theme linking specific immunologic responses to fibrosis, disease progression, decompensation, or development of HCC *(74)*.

Viral Factors

No single, unique characteristic of hepatitis C consistently predicts progression in liver disease. Viral factors that might determine outcome include the dose at the time of infection, genotype, and the presence of quasispecies (HCV genetic diversity). The effect of dose in initiating progressive disease is unknown *(75,76)*. However, several lines of evidence indicate that a large initial inoculum of hepatitis C, acquired by transfusion, may be more aggressive (*see* "Mode of Transmission" above). Most studies suggest that genotype 1 provokes more severe disease than does genotype 2 *(77,78)*, and that 1b is more harmful than 1a. But the impact of genotype on disease progression is not as evident when controlled for duration of disease. The impact of HCV quasispecies has also been studied by comparing its presence among those with acute resolving hepatitis with those who progress to chronic hepatitis *(61,79)*. Despite these observations, neither genotype, level of virus, nor quasispecies diversity have been consistently associated with disease progression.

Extraneous Factors

ALCOHOL

Most studies have suggested that chronic heavy consumption of alcohol is an important co-factor in progression of CHC to cirrhosis and hepatoma. Early epidemiological surveys *(80,81)* established the relationship between HCV infection and alcohol liver disease. Subsequent investigations indicate that chronic heavy alcohol use may promote HCV replication *(82,83)*. In numerous epidemiologic studies, alcohol is often identified as a major factor in promoting progression of liver disease *(84–88)*. An Australian study of 234 patients with CHC, who underwent liver biopsy, demonstrated cirrhosis in 21%, and that the risk of cirrhosis was related to two primary factors: patient age, and total lifetime alcohol consumption *(89)*. One could conclude that, in general, alcohol intake, especially exceeding 50 g/d, promotes progression of fibrosis, accelerates liver disease, and is also linked to an increased risk for HCC *(90)*. Two case-control studies *(91)* from Italy are consistent with the fact that both excessive alcohol consumption and hepatitis C can independently lead to cirrhosis. Excessive intake of alcohol (>50 g/d), with coexistent hepatitis C, multiplies the risk of developing cirrhosis.

IRON

Fe overload may be a risk factor for more rapid progression of fibrosis in patients with CHC *(47,54,92)*. One recent study *(93)* examined the relationships between hemochromatosis gene mutations, alcohol, and hepatic accumulation of Fe in patients with viral hepatitis. In men with chronic hepatitis, hepatic Fe concentration was independently related to only two factors: alcohol and *HFE* gene mutations (C282Y and H63D). *HFE* mutations (C282Y and H63D) were assessed in 184 patients with CHC, and in 487 controls *(94)*. Liver biopsies were done in 149 patients, and Fe was quantitated in 114 of the biopsies. The allele frequencies of C282Y in patients with CHC and controls were 7.1 and 4.8, in patients and controls, respectively. The allele frequencies of H63D were 11.6 and 11.1, respectively. Hepatic Fe overload was more common in those with *HFE* gene mutations (60 vs 33%, $P < .005$). Another study demonstrated that heterozygosity for the C282Y mutation, in patients with CHC, was not only associated an increased hepatic concentration of Fe, but also an increase in hepatic fibrosis *(95)*. Cirrhosis was found in 40% of heterozygotes for the C282Y mutation, and only 9% of those with homozygous wild-type *HFE* gene.

STEATOSIS

Hepatic steatosis is frequently observed during histology examination of liver biopsies from patients with hepatitis C, and may be another risk factor for more rapid progression of fibrosis *(47,54)*. Hourigan et al. *(96)* studied the relationship of body mass index, diabetes mellitus, alcohol consumption, hepatic Fe content, and viral load to hepatic steatosis and fibrosis, in 148 patients with CHC *(96)*. 61% had steatosis, which was highly correlated to both body mass index and degree of hepatic fibrosis. In contrast, neither steatosis nor fibrosis correlated with hepatic Fe content, alcohol intake, gender, or viral load. Thus, in subsets of patients with CHC, obesity, possibly by inducing hepatic steatosis, is a risk factor for disease progression. It has also been suggested that hepatic steatosis could be caused by inhibition of fatty acid oxidation by certain gene products of the virus, such as core protein *(97–99)*. The link between steatosis and fibrosis is less clear, but may involve lipid peroxidation, which is known to stimulate stellate cell activation and synthesis of type I collagen. Although not yet established for CHC, these pathogenetic mechanisms may be important in liver disease, because of alcohol and Fe overload or hemochromatosis *(100,101)*.

CO-INFECTION WITH HEPATITIS B

One early study *(102)* examined the impact of positive hepatitis C virus antibody on disease progression in 148 patients with chronic hepatitis B. 16 patients were co-infected with hepatitis C, and were more likely to have cirrhosis (44 vs 21%) or decompensated liver disease (24 vs 6%). Co-infection with hepatitis B also increases the risk of carcinogenesis

(103,104). Not all cases of co-infection are detected by routine serologic testing for HBsAg or hepatitis B core antibody. Cacciola et al. *(105)* examined 200 patients with chronic hepatitis for presence of HBV DNA, using a highly sensitive polymerase chain reaction assay. 100 lacked both HBsAg and hepatitis B core antibody, and the other 100 were negative for HBsAg, but positive for hepatitis B core antibody. 20% of patients negative for all HBV markers, and 46% of those with isolated hepatitis B core antibody, had positive HBV DNA. Biopsy-proven cirrhosis was more common in co-infected patients (33 vs 19%, $P < .04$).

CO-INFECTION WITH HIV

Co-infection with HCV occurs in 30–75% of patients with HIV infection, primarily in those who acquired HIV by either injection drug use or transfusion *(106)*. 90% of active injection drug users over age 45 yr are positive for HCV. Four studies *(107–110)* have demonstrated that liver disease is worse in the setting of HCV–HIV co-infection. ALT levels are higher, fibrosis is much more severe, and cirrhosis, liver failure, and hepatoma occur at an accelerated rate. Mortality rate is higher in co-infected patients (11 vs 6.8%), and nearly all of the increased mortality is related to death from liver disease (40% of deaths in the co-infected group) *(107)*. Progression of fibrosis in co-infected patients is related to consumption of >50 g/d alcohol, CD4 count <200 cells/µL, and age at onset of HCV infection of <25 yr *(111)*. It is not clear that HCV infection alters the course of HIV infection, especially in the era of highly active antiretroviral therapy.

SMOKING

One study *(103)* suggests that smoking may also promote progression of liver disease in patients with CHC. Mechanisms of this potential effect of smoking have not been defined.

RISK OF DECOMPENSATION IN CHILD'S A CIRRHOSIS

Patients who progress to cirrhosis may remain compensation without deterioration in liver function or clinical status, for many years. Fattovich et al. *(112)* reported outcomes in 384 European patients with compensated cirrhosis (Childs-Turcotte-Pugh score [CTP] <7) caused by CHC. The mean length of follow-up was 5 yr, but some patients were only followed for 6 mo and others for over 12 yr. By actuarial analysis, the risk of decompensation (ascites, variceal bleed, or encephalopathy) was 18% and risk of HCC was 7% (Fig. 5), at 5 yr follow-up (Fig. 5). 13% of the cohort died, with 71% of deaths related to liver disease. Overall survival was 91% at 5 yr, and 79% at 10 yr. Patients who experienced

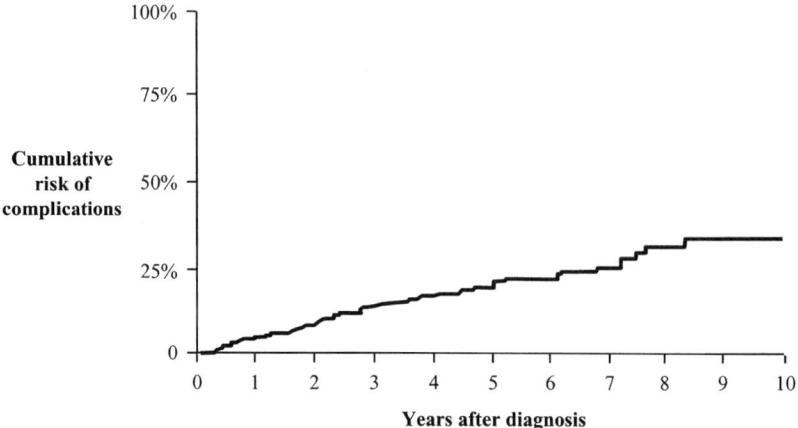

Fig. 5. Actuarial plot demonstrating risk of developing complications is shown for patients with hepatitis C and compensated cirrhosis. Risk was 18% at 5 yr and approx 35% at 10 yr. (Adapted with permission from ref. *112*.)

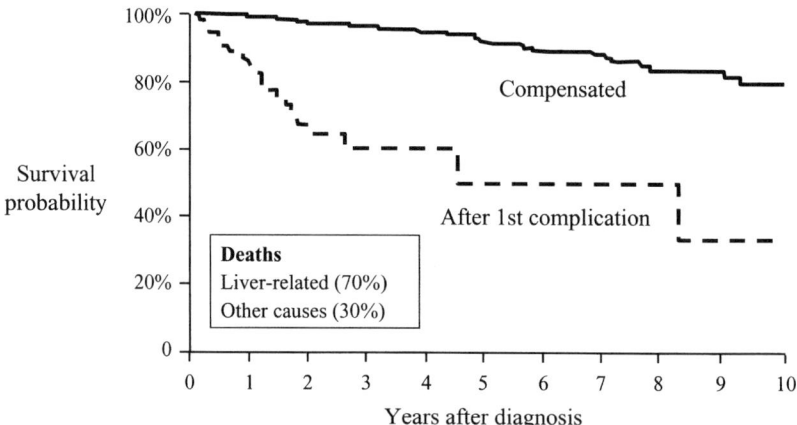

Fig. 6. Outcomes in cirrhotic patients with hepatitis C are shown. Compensated cirrhotics may enjoy a good survival for up to 10 yr. In contrast, cirrhotics who experience decompensation, manifested by a single complication, have significantly shortened survival. (Adapted with permission from ref. *112*.)

decompensation had markedly diminished survival, compared to those who remained compensated (Fig. 6). Multivariate analysis revealed that the major predictors of poor outcome were bilirubin >17 mmol/L, "hepatic stigmata" on physical examination, age >54 yr, and platelet count <130,000 × 10^6/L.

Table 4
Annual Risk of Decompensation of Liver Disease, Development of Hepatoma
(HCC), or Death in Patients with Compensated (Child's A) Cirrhosis

Ref no.	Decompensated	HCC (% patients/yr)	Death
Fattovich *(112)*	3.6	1.4	2.6
Serfaty *(113)*	5.0	3.3	4.0
Hu *(114)*	4.4	2.0	3.6
Khan *(115)*	6.0	2.4	3.8

Study of a smaller ($N = 103$), but similar cohort of patients, followed for a mean of 40 mo (range 6–72 mo), revealed a 25% risk of decompensation and 11% risk of HCC *(113)*. 16% of patients had died by 4 yr follow-up. Multivariate analysis indicated that low albumin and absence of prior treatment with interferon were the major independent predictors of poor outcome.

Hu and Tong *(114)* reported results in 112 patients, followed for a mean of 4.5 yr (range 2–7.7 yr). Decompensated occurred in 22.2%, and HCC in 10.1%. They estimated the yearly incidence of decompensation at 4.4%/yr, and risk of HCC at 2.0%/yr. Once patients deteriorated, survival diminished dramatically, from a baseline 5-yr survival of 82.8%, to a survival of 51.5% after decompensation. Survival was poorer in patients with age >55 yr, history of transfusion, albumin <3.5 g/dL, platelets <130,000 × 10^6/L, and viral load >1 × 10^6 vEq/mL. One additional series *(115)* highlighted outcome in 91 cirrhotics with compensation disease, and found that the risk of decompensation was approx 30%, and risk of HCC, 12%, at 5-yr of follow-up. 19% of the cohort either received a liver transplant or died by 5 yr.

In a patient with Child's class A cirrhosis, the overall risk of decompensation ranges from 3.6 to 6.0%/yr, the risk of HCC ranges from 1.4 to 3.3%/yr, and risk of death ranges from 2.6 to 4.0%/yr (Table 4).

OUTCOME AFTER DECOMPENSATION OF CIRRHOSIS

The natural history and the prognostic factors in hepatic cirrhosis have been extensively studied, but several aspects remain unclear, and prognostic factors have not been validated fully *(47,112–134)*.

Certain clinical problems, such as development or complications of ascites, predict a poor prognosis (Fig. 7). Patients with compensated cirrhosis who develop ascites have a 2-yr survival of 50% and 5-yr

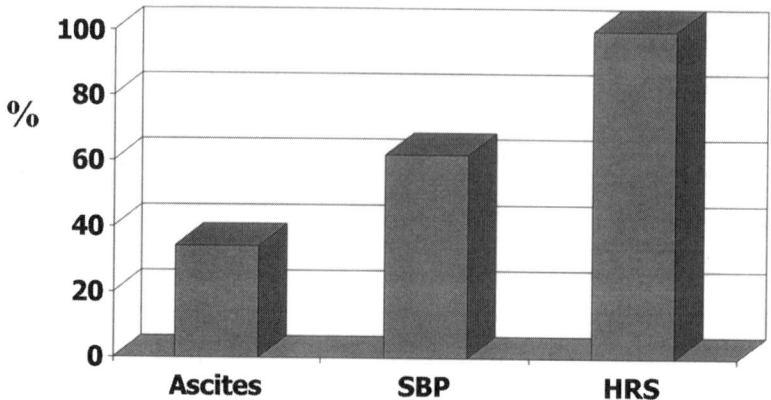

Fig. 7. Development of ascites carries an ominous prognosis. Complications of ascites, such as spontaneous bacterial peritonitis or hepatorenal syndrome, markedly shorten survival. (Adapted with permission from ref. *116.*)

survival of only 20% *(116–118)*. Various proposed scores and models combine biochemical, clinical, and histology data to give an estimate of prognosis *(119–122)*. One of these, the CTP score, is a simple and valid index for assessing the severity of disease and prognosis in patients with cirrhosis.

The majority of the clinical consequences of chronic liver disease are related to progressive hepatic fibrosis, which produces portal hypertension and progressive decline in functioning hepatic mass. Portal hypertension develops in earlier stages of cirrhosis, and the amount of functioning hepatic tissue (functional mass) progressively decreases as the disease progresses from early to advanced cirrhosis *(135,136)*. The interaction of these two consequences of progressive disease produces most clinical manifestations. Hypersplenism *(137)*, marked collateral formation (with esophageal varices), and hepatic congestion related to portal hypertension characterize the cirrhotic patient *(1,47–49)*. Progressive portal hypertension results in the major clinical events of variceal bleeding and ascites formation *(27,46–48)*. A minimum portal pressure gradient ≥12 mmHg is required to initiate these clinical events, but the average portal pressure gradient at onset of these problems is greater than this (17 ± 3 mmHg) *(138–140)*. Although most cirrhotic patients have varices, fewer than 30% have variceal bleeding. The size and appearance of varices correlates with the tendency for bleeding *(141)*. Survival after variceal hemorrhage is related to the underlying severity of liver disease, as assessed by CTP score (Fig. 8).

Ascites occurs spontaneously in moderately advanced cirrhosis, when the functional mass is less than 50% of normal *(142–144)*. The 5-yr sur-

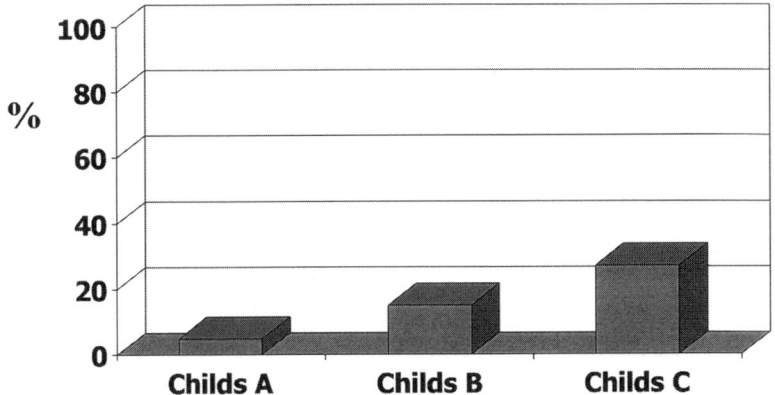

Fig. 8. Risk of dying from variceal hemorrhage is related to severity of underlying liver disease. Mortality is greatest in Child's C cirrhotics. (Adapted with permission from ref. *116.*)

vival after the onset of ascites is 20% *(116–119).* Further progression of liver disease leads to refractory ascites, hepatic encephalopathy, spontaneous bacterial peritonitis, and renal dysfunction *(145–150).* The 1-yr survival is less than 50%, in association with these clinical problems.

RISK OF HCC

HCC, complicating chronic viral hepatitis, is emerging as an increasingly important and difficult problem for programs in liver transplantation. As indicated previously, in the United States, there were 120,000–180,000 new cases of hepatitis C each year in the 1980s. Because it takes approx 20 yr to develop cirrhosis, and 30 yr to develop HCC, the clinical, social, and economic impact of the previous incident wave of cases is just now beginning to be experienced. In the year 2000, there were an estimated 8000–10,000 deaths in the United States, caused by liver disease from hepatitis C. This mortality rate is expected to double or triple by the year 2015. One cause of the projected excess mortality in these patients will be HCC.

Increasing numbers of patients are presenting for transplantation with cirrhosis and HCC, and increasing numbers of patients on the waiting list for transplantation are developing HCC while waiting on the list. The major risk factor for HCC is cirrhosis caused by chronic viral hepatitis, from both HBV and HCV. In the United States, CHC is now the most common diagnosis in patients listed for liver transplantation. Time on the waiting list prior to transplantation is increasing for newly listed patients, because of the mismatch in donor liver supply and recipient need. The risk of development of HCC in cirrhotic patients with chronic viral hepatitis ranges from 0.8 to 5.8%/yr. Patients on transplant waiting lists represent a group with more advanced cirrhosis, and are at greatest risk. Currently listed patients may wait years before being transplanted. For example, if the incidence of HCC in this population was 5%/yr, a patient on the list would have a cumulative risk of developing HCC of 14.3% at 3 yr and 22.8% at 5 yr.

HCC is the cause of death in 10–20% of cirrhotics with CHC, and nearly all of these patients are at the cirrhotic stage *(151–155)*. Fe overload, co-infection with other viruses, co-existent liver diseases, and genetic factors may increase the likelihood of HCC. Symptomatic tumors are generally large and lead to an average survival of 3–4 mo. There is no effective therapy for large tumors.

El-Serag et al. *(156)* studied the incidence of histologically proven HCC in the United States, between 1976 and 1995. Incidence of HCC was determined from the nine cancer registries that comprise the Surveillance, Epidemiology, and End Results Program of the National Cancer Institute, representing 14% of the U.S. population. Mortality statistics were determined from the National Center for Health Statistics as part of the U.S. vital statistics database. Rates of hospitalization for primary liver cancer were determined from the Patient Treatment File, a computerized database of the Department of Veteran's Affairs. Incidence of HCC increased from 1.4–2.4/100,000 population between the intervals 1976–1980 and 1990–1995. During these same periods, mortality from primary liver cancer increased by 41%, and hospitalizations for liver cancer increased by 46%. Incidence of HCC increased in younger persons in the interval 1991–1995, compared to earlier years. The increase in HCC incidence, and shift to younger persons, is consistent with the expected effect of the 1970s–1980s epidemic of hepatitis C. Similar progressive increases in HCC incidence have been noted in Japan *(157)*, United Kingdom *(158)*, and France *(159)*. Thus, developed countries, with a traditionally low-to-intermediate incidence and prevalence of HCC, are now facing an increasing number of HCC cases. This phenomenon has major implications for liver centers, transplant programs, and health care systems.

To begin to define the potential impact of HCC on a single transplant center, the author examined the annual case rate of HCC in Colorado, population approx 4 million persons, over the years 1988–1998 (Fig. 9). 1988 was chosen as the start date of analysis, because that was the beginning of the current program in liver transplantation. Data were collected from two sources: the Tumor Registry of the State of Colorado, and the Tumor Board of University of Colorado Health Sciences Center (UCHSC),

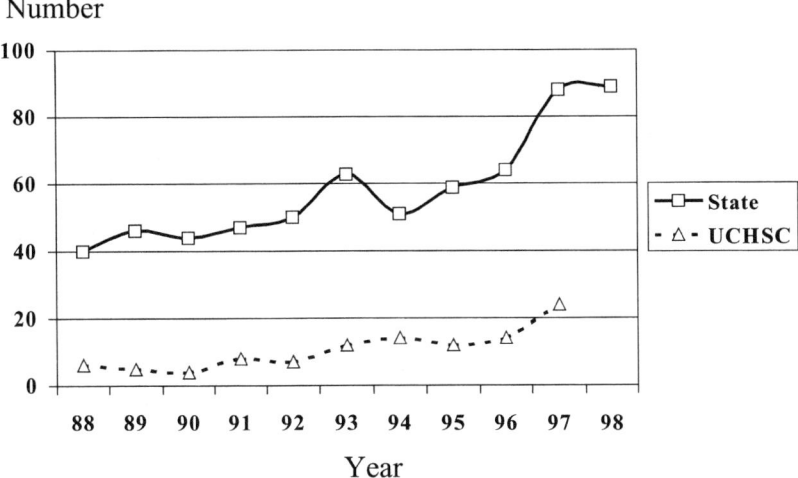

Fig. 9. Annual incidence of new cases of HCC recorded by the State of Colorado (solid line) and referred to the UCHSC (dotted line) are shown. Increasing numbers of cases of HCC will probably continue into the next 2–3 decades, overwhelm liver transplant waiting lists, and consume a high percentage of donor livers.

center's tumor registry. The annual case rate for the state at the beginning of this interval was 40–45 cases of HCC/yr, and, at the end, 85–90 cases/yr. The rise in number of new cases was nonlinear, and most dramatic for the years 1997 through 1999. During these same intervals, the number of cases of HCC evaluated and treated in this center increased approx fourfold, from 6 to 24 cases/yr. Certain characteristics of state and UCHSC cases were similar and reflective of U.S. cases in general, with male: female 2.6 and 2.7%, white 68 and 67%, and proportion of patients with local tumor 34 and 33%, respectively. However, UCHSC cases were significantly younger, with 50% of cases between ages 40 and 60 yr, compared to the state, in which 50% of cases were older than age 60 yr. Approximately 75% of UCHSC cases were HCV-positive. Thus, the relatively greater increase in cases of HCC at UCHSC resulted from younger patients with HCV referred for management and consideration of transplantation. Between 1995 and 1998, 38% of transplants performed at UCHSC were in patients with HCV, and approx one-half of new listings were HCV-positive. 21% of HCV cases had associated HCC, compared with a prevalence of 5% in non-HCV cases. Projecting these data into the near future, the author anticipates that, by the year 2010, the number of cases of HCV-related, locally confined, potentially transplantable HCC referred to this program, and developing on the waiting list, will exceed the cadaveric supply of donor livers. This emerging problem was a major stimulus for this center to move forward with living donor liver transplantation.

SUMMARY

Although much has been learned about the natural history of hepatitis C, gaps in knowledge and understanding of this chronic liver disease remain. Older, primarily retrospective studies, based in referral centers for liver disease, painted a grim picture of high rates of chronicity, moderate disease progression, and excessive rates for development of cirrhosis and HCC. Newer, prospective studies suggest a more benign outcome, with higher rates of spontaneous clearance of virus after acute infection, slower rates of progression to chronic liver disease, and reduced risk of liver cancer. Identifiable risk factors for disease progression include acquisition of infection by transfusion, long duration of disease, male gender, use of alcohol, and co-infection with hepatitis B or HIV. Cirrhotic patients, and those with HCC caused by hepatitis C, will represent an increasing burden and challenge to liver centers and programs in liver transplantation for several years to come *(160)*. The peak prevalence of persons infected for greater than 20 yr will not be reached until the year 2015. The full spectrum of the clinical, social, and economic impact of hepatitis C, both now and in the future, remains to be defined.

REFERENCES

1. Seeff LB. Natural history of hepatitis C. Hepatology 1997; 26(Suppl 1): 21S–28S.
2. Alter MJ, Kruszon-Moran D, Nainan OV, et al. Prevalence of hepatitis C virus infection in the United States, 1988 through 1994. N Engl J Med 1999; 341: 556–562.
3. Cohen J. Scientific challenge of hepatitis C. Science 1999; 285: 26–30.
4. Heintges T, Wands JR. Hepatitis C virus: epidemiology and transmission. Hepatology 1997; 26: 521–526.
5. Delage G, Infante-Rivard C, Chiavetta J, et al. Risk factors for acquisition of hepatitis C virus infection in blood donors: results of a case-control study. Gastroenterology 1999; 116: 893–899.
6. Serfaty L, Giral P, Elghouzzi MH, et al. Risk factors for hepatitis C virus infection in hepatitis C virus antibody ELISA-positive blood donors according to RIBA-2 status: a case-control survey. Hepatology 1993; 17: 183–187.
7. Williams I. Epidemiology of hepatitis C in the United States. Am J Med 1999; 107: 2S–9S.
8. Murphy EL, Bryzman SM, Glynn SA, et al., for the NHLBI Retrovirus Epidemiology Donor Study (REDS). Risk factors for hepatitis C virus infection in United States blood donors. Hepatology 2000; 31: 756–762.
9. Centers for Disease Control and Prevention. Recommendations for prevention and control of hepatitis C (HCV) infection and HCV-related chronic disease. MMWR 1998; 47: 1–38.

10. Conte D, Fraquelli M, Prati D, et al. Prevalence and clinical course of chronic hepatitis C virus (HCV) infection and rate of HCV vertical transmission in a cohort of 15,250 pregnant women. Hepatology 2000; 31: 751–755.
11. Frank C, Mohamed MK, Strickland GT, et al. Role of parenteral antischistosomal therapy in the spread of hepatitis C virus in Egypt. Lancet 2000; 355: 887–891.
12. Abdel-Aziz F, Habib M, Mohamed MK, et al. Hepatitis C virus (HCV) infection in a community in the Nile delta: population description and HCV prevalence. Hepatology 2000; 32: 111–115.
13. Kiyosawa K, Tanaka E, Sodeyama T, et al., and the South Kiso Hepatitis Study Group. Transmission of hepatitis C in an isolated area in Japan: community-acquired infection. Gastroenterology 1994; 106: 1596–1602.
14. Alter MJ. Epidemiology of hepatitis C. Hepatology 1997; 26: 62S–65S.
15. World Health Organization. Hepatitis C. Weekly Epidemiol Rec 1997; 10: 65–69.
16. Alter MJ, Mast EE. Epidemiology of viral hepatitis in the United States. Gastroenterol Clin North Am 1994; 23: 427–435.
17. Thiele DL. Viral hepatitis and acute liver failure. In: *Acute Liver Failure* (Lee WM, Williams R, eds.), Cambridge, UK: Cambridge University Press, 1997, pp. 10–18.
18. Schiodt FV, Atillasoy E, Shakil AO, et al. Etiology and outcome for 295 patients with acute liver failure in the United States. Liver Transpl Surg 1999; 5: 29–34.
19. Kenny-Walsh E for the Irish Hepatology Research Group. Clinical outcomes after hepatitis C infection from contaminated anti-D immune globulin. N Engl J Med 1999; 340: 1228–1233.
20. Wiese M, Berr F, LaFrenz M, et al., the East German Hepatitis C Study Group. Low frequency of cirrhosis in a hepatitis C (genotype 1B) single-source outbreak in Germany: a 20-year multicenter study. Hepatology 2000; 32: 91–96.
21. Yoshiba M, Dehara K, Inoue K, et al. Contribution of hepatitis C virus to non-A, non-B fulminant hepatitis in Japan. Hepatology 1994; 19: 829–835.
22. Chu CM, Sheen IS, Liaw YF. Role of hepatitis C virus in fulminant viral hepatitis in an area with endemic hepatitis A and B. Gastroenterology 1994; 107: 189–195.
23. Villamil FG, Hu KQ, Yu CH, et al. Detection of hepatitis C virus with RNA polymerase chain reaction in fulminant hepatic failure. Hepatology 1995; 22: 1379–1386.
24. Farci P, Alter HJ, Shimoda A, et al. Hepatitis C virus-associated fulminant hepatic failure. N Engl J Med 1996; 335: 631–634.
25. Hoofnagle JH. Hepatitis C: clinical spectrum of disease. Hepatology 1997; 26: 15S–20S.
26. Kiiyosawa K, Sodeyama T, Tanaka E, et al. Interrelationship of blood transfusion non-A, non-B hepatitis and hepatocellular carcinoma. Analysis by detection of antibody to hepatitis C virus. Hepatology 1990; 12: 671–675.
27. Tong MJ, El-Farra NS, Reikes AR, et al. Clinical outcomes after transfusion-associated hepatitis C. N Engl J Med 1995; 332: 1463–1466.
28. Di Bisceglie AM, Goodman ZD, Ishak KG, et al. Long-term clinical and histological follow-up of chronic posttransfusion hepatitis. Hepatology 1991; 14: 969–974.
29. Hopf U, Moller B, Kuther D, et al. Long-term follow-up of posttransfusion and sporadi chronic hepatitis non-A, non-B and frequency of circulating antibodies to hepatitis C virus (HCV). J Hepatol 1990; 10: 69–76.
30. Koretz RL, Abbey H, Coleman E, et al. Non-A, non-B post-transfusion hepatitis: looking back in the second decade. Ann Intern Med 1993; 119: 110–115.
31. Mattson L, Sonnerborg A, Weiland O. Outcome of acute symptomatic non-A, non-B hepatitis: a 13-year follow-up study of hepatitis C virus markers. Liver 1993; 13: 274–278.

32. Tremolada F, Casarin C, Alberti A, et al. Long-term follow-up of non-A, non-B (type C) post-transfusion hepatitis. J Hepatol 1992; 16: 273–281.
33. Seeff LB, Buskell-Bales Z, Wright EC, et al. Long-term mortality after transfusion-associated non-A, non-B hepatitis. N Engl J Med 1992; 327: 1906–1911.
34. Rodger AJ, Roberts S, Lanigan A, et al. Assessment of long-term outcomes of community-acquired hepatitis C infection in a cohort with sera stored from 1971 to 1975. Hepatology 2000; 32: 582–587.
35. Seeff LB, Miller RN, Rabkin CS, et al. 45-Year follow-up of hepatitis C virus infection in healthy young adults. Ann Intern Med 2000; 132: 105–111.
36. Piton A, Poynard T, Imbert-Bismut F, et al. Factors associated with serum transaminase activity in healthy subjects: consequences for the definition of normal values, for selection of blood donors, and for patients with hepatitis C. MULTIVIRC group. Hepatology 1998; 27: 1213–1219.
37. Puoti C, Magrini A, Stati T, et al. Clinical, histological, and virological features of hepatitis C virus carriers with persistently normal or abnormal alanine transaminase levels. Hepatology 1997; 26: 1393–1398.
38. NIH Consensus Statement. Management of Hepatitis C. Hepatology 1997; 15:1–41.
39. Mathurin P, Moussalli J, Cadranel JF, et al. Slow progression rate of fibrosis in hepatitis C virus patients with persistently normal alanine transaminase activity. Hepatology 1998; 27: 868–872.
40. DiBisceglie AM. Chronic hepatitis C viral infection in patients with normal serum alanine aminotransferases. Am J Med 1999; 107: 53S–55S.
41. Jamal MM, Soni A, Quinn PG, et al. Clinical features of hepatitis C-infected patients with persistently normal alanine transaminase levels in the southwestern United States. Hepatology 2000; 30: 1307–1311.
42. Persico M, Persico E, Suozzo R, et al. Natural history of hepatitis C virus carriers with persistently normal aminotransferase levels. Gastroenterology 2000; 118: 760–764.
43. Seeff LB. Natural history of hepatitis C. Am J Med 1999; 107: 10S–15S.
44. De Bac C, Stroffolini T, Gaeta GB, et al. Pathogenic factors in cirrhosis with and without hepatocellular carcinoma: a multicenter Italian study. Hepatology 1994; 20: 1225–1230.
45. Koff RS, Dienstag JL. Extrahepatic manifestations of hepatitis C and the association with alcoholic liver disease. Semin Liver Dis 1995; 15: 101–109.
46. Takahashi M, Yamada G, Miyamoto R, et al. Natural course of chronic hepatitis C. Am J Gastroenterol 1993; 88: 240–243.
47. Poynard T, Bedossa P, Opolon P. Natural history of liver fibrosis progression in patients with chronic hepatitis C. Lancet 1997; 349: 825–832.
48. Yano M, Kumada H, Hage M, et al. Long-term pathological evolution of chronic hepatitis C. Hepatology 1996; 23: 1334–1340.
49. Vaquer P, Canet R, Llompart A, et al. Histological evolution of chronic hepatitis C. Factors related to progression. Liver 1994; 14: 265–269.
50. Noda K, Yoshihara H, Suzuki K, et al. Progression of type C chronic hepatitis to liver cirrhosis and hepatocellular carcinoma: its relationship to alcohol drinking and the age of transfusion. Alcohol Exp Res 1996; 20: 92–100A.
51. Merican I, Sherlock S, McIntyre N, Dusheiko GM. Clinical, biochemical and histological features in 102 patients with chronic hepatitis C virus infection. Q J Med 1993; 86: 119–125.
52. Perasso A, Testino G, Ansaldi F, et al. r-Interferon alfa-2b/ribavirin combined therapy followed by low-dose r-interferon alfa-2b in chronic hepitis C interferon nonresponders. Hepatology 1999; 29: 297–298.

53. Friedman SL. Evaluation of fibrosis and hepatitis C. Am J Med 1999; 107: 27S–30S.
54. Gerber MA. Histopathology of HCV infection. Clin Liver Dis 1997; 1: 530–602.
55. Niederau C, Lange S, Heintges T, et al. Prognosis of chronic hepatitis C: results of a large prospective cohort study. Hepatology 1998; 28: 1687–1695.
56. Hagiwara H, Hayashi N, Mita E, et al. Quantitation of hepatitis C virus RNA in serum of asymptomatic blood donors and patients with type C chronic liver disease. Hepatology 1993; 17: 545–550.
57. Nousbaum JB, Pol S, Nalpas B, et al. Collaborative Study Group. Hepatitis C virus type 1b (II) infection in France and Italy. Ann Intern Med 1995; 122: 161–168.
58. Gretch D, Corey I, Wilson J, et al. Assessment of hepatitis C virus RNA levels by quantitative competitive RNA polymerase chain reaction: high-titer viremia correlates with advanced stage of disease. J Infect Dis 1994; 169: 1219–1225.
59. Kato N, Yokosuka O, Hosoda K, et al. Quantification of hepatitis C virus by competitive reverse transcription-polymerase chain reaction: increase of the virus in advanced liver disease. Hepatology 1993; 18: 16–20.
60. Silini E, Bono F, Cividini A, et al. Differential distribution of hepatitis C virus genotypes in patients with and without liver function abnormalities. Hepatology 1995; 21: 285–290.
61. Honda M, Kaneko S, Sakai A, et al. Degree of diversity of hepatitis C quasispecies and progression of liver disease. Hepatology 1994; 20: 1144–1151.
62. Dienstag JL. The natural history of chronic hepatitis C and what we should do about it. Gastroenterology 1997; 112: 651–655.
63. Jove J, Sanchez-Taplas M, Bruguera M, et al. Posttransfusional versus sporadic non-A, non-B chronic hepatitis: a clinicopathological and evolutive study. Liver 1988; 8: 42–47.
64. Gordon SC, Elloway RS, Long JC, Dmuchowski CF. Pathology of hepatitis C as a function of mode of transmission: blood transfusion vs intravenous drug use. Hepatology 1993; 18: 1338–1343.
65. Alter MJ, Margolis HS, Krawczynski K, et al. Natural history of community-acquired hepatitis C in the United States. N Engl J Med 1992; 327: 1899–1905.
66. Roudot-Thoraval F, Bastie A, Pawlotsky JM, Dhumeaux D, and the Study Group for the Prevalence and Epidemiology of Hepatitis C Virus. Hepatology 1997; 26: 485–490.
67. Gordon SC, Bayati N, Silverman AL. Clinical outcome of hepatitis C as a function of mode of transmission. Hepatology 1998; 28: 562–567.
68. Badizadegan K, Jonas MM, Ott MJ, et al. Histopathology of the liver in children with chronic hepatitis C viral infection. Hepatology 1998; 28: 1416–1423.
69. Guido M, Rugge M, Jara P. Chronic hepatitis C in children: the pathological and clinical spectrum. Gastroenterology 1998; 115: 1525–1529.
70. Vogt M, Lang T, Frosner G, et al. Prevalence and clinical outcome of hepatitis C infection in children who underwent cardiac surgery before the implementation of blood-donor screening. N Engl J Med 1999; 341: 866–870.
71. Jonas MM. Hepatitis C infection in children. N Engl J Med 1999; 341: 912–913.
72. Chang KM. Mechanisms of chronicity in hepatitis C virus infection. Gastroenterology 1998; 115: 1015–1018.
73. Tsai SL, Chen YM, Chen MH, et al. Hepatitis C virus variants circumventing cytotoxic T lymphocyte activity as a mechanism of chronicity. Gastroenterology 1998; 115: 954–966.
74. Cerny A, Chisari FV. Pathogenesis of chronic hepatitis C: immunological features of hepatic injury and viral persistence. Hepatology 1999; 30: 595–601.

75. Gretch D, Corey I, Wilson J, et al. Assessment of hepatitis C virus RNA levels by quantitative competitative RNA polymerase chain reaction: high-titer viremia correlates with advanced stage of disease. J Infect Dis 1994; 196: 1219–1225.
76. Kato N, Yokosuka O, Hosoda K, et al. Quantification of hepatitis C virus by competitive reverse transcription polymerase chain reaction: increase of the virus in advanced liver disease. Hepatology 1993; 18: 16–20.
77. Dusheiko G, Weiss HS, Brown D, et al. Hepatitis C virus genotypes: an investigation of type-specific differences in geographic origin and disease. Hepatology 1994; 19: 13–18.
78. Ichimura H, Tamura I, Kurimura O, et al. Hepatitis C virus genotypes, reactivity to recombinant immunoblot assay 2 antigens and liver disease. J Med Virol 1994; 43: 212–215.
79. Farci P, Melpolder JC, Shimoda A, et al. Studies of HCV quasispecies in patients with acute resolving hepatitis compared to those who progress to chronic hepatitis. Hepatology 1996; 24: 350A.
80. Coelho-Little ME, Jeffers LJ, Bernstein DE, et al. Hepatitis C virus in alcoholic patients with and without clinically apparent liver disease. Alcohol Clin Exp Res 1995; 19: 1173–1176.
81. Mendenhall CL, Seeff LB, Diehl AM, et al. Antibodies to hepatitis B virus and hepatitis C virus in alcoholic hepatitis and cirrhosis: their prevalence and clinical relevance. Hepatology 1991; 14: 581–589.
82. Oshita M, Hayashi N, Kasahara A, et al. Increased serum hepatitis C virus RNA levels among alcoholic patients with chronic hepatitis C. Hepatology 1994; 20: 1115–1120.
83. Sawada M, Takada A, Takase S, et al. Effects of alcohol on the replication of hepatitis C virus. Alcohol Alcohol 1993; 1B: 85S–90S.
84. Befrits R, Hedman M, Blomquist L, et al. Chronic hepatitis C in alcoholic patients: prevalence, genotypes, and correlation to liver disease. Scand J Gastroenterol 1995; 30: 1113–1118.
85. Jenkins PJ, Cromie SL, Roberts SK, et al. Chronic hepatitis C, alcohol and hepatic fibrosis. Hepatology 1996; 24: 153A.
86. Matsuda Y, Amuro Y, Higashino K, et al. Relation between markers for viral hepatitis and clinical features of Japanese patients with hepatocellular carcinoma: possible role of alcohol in promoting carcinogenesis. Hepatogastroenterology 1995; 42: 151–154.
87. Noda K, Yoshihara H, Suzuki K, et al. Progression of type C chronic hepatitis to liver cirrhosis and hepatocellular carcinoma: its relationship to alcohol, drinking, and the age of transfusion. Alcohol Clin Exp Res 1996; 20: 95A–100A.
88. Rosman AS, Paronetto F, Galvin K, et al. Hepatitis C virus antibody in alcoholic patients: association with the presence of portal and/or lobular hepatitis. Arch Intern Med 1993; 153: 965–969.
89. Ostapowicz G, Watson KJR, Locarnini SA, Desmond PV. Role of alcohol in the progression of liver disease caused by hepatitis C virus infection. Hepatology 1998; 27: 1730–1735.
90. Schiff ER. Alcoholic patient with hepatitis C virus infection. Am J Med 1999; 107: 95S–99S.
91. Corrao G, Arico S. Independent and combined action of hepatitis C virus infection and alcohol consumption on the risk of symptomatic liver cirrhosis. Hepatology 1998; 27: 914–919.
92. Bonkovsky HL, Banner BF, Rothman AL. Iron and chronic viral hepatitis. Hepatology 1997; 25: 759–768.

93. Piperno A, Vergani A, Malosio I, et al. Hepatic iron overload in patients with chronic viral hepatitis: role of HFE gene mutations. Hepatology 1998; 28: 1105–1109.
94. Kazemi-Shiraz L, Datz C, Maier-Dobersberger T, et al. Relation of iron status and hemochromatosis gene mutations in patients with chronic hepatitis C. Gastroenterology 1999; 116: 127–134.
95. Smith BC, Grove J, Guzail MA, et al. Heterozygosity for hereditary hemochromatosis is associated with more fibrosis in chronic hepatitis C. Hepatology 1998; 27: 1695–1699.
96. Hourigan LF, MacDonald GA, Purdie D, et al. Fibrosis in chronic hepatitis C correlates significantly with body mass index and steatosis. Hepatology 1999; 29: 1215–1219.
97. Czaja AJ, Carpenter HA, Santrach PJ, Moore SB. Host- and disease-specific factors affecting steatosis in chronic hepatitis C. J Hepatol 1998; 29: 198–206.
98. Moriya K, Fujie H, Shintani Y, et al. Core protein of hepatitis C virus induces hepatocellular carcinoma in transgenic mice. Nat Med 1998; 4: 1065–1067.
99. Schwartz KB, Larroya S, Vogler C, et al. Role of influenza B virus in hepatic steatosis and mitochondrial abnormalities in a mouse model of Reye's syndrome. Hepatology 1991; 13: 96–103.
100. Houglum K, Ramm GA, Crawford DH, et al. Excess iron induces hepatic oxidative stress and transforming growth factor beta1 in genetic hemochromatosis. Hepatology 1997; 26: 605–610.
101. Niemela O, Parkkila S, Yla-Herttuala S, et al. Sequential acetaldehyde production, lipid peroxidation, and fibrogenesis in micropig model of alcohol-induced liver disease. Hepatology 1995; 22: 1208–1214.
102. Fong TL, Di Bisceglie AM, Waggoner JG, et al. Significance of antibody to hepatitis C virus in patients with chronic hepatitis B. Hepatology 1991; 14: 64–67.
103. Chiba T, Matsuzaki Y, Abei M, et al. Role of previous hepatitis B virus infection and heavy smoking in hepatitis C virus-related hepatocellular carcinoma. Am J Gastroenterol 1996; 91: 119–203.
104. Benvegnu L, Fattovich G, Noventa F, et al. Concurrent hepatitis B and C virus infection and risk of hepatocellular carcinoma in cirrhosis: a prospective study. Cancer 1994; 27: 2442–2448.
105. Cacciola I, Pollicino T, Squadrito G, et al. Occult hepatitis B virus infection in patients with chronic hepatitis C liver disease. N Engl J Med 1999; 341: 22–26.
106. Dieterich DT. Hepatitis C virus and human immunodeficiency virus: clinical issues in coinfection. Am J Med 1999; 107: 79S–84S.
107. Monga HK, Breauz K, Rodrigues-Barradas MC, Yoffe B. Increased HCV-related morbidity and mortality in HIV patients. Hepatology 1998; 28: 565A.
108. Serfaty L, Costagliola D, Wendum D, et al. Does HIV infection aggravate chronic hepatitis C in IV drug users? A case-control study. Hepatology 1998; 28: 462A.
109. Garcia-Samaniego J, Soriano V, Castilla J, et al. Influence of hepatitis C virus genotypes and HIV infection on histological severity of chronic hepatitis C. The hepatitis /HIV Spanish Study Group. Am J Gastroenterol 1997; 92: 1130–1134.
110. Hanley JP, Jarvis LM, Andrews J, et al. Investigation of chronic hepatitis C infection in individuals with haemophilia: assessment of invasive and non-invasive methods. Br J Haematol 1996; 94: 159–165.
111. Benhamou Y, Bochet M, DiMartino V, et al., for the MULTIVIRC Group. Liver fibrosis progression in human immunodeficiency virus and hepatitis C virus coinfected patients. Hepatology 1999; 30: 1054–1058.
112. Fattovich G, Giustina G, Degos F, et al. Morbidity and mortality in compensated cirrhosis type C: a retrospective follow-up study of 384 patients. Gastroenterology 1997; 112: 463–472.

113. Serfaty L, Hugues A, Chazouilleres O, et al. Determinants of outcome of compensated hepatitis C virus-related cirrhosis. Hepatology 1998; 27: 1435–1440.
114. Hu KQ, Tong MJ. Long-term outcomes of patients with compensated hepatitis C virus-related cirrhosis and history of parenteral exposure in the United States. Hepatology 1999; 29: 1311–1316.
115. Khan MH, Farrell GC, Byth K, et al. Which patients with hepatitis C develop liver complications? Hepatology 2000; 31: 513–520.
116. Gines P, Quintero E, Arroyo V, et al. Compensated cirrhosis: natural history and prognostic factors. Hepatology 1987; 7: 122–128.
117. D'Amico G, Morabito A, Pagliaro L, et al. Survival and prognostic indicators in compensated and decompensated cirrhosis. Dig Dis Sci 1986; 31: 468–475.
118. Magliocchetti N, Torchio P, Corrao G, et al. Prognostic factors for long-term survival in cirrhotic patients after the first episode of liver decompensation. Ital J Gastroenterol Hepatol 1997; 29: 38–46.
119. Christensen E, Schlichting P, Fauerholdt L, et al. Changes of laboratory variables with time in cirrhosis: prognostic and therapeutic significance. Hepatology 1985; 5: 843–853.
120. Christensen E, Schlichting P, Fauerholdt L, et al. Prognostic value of Child-Turcotte criteria in medically treated cirrhosis. Hepatology 1984; 4: 430–435.
121. Cox DR. Regression models and life tables. J R Stat Soc 1972; 34: 187–220.
122. Christensen E. Multivariate survival analysis using Cox's regression model. Hepatology 1987; 7: 1346–1358.
123. Pugh RNH, Murray-Lyon IM, Dawson JL, et al. Transection of the esophagus for bleeding esophageal varices. Br J Surg 1973; 60: 646–664.
124. Pasualetti P, Di Lauro G, Festuccia V, et al. Prognostic value of Pugh's modification of Child-Turcotte classification in patients with cirrhosis of the liver. Panminerva Med 1992; 34: 65–68.
125. Reisman Y, Gips CH, Lavelle SM. Assessment of liver cirrhosis severity in 1015 patients of the Euricterus database with Campbell-Child, Pugh-Child and with ascites and ascites-nutritional state (ANS) related classifications. Euricterus Project Management Group. Hepatogastroenterology 1997; 44: 1376–1384.
126. Merkel C, Bolognesi M, Finucci GF, et al. Indocyanine green intrinsic hepatic clearance as a prognostic index of survival in patients with cirrhosis. J Hepatol 1989; 9: 16–22.
127. Oellerich M, Burdelski M, Lautz HU, et al. Lidocaine metabolite as a measure of liver function in patients with cirrhosis. Ther Drug Monit 1990; 12: 219–226.
128. Moreli A, Narducci F, Pelli MA, et al. Relationship between aminopyrine breath test and severity of liver disease in cirrhosis. Am J Gastroenterol 1981; 76: 110–113.
129. Finucci G, Bellon S, Merkel C, et al. Evaluation of splanchnic angiography as a prognostic index of survival in patients with cirrhosis. Scand J Gastroenterol 1991; 91: 951–960.
130. Vorobioff J, Groszmann RJ, Picabea E, et al. Prognostic value of hepatic venous pressure gradient measurements in alcoholic cirrhosis: a 10-year prospective study. Gastroenterology 1996; 11: 701–709.
131. Merkel C, Gatta A, Zoli M, et al. Prognostic value of galactose elimination capacity, aminopyrine breath test, and ICG clearance in patients with cirrhosis. Comparision with the Pugh score. Dig Dis Sci 1991; 31: 1197–1203.
132. Katsuyoshi I, Mitchell D, Hann HL, et al. Progressive viral-induced cirrhosis: serial MR imaging findings and clinical correlation. Radiology 1998; 207: 729–735.
133. Taylor KJW, Gorelick FS, Rosenfield AT, Riely CA. Ultrasonography of chronic liver disease with histological correlation. Radiology 1981; 141: 51–161.

134. Chan CC, Hwang SJ, Lee FY, et al. Prognostic value of plasma endotoxin levels in patients with cirrhosis. Scand J Gastroenterol 1997; 32: 942–946.
135. Hoefs JC, Wang F, Kanel G. Functional measurement of nonfibrotic hepatic mass in cirrhotic patients. Am J Gastroenterol 1997; 92: 2054–2058.
136. Hoefs JC, Green G, Reynolds TB, et al. Mechanism for the abnormal liver scan in acute alcoholic liver injury. Am J Gastroenterol 1984; 79: 950–958.
137. Hoefs JC, Wang FW, Walker B, Kanel G. Novel, simple method of functional spleen volume calculation by liver-spleen scan. J Nuc Med 1999; 40: 1745–1755.
138. Bosch J. Medical treatment of portal hypertension. Digestion 1998; 59: 547–555.
139. Roberts LR, Kamath PS. Pathophysiology of variceal bleeding. Gasteointest Endosc N Am 1999; 9: 167–174.
140. Hoefs JC, Jonas FM, Sarfeh IJ. Diagnosis and hemodynamic assessment of portal hypertension. Surg Clin North Am 1990; 70: 267–289.
141. North Italian endoscopic club for the study and treatment of esophageal varices. Prediction of the first variceal hemorrhage in patients with cirrhosis of liver and esophageal varices: a perspective multicenter study. N Engl J Med 1988; 319: 983.
142. Horisawa M, Goldstein G, Waxman A, Reynolds T. The abnormal hepatic scan of chronic liver disease: its relationship to hepatic hemodynamics and colloid extraction. Gastroenterology 1976; 71: 210–213.
143. Hoefs JC, Wang F, Kanel G, et al. Perfused Kupffer cell mass: correlation with histology and severity of CLD. Dig Dis Sci 1995; 20: 552–560.
144. Kodama T, Watanabe K, Hoshi H, et al. Diagnosis of diffuse hepatocellular diseases during SPECT. J Nucl Med 1986; 27: 616–619.
145. Navasa M, Rimola A, Rodes J. Bacterial infections in liver disease. Semin Liver Dis 1997; 17: 323–333.
146. Runyon BA. Care of patients with ascites. N Engl J Med 1994; Fed 3: 330: 337–342.
147. Gines P, Sort P. Patholophysiology of renal dysfunction in cirrhosis. Digestion 1998; 59: 11–15.
148. Herrera JL. Management of acute liver failure. Dig Dis 1998; 16: 274–283.
149. Butterworth RF. Pathogenesis of acute hepatic encephalopathy. Digestion 1998; 59: 16–21.
150. Hoefs JC, Runyon BA. Spontaneous bacterial peritonitis. Dis Mon 1985; 31: 1–48.
151. Cancer of the Liver Italian Program (CLIP) Investigators. A new prognostic system for hepatocellular carcinoma: a retrospective study of 435 patients. Hepatology 1998; 28: 751–755.
152. Llovet JM, Bustamente J, Castells A, et al. Natural history of untreated nonsurgical hepatocellular carcinoma: rationale for the design and evaluation of therapeutic trials. Hepatology 1999; 29: 62–67.
153. Ohnishi K, Tanabe Y, Ryu M, et al. Prognosis of hepatocellular carcinoma smaller than 5 cm in relation to treatment: study of 100 patients. Hepatology 1987; 7: 1285–1290.
154. Akashi Y, Koreeda, Enemoto S, et al. Prognosis of unresectable hepatocellular carcinoma: an evaluation based on multivariate analysis of 90 cases. Hepatology 1991; 14: 262–268.
155. Gridelli B, Remuzzi G. Strategies for making more organs available for transplantation. N Engl J Med 2000; 343: 404–410.
156. El-Serag HB, Mason AC. Rising incidence of hepatocellular carcinoma in the United States. N Engl J Med 1999; 340: 745–750.
157. Okuda K, Fujimoto I, Hanai A, Urano Y. Changing incidence of hepatocellular carcinoma in Japan. Cancer Res 1987; 47: 4967–4972.

158. Taylor-Robinson SD, Foster GR, Arora S, et al. Increase in primary liver cancer in the UK, 1979–1994. Lancet 1997; 350: 1142–1143.
159. Deuffic S, Poynard T, Buffat L, Valleron AJ. Trends in primary liver cancer. Lancet 1998; 351: 214–215.
160. Armstrong GL, Alter MJ, McQuillan GM, Margolis HS. Past incidence of hepatitis C virus infection: implications for the future burden of chronic liver disease in the United States. Hepatology 2000; 31: 777–782.

5 Hepatitis C and HIV Co-Infection

Michael A. Poles, MD
and Douglas T. Dieterich, MD

CONTENTS

> INTRODUCTION
> HCV IS PREDOMINANTLY TRANSMITTED PARENTERALLY
> HIV CO-INFECTION ACCELERATES NATURAL HISTORY
>   OF HCV DISEASE
> HEPATITIS C INFECTION LIMITS ABILITY TO TREAT HIV
> PRESENCE OF HIV DOES NOT ALTER EFFICACY
>   OF ANTI-HCV THERAPY
> CONCLUSIONS
> REFERENCES

INTRODUCTION

The use of highly active antiretroviral therapy (HAART) has extended the healthy life-span of human immune deficiency virus (HIV)-infected patients; deaths among people with acquired immune deficiency syndrome (AIDS) declined for the first time in 1996, after the institution of this therapeutic approach. As the life expectancy of HIV-infected patients increases, greater attention will need to be focused on the recognition and management of potentially severe concurrent illnesses that may increase their mid- to long-range morbidity and mortality. Infection with hepatitis C virus (HCV) is many times more prevalent than that of HIV: According to the Centers for Disease Control (CDC), the prevalence of anti-HCV antibodies in the general population of the United States in early 1999 was 1.8%, corresponding to an estimated 3.9 million Americans infected with HCV. In comparison, the prevalence of HIV in the

From: *Clinical Gastroenterology: Diagnosis and Therapeutics*
Edited by: R. S. Koff and G. Y. Wu © Humana Press Inc., Totowa, NJ

United States was estimated, by the CDC, to be 800,000–900,000. HCV may not only impact upon the health status of HIV-infected patients, but also may decrease their quality of life and increase health care costs. The CDC estimates that the economic burden of HCV infection in the United States is $600 million/yr (CDC home page: www.cdc.gov). In terms of mortality, a recent European study showed that chronic liver disease, especially that caused by hepatotropic viruses, was the fifth leading cause of death among HIV patients admitted to the hospital *(1)*. Further, data from a postprotease database of almost 4000 patients (CHORUS) suggests that 39-yr-old HIV-infected patients, with CD4 cell count over 200, have almost matched survival, compared to age-matched non-HIV patients, but that the leading cause of non-AIDS-related death in these patients was liver disease *(2)*. Physicians caring for patients with HIV require up-to-date information to make rational decisions regarding HCV co-infection, to ensure that morbidity and mortality are minimized and quality of life and medical care costs are optimized.

In addition to both being major health issues, there are many other important similarities between HIV and HCV infection. Both viruses possess a single-stranded RNA genome, and result in a subclinical, chronic infection. Each of these viruses is able to evade the host's immune system, and each is naturally resistant to eradication through use of present therapeutic approaches. Additionally, the replication rate of each virus is extraordinarily high, with billions of HIV virions produced each day, and trillions of HCV virions being produced daily.

HCV IS PREDOMINANTLY TRANSMITTED PARENTERALLY

The risk of HCV transmission is far greater in patients who acquire HIV infection through the parenteral, compared to the sexual, route. It is estimated that 50–98% of patients who acquired HIV though intravenous drug use are co-infected with HCV *(3)*. The incidence of HCV infection is also high in HIV-infected hemophiliac patients, who, in the past, were treated with nonviral attenuated-clotting products (60–85%).

Only half of all patients infected with hepatitis C admit to a history of percutaneous exposure; sexual transmission is thought to play a role in some of the remaining cases. Despite the fact that a number of studies have addressed this issue, the role of homosexual and heterosexual transmission of HCV is still controversial; it is believed to occur, but with low efficiency. Nevertheless, the prevalence of HCV antibodies in HIV-positive homosexual males is ~4–8%, which is no different from HIV negative homosexuals *(4)*. However, this is still greatly increased over the

Table 1
Reported Effect of HIV Infection on HCV Infection

Increased sexual and vertical transmission of HCV
Increased HCV viral load
Accelerated natural history of HCV disease
Worsened hepatic damage caused by HCV
Increased genomic of HCV (development of quasispecies)
Increased risk of hepatotoxicity with HAART
No change in the efficacy of IFN-based therapy

prevalence in the general population. HCV may also be transmitted, though likely less frequently, through heterosexual sex. Some studies have suggested that the presence of HIV also increases heterosexual transmission of HCV, with one study showing male-to-female sexual transmission to be 5× more likely in the presence of HIV (5). Higher HCV viral loads, as has been reported in HIV co-infected patients, may be responsible for this increased transmissibility.

Vertical transmission of HCV, which also appears to occur with low efficiency, may be facilitated by HIV co-infection (6) (Table 1). In one study of 155 mothers infected with HCV, the risk of vertical transmission of HCV was 3.2× greater in mothers co-infected with HIV than those with HCV alone (7). The risk of vertical transmission of HCV may be proportional to the maternal HCV viral load that may be correlated with her degree of HIV-related immunosuppression. Some studies have not revealed an increased rate of vertical transmission in co-infected patients.

HIV CO-INFECTION ACCELERATES NATURAL HISTORY OF HCV DISEASE

Greater than half of immunocompetent, HCV-infected patients develop chronic hepatitis, and about 20% develop cirrhosis after 10–20 yr of infection. Approximately 15% of patients with HCV-related cirrhosis will develop hepatocellular carcinoma. Immunosuppression caused by HIV significantly alters the natural history of HCV infection. Hepatic damage resulting from HCV infection is believed to be predominantly caused by direct viral cytotoxicity, with contributions from the host immune response. Cell-mediated immunity, T-helper 1 (TH1) clones that recognize multiple core epitopes of HCV, are important in immune clearance of HCV, through elimination of virally infected hepatocytes (8–10). The decline in CD4 cells associated with progressive HIV infection appears to permit greater HCV replication, with more hepatic spread of HCV, and therefore vast hepatocyte injury. Co-infection with HIV also probably alters the response of immune cells to HCV; when CD3$^+$/CD30$^+$ cells are infected with both HIV and HCV, their cytokine production is skewed toward an anti-inflammatory TH2 response, rather than the protective TH1 response seen when cells are infected with HCV alone *(11)*. HCV can also escape from immunologic control through mutation of its hypervariable region, which is a major target of cell-mediated and humoral immune mechanisms *(12)*; thus, heterogeneity of this region, as seen to a greater degree in HIV-infected patients, may permit increased viral replication *(13)*. Although there is not a direct correlation between the plasma titers of HCV RNA and disease course, co-infected patients harbor greater amounts of HCV than immunocompetent patients, both in their plasma *(14,15)* and in their liver *(16)*.

A number of studies have suggested that the presence of HIV infection accelerates the course of HCV-related liver disease. When compared to HIV-negative patients, co-infected patients have a greater degree of piecemeal necrosis, portal inflammation, and fibrosis, which is the most important prognostic factor *(17,18)*. These pathologic findings appear to be clinically significant. Studies comparing HCV singly infected patients with HCV–HIV co-infected patients have shown that progression to cirrhosis occurs more commonly and more rapidly in those patients with HIV *(19,20)*. Studies comparing HCV and HCV–HIV co-infected hemophiliacs showed a significantly greater risk of hepatic decompensation and liver failure in the co-infected patients *(21,22)*. Another explanation for worsened hepatic damage in these patients is the greater use of hepatotoxic medications by HIV-infected patients, which may exacerbate the HCV-related hepatic disease. Some studies have suggested that HIV infection does not effect progression of HCV infection *(23)*, and all of these natural history studies are limited by the inability to precisely pinpoint the onset of HCV infection.

Less clear is what effect HCV infection has on the natural history of HIV infection. Most cross-sectional and longitudinal studies have not shown an effect of HCV infection on the course HIV disease, but controversy remains. For instance, one study showed that HIV–HCV co-infected patients, with CD4 cell counts greater than 500, experienced a greater progression to AIDS, wasting, and death *(24)*, and others have shown faster progression to AIDS and death in subjects infected with HCV genotype 1 *(25)*.

HEPATITIS C INFECTION LIMITS ABILITY TO TREAT HIV

A number of studies have attempted to address the question of whether protease inhibitors and other anti-HIV drugs affect HCV replication, and, conversely, whether HCV effects the development of hepatic damage caused by antiviral agents.

HIV protease inhibitors have not been found to inhibit HCV replication *(26)*. Additionally, the control of HIV to less than 400 copies by anti-HIV medications has no effect on the HCV viral load. Instead, initiation of HAART may transiently increase the level of aminotransferases, and even the HCV viral load for the first 3–4 mo of treatment, typically returning to baseline over the ensuing 3–8 mo *(27)*. A number of studies have addressed whether the presence of HCV infection increases the liver toxicity associated with HAART. Many antiretroviral drugs are hepatotoxicity; according to data found in the physicians' desk reference, the risk of hepatotoxicity of antiretroviral drugs is between 3 and 12%, depending on the therapeutic agent. Perhaps the earliest evidence of the true hepatotoxicity potential of these drugs was observed in 1995, when a hepatitis B treatment trial, using a fluorinated uridine nucleoside analog, fialuridine (FIAU), similar to those used in HIV treatment, resulted in hepatic failure and death in the majority of treated patients *(28)*. The mechanism has been found to be mitochondrial toxicity. Nucleoside analogs do not bind to nuclear DNA, but will bind to mitochondrial DNA and cause mitochondrial damage. The FIAU story was the worst reported to date, because FIAU is an irreversible binder of the mitochondrial DNA. All nucleoside analogs have the capacity to do this, and it is cumulative over time. FIAU toxicity was seen with 9 wk of exposure to the drug; other nucleoside analogs could take years to result in lactic acidosis. When over 70% of mitochondria are incapacitated, severe disease results. This is usually manifested by rising alanine aminotransferase (ALT) and bilirubin, liver failure (microvesicular steatosis on liver biopsy), lactic acidosis, and often pancreatitis, myopathy, and neuropathy. It appears that dideoxyinosine, stavvdine (d4T), and dideoxycytidine have much more affinity for mitochondria than do azidothymidine, abacavir, and 3TC (lamivudine). A normal lac-tic acid is <2.0 mmol/L, and any level over 10 is significantly associated with mortality. Monitoring the anion gap in these patients is not sufficient, because elevated anion gaps may be absent. It is important to think about mitochondrial toxicity in the care of HIV patients, when the patients complain of abdominal pain, nausea, vomiting, and rising ALT levels, especially for those infected with HCV or HBV. HC may also cause mitochondrial toxicity. A recent finding *(29)* on electron microscopy, in HC patients who do not have HIV, was mitochondrial damage in 92% of genotype 1 HC, 62% of genotype 2, and less commonly in genotype 3. This may explain why co-infected patients are more likely to have mitochondrial toxicity from nucleoside analogs. Hernandez et al. *(30)* found that co-existing HCV infection, older age, and a lower CD4 cell count contributed to nucleoside analog-related hepatotoxicity.

Protease inhibitors are also hepatotoxicity. In the largest study to date, Sulkowski et al. *(31)* studied approx 300 patients who were prescribed new antiretroviral therapy between 1996 and 1998. During therapy, aminotransferase levels increased in all patients, although severe hepatotoxicity (aminotransferase levels over 5× the upper limit of normal) was present in only 10% of patients, with the highest incidence occurring in patients given ritonavir (30%). The incidence of hepatotoxicity of any grade was greater in patients infected with HCV (54 vs 39%). Overall, in patients receiving antiretrovirals, excluding ritonavir, severe hepatotoxicity was seen in 9.4% of patients with chronic viral hepatitis, compared to 2.7% without viral hepatitis. However, most patients with chronic hepatitis did not experience hepatotoxicity (88%). Multivariate logistic analysis suggests that only ritonavir, and a CD4 cell count increase of more than 0.05×10^9 cells, was associated with severe hepatotoxicity. In this study, 60% of instances of severe hyperbilirubinemia resulted from indinavir usage. Again, the incidence of severe hyperbilirubinemia was elevated in patients with HCV co-infection (5.1 vs 1.4%). The increased incidence of hepatotoxicity in HCV patients receiving HAART may be caused by enhanced CD8 cell activity with CD4 reconstitution; studies have not shown that the increase in hepatotoxicity results from increased HCV replication *(32)*.

Clinicians may be reluctant to prescribe antiretroviral medications in the presence of chronic viral hepatitis, with or without elevations in liver-associated enzymes. Therefore, the presence of HCV infection limits the ability to care for HIV-infected patients. Normalizing ALT levels, and/or reducing HCV titer through anti-HCV treatment, may increase the tolerance of co-infected patients to antiretroviral therapy, although this remains untested.

PRESENCE OF HIV DOES NOT ALTER EFFICACY OF ANTI-HCV THERAPY

Given the effect that HIV has on the natural history of HCV disease, infection with HCV should be treated as any other opportunistic disease *(33)*, as has been suggested in the U.S. Public Health Service/Infections Disease Society of America 1999 guidelines. Until recently, the only FDA-approved treatment for chronic hepatitis C was α-interferon (IFN-α) monotherapy. A standard dosing regimen of 3 million units, thrice weekly for 6 mo, induces normalization of aminotransferase levels and histological improvement in up to 50% of treated patients. However, of these initial responders, more than one-half relapse within 6 mo after termination of treatment. In all, IFN-α therapy induces a sustained response, with eradication of the virus and stable improvement of liver histology in less than 20% of treated patients. The rate is even lower in patients infected with HCV genotype 1b, who make up the majority of the infected patients in the United States. There are few studies that have reported long-term results of the so-called sustained responders, raising the question of how IFN-α affects the future development of the sequelae of hepatitis C, e.g., cirrhosis, end-stage liver disease. The incidence of hepatocellular carcinoma is reduced, even if treatment fails *(34,35)*. Patients who clear HCV RNA after 6 mo of IFN-α, and whose HCV is genotype 1a or 1b, should be treated for at least 12, and perhaps 18 mo.

Several factors may help predict which patients may respond to IFN-α, including low pretreatment levels of HCV RNA, low genomic diversity, infection with non-1b genotype, and low-grade pretreatment hepatic fibrosis. The latest hypothesis advanced for the low treatment success rate in the genotype 1 patients is the observation that the E2 protein of genotype 1 HCV envelope has sequence homology with the protein kinase, PKR. This enzyme is responsible for the actions of IFN. The E2 protein of genotype 1 is a blocker of IFN's action *(36)*. Another theory postulates that patients who fail to respond to IFN are genetically predisposed to a TH2 cytokine response to HCV, which is ineffective in inhibiting HCV replication *(37)*. A much simpler epidemiologic explanation for lack of response would be an increased incidence of occult HBV co-infection, as shown by Cacciola *(38)*. It is unknown whether the newly described transfusion-transmitted virus, found with an increased prevalence in HIV patients and those with HCV, also increases hepatic toxicity in these patients *(39)*. It appears likely that TTV, like hepatitis G virus, does not influence the severity of liver disease although this remains to be determined.

It is widely believed that HIV co-infected patients respond poorly to IFN-α monotherapy, given the higher HCV viral titers in these patients. Several studies, however, have shown that the biologic and histologic benefit of IFN-α therapy in co-infected patients is not significantly different from that noted in HIV-negative patients (i.e., normalization of aminotransferase levels in 50% of treatment patients). Most of the patients in these studies were parenteral drug users, with high CD4 lymphocyte counts, and without a diagnosis of AIDS. One study *(40)* showed an initial complete response in almost 45% of co-infected patients treated with IFN-α therapy, which was sustained in 80%. The majority of studies have not been as encouraging. In one study of 12 patients who had high CD4 lymphocyte counts *(41)* and who were treated with IFN-α, only one patient (8.3%) had a sustained complete response after a 12-mo follow-up. Another prospective, controlled trial *(42)*, which included 78 patients, showed a complete response after 8 mo of therapy in 38% of co-infected patients, compared to a 47% response rate in HIV-negative patients. That study, in addition to others, demonstrated a positive correlation between CD4 cell count and response to therapy. Alternatively, a comparative study *(43)* examined treatment of HCV-infected, HIV-seropositive (IFN dose 5 MU thrice weekly), and HIV-seronegative patients (IFN dose 5 MU thrice weekly), for 6 mo, showed comparable complete response (44.1 vs 47.4%) immediately after completion, and complete biologic response 12 mo after cessation (23.2 vs 24.3%). However, a sustained virologic response was observed in only 50% HIV responders and 89.5% non-HIV responders. In the majority of these studies, the side-effect profile and tolerance of treatment was found to be no different between the co-infected patients and the HIV-negative patients. Use of IFN-α may result in a fall in the CD4 cell count of HIV patients, although this decline is transient and reversible upon discontinuation of treatment, reflecting neutropenia, and does not appear to increase the risk of opportunistic infections.

Given the low sustained response rate, use of IFN-α monotherapy has been mostly abandoned in favor of combination therapy with ribavirin. Ribavirin, a guanosine analog, is a broad-spectrum antiviral agent that targets both DNA and RNA viruses. When used alone, ribavirin will reduce ALT levels without significantly changing viral HCV-RNA levels, suggesting that it does not affect viral replication. However, when used in combination with IFN-α, ribavirin reduces the rate of hepatitis relapse, suggesting an enhancement of IFN-α's antiviral activity. Ribavirin may act on IFN-α-resistant subpopulations of virus, or on intracellular reservoirs of HCV that are not accessible to IFN-α. Other postulated mechanisms include inhibition of viral-dependent RNA polymerase, inhibition of the 5'-Cap structure of viral messenger RNA, and inhibition of inosine monophosphate dehydrogenase. The most likely mechanism of action is that ribavirin increases production of TH1 cytokines and decreasing TH2 cytokines. Combination therapy appears to be safe and more efficacious than IFN-α monotherapy, when given to immunocompetent patients. A recent, large, randomized study demonstrated a superior sustained response of naïve, HIV-seronegative patients to combination therapy for either 24 or 48 wk, compared to those patients treated with extended-duration IFN-α monotherapy *(44)*. Combination ribavirin with IFN may raise the sustained response rate to closer to 50%. This superior response has been demonstrated in all subgroups, including those infected with genotype 1, with high baseline viral load, or those with pretreatment cirrhosis or bridging fibrosis.

The effect of IFN and ribavirin combination therapy has been encouraging to date, in small series of HIV patients. In a recent report, Dieterich et al. *(45)* reported on 24 patients who were treated with combined IFN and ribavirin. They showed that, after only 3 mo, patients receiving combination therapy had decreased HCV RNA, from a median of 350,000 to 600 copies/mL. By 6 mo, the median HCV viral load remained at 600, and had become undetectable in 5/8 patients (62.5%) of combination-treated patients. Anemia was seen in 21% of combination-treated patients, but was successfully treated with erythropoietin *(46)*. In a report presented at the same conference, Landau et al. *(47)* reported that combination IFN-ribavirin rendered HCV RNA undetectable in 50% of 20 patients, after 6 mo. In the majority of these patients, HCV RNA was undetectable by 3 mo of treatment. In a Spanish study, Sauleda et al. *(48)* also showed a complete virologic response in 50% of HIV-positive patients treated with combination therapy. In a study of 37 patients with HIV, eight of whom had cirrhosis, Sulkowski *(31)* showed that combination IFN–RBV resulted in 50% HCV RNA <100 copies at 12 wk, with only seven dropouts for adverse events. There has been some concern about using ribavirin in HIV-infected individuals, because of the potential inhibition of the phosphorylation of AZT and d4T *(49)*, although phosphorylation of dideoxyinosine increases *(50)*. In all of the studies, combination therapy did not have a significant effect on the patient's HIV viral load or CD4 cell count.

When embarking on a course of treatment of HCV, using IFN-based therapy, the high incidence of adverse events is an important consideration. In a large percentage of patients, therapy is associated with mild-to-moderate adverse effects. Patients should be prepared for a decrease in their quality of life, prior to starting treatment. The majority of patients receiving the drug will experience a self-limited, dose-dependent, flu-like illness that usually begins 2–4 h following the dose of IFN. The syndrome consists of mild fever, chills, headache, lethargy, arthralgias, and myalgias. These symptoms usually respond to treatment with acetaminophen and/or prednisone, and the severity appears to decrease after repeated dosing. These early side effects rarely limit the use of IFN. Less-common adverse events represent later manifestations of IFN therapy, appearing 2–6 wk after initiation of treatment. They occur more commonly with high-dose therapy, and include irritability, fatigue, depression, headaches, anorexia, nausea, rashes, and alopecia. Thrombocytopenia and leukopenia associated with this medication necessitate monitoring of blood cell counts, but are generally reversible, and granulocyte colony-stimulating factor may be used as prophylaxis for neutropenia. Bacterial infection associated with the immunosuppression induced by IFN therapy is one of the most worrisome effects of therapy. Urinary tract infection, sinusitis, and bronchitis are seen with increased frequency in patients receiving this drug. More serious infections have also been noted; thus, any sign of fever should be promptly evaluated. Despite the high incidence of adverse effects associated with the use of this agent, there does not seem to be an increase in the incidence of intolerance among the patients who are HIV-infected. One area of concern in using combination therapy in HIV-infected individuals is the tolerance of potential side effects of anemia, and decreasing leukocyte count in this immunosuppressed population. The most serious side effect of combination therapy is hemolytic anemia (ribavirin-related), which can be managed by dose reduction of ribavirin. A decline in leukocyte and platelet counts is also noted. Erythropoeitin may prevent or reverse the anemia associated with this regimen.

Other modalities may replace typical IFN-α-based therapy. IFN-α monotherapy may be replaced with longer-acting pegylated IFN (polyethylene glycol [PEG]-IFN). Modification of IFN-α, by attachment of a 43 or a 12 kDA branched PEG moiety, has resulted in pegylated (PEG-IFN), which has a more sustained delivery, and reduced clearance. PEG-IFN therefore has a half-life of approx 54–100 h, compared to 8 h for routine IFN-α, and may be administered once weekly. One early study suggested that, in HIV-seronegative patients, PEG-IFN's-safety profile was similar to routine IFN, and appears to have an efficacy equivalent, or slightly superior, to routine IFN monotherapy *(51)*. That initial study suggested that, in HIV-seronegative patients, PEG-IFN's-safety profile was similar to routine IFN, and appears to have an efficacy equivalent, or slightly superior, to routine IFN monotherapy. Further controlled studies of this antiviral agent will be needed before further conclusions can be drawn, but, regarding HIV, the potential inhibition of AZT and D4T phosphorylation, by ribavirin, makes use of PEG-IFN monotherapy very appealing. Studies of PEG-IFN have not been completed in an HIV-positive population, but research is currently underway, in the form of a phase III, prospective multicenter trial examining PEG-IFN alone, compared to PEG-IFN plus ribavirin and IFN plus ribavirin.

Despite the advances in IFN-based therapy, other unique therapeutic modalities are sorely needed. In one recent study, Schlaak et al. *(52)* showed that, when 2/7 (28.6%) HIV–HCV co-infected patients were treated with IL-2, they cleared their HCV RNA for 6 and 11 mo. Although the proinflammatory effects of IL-2 therapy may theoretically have up-regulated anti-HCV immune responses in these patients, large studies will be necessary to determine whether other immunomodulatory therapy, in addition to IFN, should be considered in the treatment of HCV infection. IL 10 has been shown to reduce fibrosis in preliminary studies, but may downregulate TH1 cytokines, and may not be the best choice in HIV-infected individuals. Other new approaches that will soon be tested include antisense technology, ribozymes, HCV-specific protease inhibitors, and helicase inhibitors. Future anti-HCV therapy will probably entail multiple combinations of medications with IFN-α, similar to the multiple drug regimens used in HIV therapy today. The future is bright for antiviral and immunologic therapy of hepatitis C, both with and without co-infection with HIV, and much of the technology that has moved the field forward has been, and continues to be, translated from the field of HIV.

CONCLUSIONS

In the preprotease era, the presence of hepatitis virus infection was not viewed with concern, but now that the healthy life-span of these patients has increased substantially, many patients with concurrent hepatitis C will die of liver disease before succumbing to the effects of HIV. Realistic expectations of long-term survival with HIV disease, especially with early diagnosis and combination antiretroviral therapy, demands consideration of therapy for concurrent chronic viral hepatitis, especially given the large population at risk. The presence of HCV infection not only affects the health status of HIV-infection patients, leading to enhanced risk of mortality and mortality, but the accompanying elevation of liver-associated enzymes limits use of many medications useful in the treatment of HIV disease, because of the threat of worsened liver disease. Research in the past 5 yr has yielded new agents with greater efficacy, greater ease of use, and a lower incidence of adverse events for patients with hepatitis C. The next years are likely to be just as fruitful, with development of many more agents, which opens the possibility of dramatically more effective combination therapy of HCV in the near future.

REFERENCES

1. Soriano V, Garcia Samaniego J, Valencia E, et al. Impact of chronic liver disease due to hepatitis viruses as a cause of hospital admission and death in HIV-infected drug users. Eur J Epidemiol 1999; 15: 1–4.
2. Justice AC, Chang CH, Fusco J, West N. Extrapolating long-term HIV/AIDS survival in the post-HAART era. 39th Annual ICAAC, San Francisco, CA, 1999 (abstract 1158), p. 156.
3. Zylberberg H, Pol S. Reciprocal interaction between human immunodeficiency virus and hepatitis C virus infections. Clin Infect Dis 1996; 23: 1117–1125.

4. Ndimbie OK, Kingsley LA, Nedjar S, et al. Hepatitis C virus infection in a male homosexual cohort: risk factor analysis. Genitourin Med 1996; 72: 213–216.
5. Eyster ME, Alter HJ, Aledort LM, et al. Heterosexual co-transmission of hepatitis C virus (HCV) and human immunodeficiency virus (HIV). Ann Intern Med 1991; 115: 764–768.
6. Thomas DL, Villano SA, Nedjar S, et al. Perinatal transmission of hepatitis C virus from human immunodeficiency virus type 1. J Infect Dis 1998; 177: 1480–1488.
7. Granovsky MO, Minkoff HL, Tess BH, et al. Hepatitis C virus infection in the mothers and infants cohort study. Pediatrics 1998; 102: 355–359.
8. Gerlach JT, Diepolder HM, Jung M-C, et al. Recurrence of hepatitis C virus after loss of virus-specific $CD4^+$ T-cell response in acute hepatitis C. Gastroenterology 1999; 117: 933–941.
9. John M, Flexman J, French MA. Hepatitis C virus-associated hepatitis following treatment of HIV-infected patients with protease inhibitors: an immune restoration disease? AIDS 1998; 12: 2289–2293.
10. Rosen HR, Hinrichs DJ, Gretch DR, et al. Association of multispecific $CD4^+$ response to hepatitis C and severity of recurrence after liver transplantation. Gastroenterology 1999; 117: 926–932.
11. Woitas RP, Rockstroh JK, Beier I, et al. Antigen-specific cytokine response to hepatitis C virus core epitopes in HIV/hepatitis C virus-coinfected patients. AIDS 1999; 13: 1313–1322.
12. Puntoriero G, Meola A, Lahm A, et al. Towards a solution for hepatitis C virus hypervariability: mimotopes of the hypervariable region 1 can induce antibodies cross-reacting with a large number of viral variants. EMBO J 1998; 17: 3521–3533.
13. Dove LM, Phung Y, Wrock J, et al. HCV quasispecies as a mechanism of rapidly progressive liver disease in patients infected with the human immunodeficiency virus. 50th Annual Meeting of the American Association for the Study of Liver Diseases. Dallas, TX, 1999 (abstract 1183), p. 456A.
14. Cribier B, Rey D. High hepatitis viremia and impaired antibody response in patients co-infected with HIV. AIDS 1995; 9: 113–116.
15. Dragoni F, Caffolla A, Gentile G. HIV-HCV RNA loads and liver failure in coinfected patients with coagulopathy. Haematologica 1999; 84: 525–529.
16. Bonacini M, Govindarajan S, Blatt LM, et al. Patients co-infected with human immunodeficiency virus and hepatitis C virus demonstrate higher levels of hepatic HCV RNA. J Viral Hepat 1999; 6: 203–208.
17. Bierhoff E, Fischer HP, Willsch E, et al. Liver histopathology in patients with concurrent chronic hepatitis C and HIV infection. Virchows Arch 1997; 430: 271–277.
18. Garcia-Samaniego J, Soriano V, Castilla J. Influence of hepatitis C virus genotypes and HIV infection on histological severity of chronic hepatitis C. The Hepatitis/HIV Spanish Study Group. Am J Gastroenterol 1997; 92: 1130–1134.
19. Sanchez-Quijano A, Andreu J, Gavilan F, et al. Influence of human immunodeficiency virus type 1 infection on the natural course of chronic parenterally acquired hepatitis C. Eur J Clin Microbiol Infect Dis 1995; 14: 949–953.
20. Soto B, Sanchez-Quijano A, Rodrigo L, et al. Human immunodeficiency virus infection modifies the natural history of chronic parenterally-acquired hepatitis C with an unusually rapid progression to cirrhosis. J Hepatol 1997; 26: 1–5.
21. Makris M, Preston FE, Rosendaal FR, et al. Natural history of chronic hepatitis C in haemophiliacs. Br J Haematol 1996; 94: 746–752.
22. Telfer P, Sabin C, Devereux H, et al. Progression of HCV-associated liver disease in a cohort of haemophilic patients. Br J Haematol 1994; 87: 555–561.

23. Wright TL, Hollander H, Pu X, et al. Hepatitis C in HIV-infected patients with and without AIDS: prevalence and relationship to patient survival. Hepatology 1994; 20: 1152–1155.
24. Piroth L, Duong M, Quantin C, et al. Does hepatitis C virus co-infection accelerate clinical and immunological evolution of HIV-infected patients? AIDS 1998; 12: 381–388.
25. Berger A, Depka Prondzinski MV, Doerr HW. Hepatitis C plasma viral load is associated with HCV genotype but not with HIV coinfection. J Med Virol 1996; 48:339–343.
26. Gavazzi G, Richallet G, Morand P, et al. Effects of double and triple antiretroviral agents on the HCV viral load in patients co-infected with HIV and HCV. Pathol Biol 1998; 46: 412–415.
27. Rutschmann OT, Negro F, Hirschel B, et al. Impact of treatment with human immunodeficiency virus (HIV) protease inhibitors on hepatitis C viremia in patients co-infected with HIV. J Infect Dis 1998; 177: 783–785.
28. McKenzie R, Fried MW, Sallie R, et al. Hepatic failure and lactic acidosis due to fialuridine (FIAU), an investigational nucleoside analogue for chronic hepatitis B. N Engl J Med 1995; 333: 1099–1105.
29. Barbaro G, Di Lorenzo G, Asti A, et al. Hepatocellular mitochondrial alterations in patients with chronic hepatitis C: ultrastructural and biochemical findings. Am J Gastroenterol 1999; 94: 2198–2205.
30. Hernandez LV, Vincents DJ, Jerold JJ, Ian G. 50th Annual Meeting of the American Association for the Study of Liver Diseases. Dallas, TX, 1999 (abstract 684), p. 331A.
31. Sulkowski MS, Thomas DL, Chaisson RE, et al. Hepatotoxicity associated with antiretroviral therapy in adults infected with human immunodeficiency virus and the role of hepatitis C or B virus Infection. JAMA 2000; 283: 74–80.
32. Zylberberg H, Chaix M-L, Rabian C, et al. Tri-therapy for human immunodeficiency virus does not modify replication of hepatitis C in coinfected patients. Clin Infect Dis 1998; 26: 1104–1106.
33. USPHS/IDSA Prevention of Opportunistic Infections Working Group. Infectious Diseases Society of American (1999). USPHS/IDSA guidelines for the prevention of opportunistic infections in persons infected with human immunodeficiency virus. Ann Intern Med 1999; 131: 873–908.
34. Kowdley KV. Does interferon therapy prevent hepatocellular carcinoma in patients with chronic hepatitis C? Gastroenterology 1999; 117: 738–739.
35. Shiratori Y, Moriyama M, Arakawa Y, et al. Interferon therapy reduces the risk for hepatocellular carcinoma: national surveillance program of cirrhotic and noncirrhotic patients with chronic hepatitis C in Japan. Ann Intern Med 1999; 131: 174–181.
36. Taylor DR, Shi ST, Romano PR, et al. Inhibition of the interferon-inducible protein kinase PKR by HCV E2 protein. Science 1999; 285: 107–110.
37. Edwards-Smith CJ, Jonsson JR, Purdie DM, et al. Interleukin-10 promoter polymorphism predicts initial response of chronic hepatitis C to interferon alfa. Hepatology 1999; 30: 526–530.
38. Cacciola I, Pollicino T, Squadrito G, et al. Occult hepatitis B virus infection in patients with chronic hepatitis C liver disease. N Engl J Med 1999; 341: 22–26.
39. Sherman KE, Rouster SD. Increased prevalence of TTV in HIV infected patients. 50th Annual Meeting of the American Association for the Study of Liver Diseases. Dallas, TX, 1999 (abstract 513), p. 289A.
40. Marriott E, Navas S, del Romero J, et al. Treatment with recombinant alpha-interferon of chronic hepatitis C in anti-HIV positive patients. J Med Virol 1993; 40: 107–111.

41. Boyer N, Marcellin P, Degott C, et al. Recombinant interferon-alpha for chronic hepatitis C in patients positive for antibody for human immunodeficiency virus. J Infect Dis 1992; 165: 723–726.
42. Soriano V, Garcia-Samaniego J, Bravo R, et al. Efficacy and safety of interferon-alpha treatment for chronic hepatitis C in HIV-infected patients. J Infect 1995; 31: 9–13.
43. Coll S, Sola R, Vila MC, et al. Treatment of hepatitis C HIV-coinfected patients with interferon: controlled study. 50th Annual Meeting of the American Association for the Study of Liver Diseases. Dallas, TX, 1999 (abstract 153), p. 199A.
44. Reichard O, Norkrans G, Fryden A, et al. Randomised, double-blind, placebo-controlled trial of interferon alpha-2b with and without ribavirin for chronic hepatitis C. Lancet 1998; 351: 83–87.
45. Dieterich DT, Weisz KB, Goldman DJ, Malicdem ML. Combination treatment with interferon and ribavirin for hepatitis C in HIV Co-infection patients. 50th Annual Meeting of the American Association for the Study of Liver Diseases. Dallas, TX, 1999 (abstract 422), p. 266A.
46. Weisz K, Kreiswirth S, McMeeking M, et al. Erthyropoetin use for ribavirin/interferon induced anemia in patients with hepatitis C. Proc ICAAC, San Diego, CA, 1998, p. 325.
47. Landau AO, Batisse DP, Van Huen JPD, et al. Efficacy and safety of combination therapy with interferon-alpha 2B and ribavirin for severe chronic hepatitis C in HIV-infected patients. 50th Annual Meeting of the American Association for the Study of Liver Diseases. Dallas, TX, 1999 (abstract 828), p. 367A.
48. Sauleda S, Esteban JI, Altisent C, et al. Impact of interferon plus ribavirin combination treatment on HIV infection in hemophiliacs with chronic hepatitis C and under HAART. 50th Annual Meeting of the American Association for the Study of Liver Diseases. Dallas, TX, 1999 (abstract 134), p. 194A.
49. Sim SM, Hoggard PG, Sales SD, et al. Effect of ribavirin on zidovudine efficacy and toxicity in vitro: a concentration-dependent interaction. AIDS Res Hum Retroviruses 1998; 14: 1661–1667.
50. Hoggard PG, Kewn S, Barry MG, et al. Effects of drugs on 2',3'-dideoxy-2',3'-didehydrothymidine phosphorylation in vitro. Antimicrob Agents Chemother 1997; 41: 1231–1236.
51. Glue P, Fang JWS, Sabo R, et al. PEG-interferon-alpha2B: pharmacokinetics, safety, and preliminary efficacy data. 50th Annual Meeting of the American Association for the Study of Liver Diseases. Dallas, TX, 1999 (abstract 116), p. 189A.
52. Schlaak JF, zum Bueschenfelde, Gerken G, Galle PR. Sustained HCV eradication after interleukin-2 therapy in patients with HIV/HCV coinfection. 50th Annual Meeting of the American Association for the Study of Liver Diseases. Dallas, TX, 1999 (abstract 431), p. 268A.

6 HBV and HCV Co-Infection

Terence L. Angtuaco, MD
and Donald M. Jensen, MD

CONTENTS
INTRODUCTION
VIRAL REPLICATION IN HBV AND HCV CO-INFECTION
CLINICAL AND HISTOLOGIC PRESENTATIONS OF HBV
 AND HCV CO-INFECTION
RESPONSE OF PATIENTS WITH DUAL INFECTION TO IFN
 THERAPY
OUTCOME OF LIVER TRANSPLANT IN HBV AND HCV
 CO-INFECTION
SUMMARY
REFERENCES

INTRODUCTION

Patients at risk for hepatitis B virus (HBV) infection are similarly at risk for hepatitis C virus (HCV) infection. They both may be acquired via the parenteral route, such as blood transfusion, injection drug use, and hemodialysis, although inoculation via the percutaneous and mucosal routes have also been reported. Injection drug use has been associated with the highest risk of HBV and HCV co-infection, compared to other risk groups *(1,2)*. Because of their common mode of transmission, dual infection with HBV and HCV occurs in at-risk patients.

In an analogous situation, co-infection or super-infection of HBV with hepatitis D virus (HDV) is associated with fulminant hepatic failure (FHF), rapid evolution to cirrhosis *(3,4)*, and poor response to interferon (IFN) treatment *(5)*. Moreover, there is evidence that HDV suppresses the replication of HBV *(6,7)*.

From: *Clinical Gastroenterology: Diagnosis and Therapeutics*
Edited by: R. S. Koff and G. Y. Wu © Humana Press Inc., Totowa, NJ

This chapter discusses the effect of HCV on HBV replication, as well as the effect of HBV on HCV replication. Included in the discussion are the effects of this dual infection on the clinical course of these patients, and the risk for early progression to cirrhosis and hepatocellular carcinoma (HCC). Treatment issues and outcomes of liver transplantation are likewise addressed.

VIRAL REPLICATION IN HBV AND HCV CO-INFECTION

Mutual suppression of viral replication occurs in hepatitis B and HCV co-infection, with HCV exerting a negative effect on HBV replication. Likewise, HBV exerts a negative effect on HCV replication. Studies investigating the relationship of viral replication markers in co-infected patients have demonstrated that HBV DNA and hepatitis B surface antigen (HBsAg) titers are lower in those individuals with concurrent HCV infection, compared to those with HBV infection alone, implying an interference of HCV on HBV replication. Lower HCV RNA titers have also been noted in patients with concurrent HBV infection, compared to those with HCV infection alone, implying HBV interference with HCV replication *(8,53)*. This phenomena of viral interference involves a complex interplay between the host's immune system and virus-specific replication properties, but the exact mechanism remains unknown.

Effect of HCV on HBV Replication

HCV suppression of HBV replication has been demonstrated in several animal and human studies. In experiments using chimpanzees with chronic HBV infection, inoculation with a non-A, non-B hepatitis agent resulted in an acute elevation of alanine aminostransferase (ALT), and a precipitous decline in HBsAg titers. The loss of HBsAg during the acute phase of non-A, non-B virus super-infection was thought to result from viral interference by the HCV. This may have resulted from an alteration in the mechanisms responsible for virus absorption, penetration, and replication *(9)*. An in vitro study in human hepatoma cell line, HuH-7, has demonstrated the potential role of the HCV core protein in the suppression of HBV gene replication and expression *(10)*. Liaw *(11)* postulated that liver injury induced by HCV, and its accompanying cell renewal, increases the expression of HBV epitopes on the hepatocyte surface, leading to cytotoxic T-cell clearance of HBV-infected hepatocytes, which may explain the lower HBV load in the presence of co-existing HCV infection. De novo synthesis of IFN or IFN-like substances *(9)*, tumor necrosis factor-α and interleukin-6 have also been implicated *(12)* in HCV interference on HBV replication.

In patients co-infected with hepatitis C virus genotype 1, either 1a or 1b, HBV replication seems to be inhibited. The same is not true, however, for those co-infected with hepatitis C virus genotype 2, in whom active HBV replication may persist, and thus contribute to the severity of liver damage. Hepatitis C virus genotype 1, but not hepatitis C virus genotype 2, induces strong activation of the hepatic IFN system, but is itself insensitive to its effect, which may explain why HBV is suppressed or cleared only in hepatitis C virus genotype 1 co-infection *(13)*. Another study *(13a)*, looking into the effects of HCV genotypes on HBV replication, failed to demonstrate a significant difference in the HBV DNA levels between patients with hepatitis C virus genotype 1 and those with other genotypes. These data are inconclusive, however, given the small number of patients in these studies.

Effect of HBV on HCV Replication

HBV replication status, as measured by the HBV DNA polymerase (DNA-p) activity, has been shown to affect the HCV RNA titer. This represents reciprocal viral suppression of HCV by HBV, but the mechanism that governs this interaction remains speculative. HCV RNA in serum was detected less frequently in patients with highly replicating HBV (DNA-p >100 cpm). Higher titers of HCV RNA were measured in those with low-replicating HBV (DNA p <100 cpm). HCV RNA titers in co-infected patients with DNA-p <100 cpm were still lower than those in patients with anti-HCV but without HBsAg *(8)*. In an in vitro co-transfection experiment, wild-type HBV DNA was shown to suppress the secretion of HCV RNA. However, co-transfection of HCV RNA with the HBV DNA silent mutant, (i.e., HBV DNA with eight-nucleotide deletion in the region encoding the X gene) resulted in the release of higher levels of HCV RNA *(14)*.

HBV and HCV Latency

The mutual suppression of viral replication in HBV and HCV co-infection may lead to the development of both HBV and HCV latency. In one study, co-infected patients with active HCV infection lost their HBsAg, and had undetectable serum HBV DNA. However, histologic evaluation of tumorous and nontumorous liver tissues from these patients revealed the presence of HBV DNA (HBV latency). Likewise, some patients with dual infection who had active HBV replication had undetectable serum

HCV RNA, and yet were found to have HCV RNA in liver biopsy specimens (HCV latency) *(15)*.

HCV Usurpation of HBV

HBsAg seroconversion is usually followed by normalization of serum ALT. However, in some patients co-infected with HBV and HCV, elevated ALT and histologic evidence of hepatitis activity persist. There is evidence that active HCV infection is the major cause of persistent hepatitis or ALT elevation after HBsAg clearance in patients co-infected with the HBV *(16)*. HCV may have suppressed or eliminated the HBV, but it then takes over the role of HBV in eliciting continuing chronic inflammation (HCV usurpation of HBV).

Alternating Dominance of HBV and HCV

Alternating appearance of serum HBV DNA and HCV RNA, with concomitant disappearance of the other virus, has been described *(11,13a, 17)*. During the clinical course of patients with dual infection, either HBV or HCV becomes the dominant replicator. This continuous alternating pattern may be responsible for the more unfavorable clinical course of some patients with HBV and HCV co-infection, because of the unrelenting inflammation of the liver.

Some authors *(18,19)* believe that, in co-infected patients, HCV plays the lead role in the maintenance and progression of liver damage, with elimination or suppression of HBV replication. A biphasic pattern of ALT activity was observed in patients with dual infection *(20,21)*, which may represent the sequential alternating expression of HBV and HCV. HCV was thought to be responsible for the second peak of the serum ALT, because it occurred when HBV DNA was undetectable by polymerase chain reaction (PCR), and anti-HBs was detected. Immunoglobulin A anti-HBc is associated with active immune response against HBV-infected hepatocytes, and, therefore, indicates HBV-induced liver injury. In patients with positive HCV RNA, immunoglobulin A anti-HBc levels were found to be low, and equivalent to levels seen in asymptomatic HBV carriers, which implies that, in the presence of active HCV replication and low immunoglobulin A anti-HBc, the on-going liver damage is probably caused by HCV, and not HBV *(19)*.

Spontaneous HBsAg Seroconversion in Co-Infection with HCV

In co-infected patients, HBsAg appearance may be delayed, its level lower, and the duration of hepatitis B surface antigenemia shorter than in non-co-infected patients *(20)*. Spontaneous HBsAg seroconversion is higher in HBV and HCV co-infection. In one series *(22)*, the actuarial cumulative probability of spontaneous serum HBsAg seroconversion, at 5 and 10 yr, was 9.1 and 17.6% in HBV and HCV co-infected patients, respectively, compared to 1.2 and 5.6% in patients with chronic hepatitis B with no evidence of super-infection with HCV. Using Cox multivariate regression analysis, older age (i.e., >35 yr old) and HCV super-infection were the only independent factors related to a significantly higher HBsAg clearance rate. Co-infection with HDV had no additive suppressive effect.

CLINICAL AND HISTOLOGIC PRESENTATIONS OF HBV AND HCV CO-INFECTION

There are conflicting data on the pathogenic effects of double infection with HBV and HCV, compared to infection with a single virus. Patients with dual infection may have a worse clinical presentation and a more rapidly evolving form of chronic liver disease *(8,11,18,23–30)*. Aminotransferase levels are higher and liver disease more severe, both histologically and in the degree of clinical decompensation, in co-infected patients *(18,28,30,31)*.

Contrasting views have been reported by others, who found no significant difference in the clinical and histologic presentation of HBV and HCV co-infected patients, compared to those with single infection. Furthermore, they described the liver injury in a majority of co-infected patients as only mild to moderate in severity, similar to those seen in patients infected with either HBV or HCV alone *(20,25,32–34)*.

Risk of FHF

HCV and HBV co-infection and HCV super-infection in HBV carriers have been implicated in several cases of fulminant and subfulminant hepatitis *(11,21,23,24,26,29)*. It was suggested that this is more likely to happen in dual infection than in single-virus infection. In Taipei, viral super-infection is the most common cause of fulminant viral hepatitis, and 10–20% of these were caused by HCV super-infection of HBV-infected patients *(24,29)*. In one study *(11)*, there was a significantly higher proportion of patients with HBV and HCV co-infection in those with FHF or sub-FHF, compared to those with moderate or mild liver injury. It is still unclear whether the increased risk of developing FHF in HBV and HCV co-infection results from a summing up of the individual pathogenic effects of the viruses, potentiation of these effects, or the result of some as-yet-unknown mechanism.

Rate of Progression to Cirrhosis

HBV co-infection in chronic hepatitis C has been associated with a higher prevalence of cirrhosis, as well as an accelerated evolution to cirrhosis *(8,23,30,53)*. A similar observation was noted in those with occult HBV co-infection *(25)*. Patients with hepatitis C infection, who were HBV DNA-positive, had worse Knodell scores, attributed to more severe piecemeal necrosis and fibrosis, compared to those who were HBV DNA-negative *(15,23)*. This implies that the persistence of HBV replication plays an important role in disease progression. On the contrary, Colombari et al. *(33)* and Liaw et al. *(34)* reported that the prevalence and time to development of cirrhosis in co-infected patients were not different from those who were infected with only a single virus. Furthermore, the effect of dual infection with HBV and HCV on the long-term outcome of the disease was thought to be insignificant.

Risk for Development of HCC

Dual infection with HBV and HCV may accelerate the progression of chronic liver disease to cirrhosis and HCC *(35–38)*. In one study of patients with HCC, the presence of both anti-HCV and HBsAg was found in 12% of cases *(38)*. 45% did not have HBsAg, but integrated HBV DNA was detected in the tumor tissue. The relative risk of developing HCC was highest in those with HBsAg and anti-HCV positivity (RR = 40.05), compared to those who are positive for only anti-HCV (RR = 27.12) or HBsAg (RR = 13.96), and those who were negative for both markers (RR = 1.00). In a multivariate analysis of cirrhotic patients, male gender, older age, alcohol abuse, and dual positivity for HBsAg and anti-HCV were determined to be independent risk factors for the development of HCC. Benvegnu et al. *(35)* suggested that HBV might act as the "initiating" factor, by altering the arrangement of the hepatocyte genome, and that HCV is the "promoting" factor, by virtue of its contribution to continuing liver injury and regeneration.

Risk for HCC
in those with Hepatitis C and past HBV Infection

Prior infection with HBV, even in those who have undergone HBsAg seroconversion, has been linked to the development of HCC in the setting of co-infection with HCV *(39–41)*. The risk for hepatocarcinogenesis increased twofold in those with anti-HBs and anti-HBc, compared to those who were only anti-HCV-positive *(42)*. These patients with inapparent HBV infection were found to have low-level viremia that was detected only with the highly sensitive (PCR) assay *(41,43)*. Therefore, anti-HBs positivity does not exclude the possibility of low-level replication. Moreover, the time to development of HCC from the introduction of a risk factor (i.e., blood transfusion) was shorter in patients with HCV and anti-HBc (without HBsAg) than for those with HCV alone *(39)*. On the other hand, other studies did not find an increased frequency of HCC in anti-HCV-positive patients with antibodies to HBV; and only those with apparent chronic hepatitis B infection were found to be at increased risk for HCC *(35)*. Further controversy was raised by Shiratori et al. *(36)*, who found no evidence of synergistic effect of either past or active HBV and HCV infection on the progression to HCC. Instead, they suggested that HBV and HCV act as independent risk factors for HCC. Moreover, because viral replication in co-infected patients is mutually exclusive, the virologic and clinicopathological features of HCC are determined by the dominant virus.

There is a higher incidence of HCC, without underlying cirrhosis, in those who had past HBV infection, compared to those who only had HCV mono-infection, without any evidence of infection with HBV *(39)*. Because HCC is known to develop occasionally in the absence of cirrhosis in chronic hepatitis B, it is possible that past HBV infection may have a role, as well, in the development of HCC, in the absence of cirrhosis, in patients with HCV. Moreover, the HCC found in patients with hepatitis C, who had past HBV infection, had a more aggressive histopathology, compared to those without past HBV infection *(39)*.

Outcomes of Surgical Resection of HCC

Surgical resection of HCC in co-infected patients was associated with only a slight increase in postoperative morbidity and mortality, compared to those with either infection alone *(44)*. The incidence of liver failure, ascites, and infection was higher in co-infected patients, although the differences were not statistically significant. The long-term survival rate after resection was lower in those with dual infection, but this was not statistically significant. Recurrence rate after surgery, however, was significantly lower in those with HBV and HCV co-infection, compared to the HBV mono-infected patients with HCC, but was significantly higher, compared to those with HCV-related HCC.

It is evident from available data that concurrent HCV, and active or past HBV infection, increases the risk for the development of HCC, and the overall prognosis of these patients may be worse, compared to those with either infection alone.

RESPONSE OF PATIENTS
WITH DUAL INFECTION TO IFN THERAPY

Approximately 30–45% of patients with chronic HCV respond to IFN therapy by clearance of serum HCV RNA and normalization of transaminases, and half of these may achieve a sustained response. In patients with chronic hepatitis B, a higher dose of IFN is used, and this leads to hepatitis B-sensitive antigen seroconversion and loss of HBV DNA, in about 30–40% of cases. The efficacy of IFN, in chronic HCV patients co-infected by HBV, has been poor *(31,45,46)*. Using the standard treatment regimen for hepatitis C, of 3 million units of recombinant IFN-α-2a 3× weekly for 12 mo, less than one-third of patients had normalization of their transaminases, and all of them relapsed after withdrawal of therapy *(45)*. The ALT elevation during relapse was associated with an isolated HBV viremia, and not with HCV or combined HBV and HCV viremia. Treatment of co-infected patients with the standard dose used for chronic hepatitis C may be inadequate. Apparently, this approach favored HBV replication and persistence. Higher doses, similar to that required for hepatitis B infection, may be needed in the treatment of co-infected patients. Villa et al. *(47)* suggested that the dose and duration of IFN treatment for co-infected patients should be directed against the more actively replicating virus.

Caution must be exercised in the treatment of co-infected patients, because there is a potential risk for hepatic decompensation *(46)*. Studies have demonstrated that IFN therapy may decrease the replication of one virus, resulting in reduction of its suppressive effect on the co-infecting virus, to a level that allows reactivation of the latter and induction of hepatitis *(46,47)*. The use of combination therapy, e.g., IFN plus lamivudine, in co-infected patients, deserves to be studied. However, until the safety of antiviral medication use in co-infected patients is proven by further clinical trials, and its efficacy improved by determination of the appropriate dosage and duration of therapy, institution of treatment in these patients must be done with great caution.

OUTCOME OF LIVER TRANSPLANTATION
IN HBV AND HCV CO-INFECTION

Although recurrence of HCV after orthotopic liver transplantation (OLT) in patients with HCV mono-infection is common *(48)*, the hepatic damage associated with this is usually mild, and long-term graft survival is not reduced *(49)*. In those co-infected with HBV and HCV, virologic recurrence of HCV is less frequent, but histologic liver injury is thought to be possibly more severe. In one series, only 41% of patients with dual infection (vs 59% of patients with HCV mono-infection) had detectable HCV RNA by PCR in both serum and liver, during post-OLT follow-up. However, there was evidence of ongoing necroinflammatory activity, by histologic in some patients with negative serum HCV RNA *(50)*. It was suggested that HBV may be masking the HCV, and the presence of both viruses led to more injury, and to development of a more severe liver disease. Two patients (5%) in this study had severe liver damage histologically, and both were co-infected with HBV and HCV *(50)*.

Caccamo et al. *(51)* reported that HCV-related graft failure was more common in patients with HCV mono-infection, compared to those with dual infection. The occurrence of graft loss was 20% in those with mono-infection, which also happened relatively early during follow-up; none of those with dual infection had graft failure.

Rejection leading to graft loss was more frequent in dual HBV and HCV infection. This occurred in 21% of co-infected patients, compared to none in those with single infection with HBV *(52)*. The underlying mechanism for this increased incidence of rejection, leading to graft failure, is unknown.

Post-OLT survival outcome of co-infected patients was significantly better, compared to those with HBV re-infection of the graft (i.e., 5-yr survival rate of 80 vs 30%, respectively) *(52)*, and was similar to those with HCV re-infection *(49)*. In the study by Huang et al. *(52)*, there were two distinct histopathological patterns described in co-infected patients: One had predominantly HCV features, and the other one had predominantly HBV features. Rarely did they have a mixed histologic picture. It was suggested that the better outcome in co-infected patients may result from predominance of the HCV histopathological pattern, which is believed to have a more benign clinical course. Moreover, fibrosing cholestatic hepatitis, a histopathological entity described in recurrent HBV post-OLT associated with severe injury and poor outcome, was less frequent in the HBV and HCV dual-infection subgroup *(52)*.

SUMMARY

Mutual suppression of HBV and HCV occurs in co-infected patients, which leads to lower levels of either HBV DNA or HCV RNA, compared to patients with mono-infection of either virus. The exact mechanism of this interaction is unknown, although several hypotheses have been proposed. Co-infection with HBV and HCV results in HBV and HCV latency, HCV usurpation of HBV, lower titer of HBsAg, and higher incidence of spontaneous HBsAg seroconversion. There may be alternating dominance of either virus during the clinical course of patients with concurrent HBV and HCV infection, which may lead to more hepatic injury caused by unrelenting inflammation of the liver. The clinical and histologic presentations of these patients are determined by whichever virus is the dominant replicator.

Co-infection with HBV and HCV is associated with more aggressive chronic hepatitis, including fulminant or subfulminant hepatitis, and rapid progression to cirrhosis and development of HCC. However, there are also reports challenging this view. Patients with hepatitis C, who only have evidence of past HBV infection, may also behave similarly as those with HCV and active HBV co-infection. Morbidity and mortality associated with surgical resection of HCC, in co-infected patients, was only slightly higher, compared to those with single infection.

Response of co-infected patients to IFN therapy is poor, and may potentially lead to hepatic decompensation. The optimal effective dose and duration of treatment is yet to be determined.

The rate of virologic HCV recurrence post-OLT may be low in co-infected patients, however, histologic liver injury may possibly be more severe, and graft failure more frequent. Allograft rejection was likewise more com-mon in co-infected patients. Overall survival post-OLT was significantly better in co-infected patients, compared to those with HBV re-infection of the graft, and similar to those with HCV graft re-infection.

REFERENCES

1. Rodriguez M, Navascues A, Martinez A, et al. Prevalence of antibody to hepatitis C virus in chronic HBsAg carriers. Arch Virol 1992; 4(Suppl): 327–328.
2. Pallas J, Farinas-Alvarez C, Prieto D, et al. Risk factors for monoinfections and coinfections with HIV, hepatitis B and hepatitis C in northern Spanish prisoners. Epidemiol Infect 1999; 123: 95–102.
3. Smedile A, Farci P, Verme G, et al. Influence of delta infection on severity of hepatitis B. Lancet 1982; 2: 945–947.
4. Rizzetto M, Verme G, Recchia S, et al. Chronic hepatitis in carriers of hepatitis B surface antigen, with intrahepatic expression of delta antigen: an active and progressive disease unresponsive to immunosuppressive treatment. Ann Intern Med 1983; 98: 437–441.
5. Farci P, Mandas A, Coiana A, et al. Treatment of chronic hepatitis D with interferon alfa-2a. N Engl J Med 1994; 330: 88–94.
6. Lok AS, Lindsay I, Scheuer J, et al. Clinical and histological features of delta infection in chronic hepatitis B virus carriers. J Clin Pathol 1985; 38: 530–533.
7. Fattovich G, Boscaro S, Novena F, et al. Influence of hepatitis delta virus infection on progression to cirrhosis in chronic hepatitis type B. J Infect Dis 1987; 155: 931–935.
8. Tsuji H, Shimomura H, Fujio K, et al. Relationship of serum markers of hepatitis B and C virus replication in coinfected patients. Acta Med Okayama 1998; 52: 113–118.

9. Bradley D, Maynard J, McCaustland K, et al. Non-A, non-B hepatitis in chimpanzees: interference with acute hepatitis A virus and chronic hepatitis B virus infection. J Med Virol 1983; 11: 207–213.
10. Shih CM, Lo S, Miyamura T, et al. Suppression of hepatitis B virus expression and replication by hepatitis C virus core protein in HuH-7 cells. J Virol 1993; 67: 5823–5832.
11. Liaw YF. Role of hepatitis C virus in dual and triple hepatitis virus infection. Hepatology 1995; 22: 1101–1108.
12. Gilles PN, Fey G, Chisari FV. Tumor necrosis factor alpha negatively regulates hepatitis B virus gene expression in transgenic mice. J Virol 1992; 66: 3955–3960.
13. Pontisso P, Gerotto M, Ruvoletto MG, et al. Hepatitis C genotypes in patients with dual hepatitis B and C virus infection. J Med Virol 1996; 48: 157–160.
13a. Mathurin P, Thibault V, Kadidja K, et al. Replication status and histological features of patients with triple (B,C,D) and dual (B,C) hepatic infections. J Viral Hepatitis 2000; 7: 15–22.
14. Uchida T, Kaneita Y, Gotoh K, et al. Hepatitis C virus is frequently coinfected with serum marker-negative hepatitis B virus: probable replication promotion of the former by the latter as demonstrated by in vitro cotransfection. J Med Virol 1997; 52: 399–405.
15. Pontisso P, Ruvoletto MG, Fattovich G, et al. Clinical and virological profiles in patients with multiple hepatitis virus infections. Gastroenterology 1993; 105: 1529–1533.
16. Liaw YF, Tsai SL, Chang JJ, et al. Displacement of hepatitis B virus by hepatitis C virus as the cause of continuing chronic hepatitis. Gastroenterology 1994; 106: 1048–1053.
17. Koike K, Yasuda K, Yotsuyanagi H, et al. Dominant replication of either virus in dual infection with hepatitis viruses B and C. J Med Virol 1995; 45: 236–239.
18. Crespo J, Lozano J, Cruz F, et al. Prevalence and significance of hepatitis C viremia in chronic active hepatitis B. Am J Gastroenterol 1994; 89: 1147–1151.
19. Sato S, Fujiyama S, Tanaka M, et al. Coinfection of hepatitis C virus in patients with chronic hepatitis B infection. J Hepatol 1994; 21: 159–166.
20. Mimms L, Mosley J, Hollinger F, et al. Effect of concurrent acute infection with hepatitis C virus on acute hepatitis B virus infection. B Med J 1993; 307: 1095–1097.
21. Chu CM, Liaw YF. Simultaneous acute hepatitis B virus and hepatitis C virus infection leading to fulminant hepatitis and subsequent chronic hepatitis C. Clin Infect Dis 1995; 20: 703–705.
22. Sheen IS, Liaw YF, Lin DY, et al. Role of hepatitis C and delta viruses in the termination of chronic hepatitis B surface antigen carrier state: a multivariate analysis in a longitudinal follow-up study. J Infect Dis 1994; 170: 358–361.
23. Zarski JP, Bohn B, Bastie A, et al. Characteristics of patients with dual infection by hepatitis B and C viruses. J Hepatol 1998; 28: 27–33.
24. Chu CM, Sheen IS, Liaw YF. Role of hepatitis C virus in fulminant viral hepatitis in an area with endemic hepatitis A and B. Gastroenterology 1994; 107: 189–195.
25. Cacciola I, Pollicino T, Squadrito G, et al. Occult hepatitis B virus infection in patients with chronic hepatitis C liver disease. N Engl J Med 1999; 341: 22–26.
26. Feray C, Gigou M, Samuel D, et al. Hepatitis C virus RNA and hepatitis B virus DNA in serum and liver of patients with fulminant hepatitis. Gastroenterology 1993; 104: 549–555.
27. Ohkawa K, Hayashi N, Yuki N, et al. Hepatitis C virus antibody and hepatitis C virus replication in chronic hepatitis B patients. J Hepatol 1994; 21: 509–514.
28. Fukuda R, Ishimura N, Niigaki M, et al. Serologically silent hepatitis B virus coinfection in patients with hepatitis C virus-associated chronic liver disease: clinical and virological significance. J Med Virol 1999; 58: 201–207.

29. Wu JC, Chen CL, Hou MC, et al. Multiple viral infection as the most common cause of fulminant and subfulminant viral hepatitis in an area endemic for hepatitis B: application and limitations of the polymerase chain reaction. Hepatology 1994; 19: 836–840.
30. Fong TL, DiBisceglie A, Waggoner J, et al. Significance of antibody to hepatitis C virus in patients with chronic hepatitis B. Hepatology 1991; 14: 64–67.
31. Weltman M, Brotodihardjo A, Crewe E, et al. Coinfection with hepatitis B and C or B, C and delta viruses results in severe chronic liver disease and responds poorly to interferon-alpha treatment. J Viral Hepatitis 1995; 2: 39–45.
32. Villari D, Pernice M, Spinella S, et al. Chronic hepatitis in patients with active hepatitis B virus and hepatitis C virus combined infections: a histological study. Am J Gastroenterology 1995; 90: 955–958.
33. Colombari R, Dhillon A, Piazzola E, et al. Chronic hepatitis in multiple virus infection: histopathological evaluation. Histopathology 1993; 22: 319–325.
34. Liaw YF, Chien RN, Chen TJ, et al. Concurrent hepatitis C virus and hepatitis delta virus superinfection in patients with chronic hepatitis B virus infection. J Med Virol 1992; 37: 294–297.
35. Benvegnu L, Fattovich G, Noventa F, et al. Concurrent hepatitis B and C virus infection and risk of hepatocellular carcinoma in cirrhosis. A prospective study. Cancer 1994; 74: 2442–2448.
36. Shiratori Y, Shiina S, Zhang P, et al. Does dual infection by hepatitis B and C viruses play an important role in the pathogenesis of hepatocellular carcinoma in Japan? Cancer 1997; 80: 2060–2067.
37. Sun CA, Farzadegan H, You SL, et al. Mutual confounding and interactive effects between hepatitis C and hepatitis B viral infections in hepatocellular carcinogenesis: a population-based case-control study in Taiwan. Cancer Epidemiol Biomarkers Prev 1996; 5: 173–178.
38. Chuang WL, Chang WY, Lu SN, et al. Role of hepatitis B and C viruses in hepatocellular carcinoma in a hepatitis B endemic area. A case-control study. Cancer 1992; 69: 2052–2054.
39. Kubo S, Nishiguchi S, Tamori A, et al. Development of hepatocellular carcinoma in patients with HCV infection, with or without past HBV infection, and relationship to age at the time of transfusion. Vox Sang 1998; 74: 129.
40. Kubo S, Nishiguchi S, Hirohashi K, et al. Clinical significance of prior hepatitis B virus infection in patients with hepatitis C virus-related hepatocellular carcinoma. Cancer 1999; 86: 793–798.
41. Liang T, Jeffers L, Reddy K, et al. Viral pathogenesis of hepatocellular carcinoma in the United States. Hepatology 1993; 18: 1326–1333.
42. Chiba T, Matsuzaki Y, Abei M, et al. Role of previous hepatitis B virus infection and heavy smoking in hepatitis C virus-related hepatocellular carcinoma. Am J Gastroenterol 1996; 91: 1195–1203.
43. Paterlini P, Gerken G, Nakajima E, et al. Polymerase chain reaction to detect hepatitis B virus DNA and RNA sequences in primary liver cancers from patients negative for hepatitis B surface antigen. N Engl J Med 1990; 323: 80–85.
44. Chen MF, Jeng LB, Lee WC, et al. Surgical results in patients with dual hepatitis B- and C-related hepatocellular carcinoma compared with hepatitis B- or C-related hepatocellular carcinoma. Surgery 1998; 123: 554–559.
45. Zigneno AL, Fontana R, Puliti S, et al. Relevance of inapparent coinfection by hepatitis B virus in alpha interferon-treated patients with hepatitis C virus chronic hepatitis. J Med Virol 1997; 51: 313–318.

46. Liaw YF, Chien RN, Lin SM, et al. Response of patients with dual hepatitis B virus and C virus infection to interferon therapy. J Interferon Cytokine Res 1997; 17: 449–452.
47. Villa E, Grottola A, Trande P, et al. Reactivation of hepatitis B virus infection induced by interferon (IFN) in HBSAg-positive, anti-HCV-positive patients. Lancet 1993; 341: 1413.
48. Lake J, Wright T, Ferrell L, et al. Hepatitis C and B in liver transplantation. Transplant Proc 1993; 25: 2006–2009.
49. Ferrell L, Wright T, Roberts J, et al. Hepatitis C viral infection in liver transplant recipients. Hepatology 1992; 16: 865–876.
50. Loda M, Fiorentino M, Meckler J, et al. Hepatitis C virus reinfection in orthotopic liver transplant patients with or without concomitant hepatitis B infection. Diagn Mol Pathol 1996; 5: 81–87.
51. Caccamo L, Maggi U, Rossi G, et al. Mild course of C hepatitis after long-term follow-up in hepatitis B and C coinfected liver transplant recipients. Transplant Proc 1998; 30: 2073–2075.
52. Huang E, Wright T, Lake J, et al. Hepatitis B and C coinfections and persistent hepatitis B infections: clinical outcome and liver pathology after transplantation. Hepatology 1996; 23: 396–404.

7 Treatment of Chronic Hepatitis B

*Eng-Kiong Teo, MB, BS
and Anna Suk-Fong Lok, MD*

CONTENTS

INTRODUCTION
INTERFERON THERAPY
LAMIVUDINE (EPIVIR™-HBV, 3TC)
OTHER TREATMENT OPTIONS
IMMUNOMODULATORY THERAPIES
MOLECULAR APPROACHES
TREATMENT STRATEGIES IN THE NEW MILLENNIUM
REFERENCES

INTRODUCTION

Chronic hepatitis B is the commonest cause of chronic liver disease worldwide. Although vaccination has been successful in preventing new infections, there are still 350 million individuals, or approx 5% of the world's population, with chronic hepatitis B virus infection *(1)*. These individuals are at risk of developing liver cirrhosis, liver failure, and hepatocellular carcinoma. Thus, treatment that can arrest the disease, before irreversible damage to the liver occurs, is urgently needed. The aims of treatment are to achieve sustained suppression of HBV replication, and remission of liver disease (Table 1). The end points of treatment include clearance of HBV DNA in serum, loss of hepatitis B e antigen (HBeAg), development of hepatitis B e antibody (anti-HBe), and normalization in alanine aminotransferase (ALT) levels. Currently, two therapeutic agents have been approved by the FDA for the treatment of chronic hepatitis B. Many new antiviral and immunomodulatory therapy are being evaluated, some of them with very promising results.

From: *Clinical Gastroenterology: Diagnosis and Therapeutics*
Edited by: R. S. Koff and G. Y. Wu © Humana Press Inc., Totowa, NJ

Table 1
Aims of Antiviral Treatment of Chronic Hepatitis B Virus Infection

Sustained suppression of HBV replication
   HBV DNA undetectable in serum (on non-PCR-based assay)
   HBeAg to anti-HBe seroconversion
   HBsAg to anti-HBs seroconversion
Remission of liver disease
   Normalization of serum ALT levels
   Decrease in necroinflammation of the liver on histology
Improvement in clinical outcome
   Decrease risk of developing cirrhosis, liver failure and hepatocellular carcinoma
   Increase survival

INTERFERON THERAPY

Interferon (IFN) is the first therapeutic agent that was approved for the treatment of chronic hepatitis B. IFNs are proteins that have antiviral, antiproliferative, and immunomodulatory effects. Interferon α (IFN-α) has been extensively studied in patients with chronic hepatitis B, and has been shown to be effective in suppressing HBV replication, and in inducing remission of liver disease. However, IFN-α is expensive, is associated with many side effects, and its efficacy is limited to a small percent of highly selected patients.

Patient Selection

1. HBeAg-positive, HBV-DNA-positive, elevated ALT. These are the typical chronic hepatitis B patients. They have active virus replication and some immune reactivity to the virus. Wong et al. *(2)* analyzed a total of 837 adult patients with HBeAg-positive chronic hepatitis B from 15 randomized, controlled studies, who were treated with IFN-α for at least 3 mo, and followed for at least 6 mo after cessation of therapy *(2;* Fig. 1). The result from this meta-analysis showed that, compared to untreated controls, a significantly higher percent of IFN-α treated patients cleared HBeAg and hepatitis B surface antigen (HBsAg), and had normalization in ALT level.
2. HBeAg-positive, HBV-DNA-positive, normal ALT. This profile is usually seen in patients with perinatally acquired HBV infection, who are still in the immune-tolerant phase, with minimal liver disease, despite active viral replication. Response to IFN-α therapy is observed in less than 10% of these patients *(3,4)*. IFN-α treatment is therefore not recommended.
3. HBeAg-negative, HBV-DNA-positive, elevated ALT. Traditionally, patients who are HBeAg-negative are considered to have nonreplicative

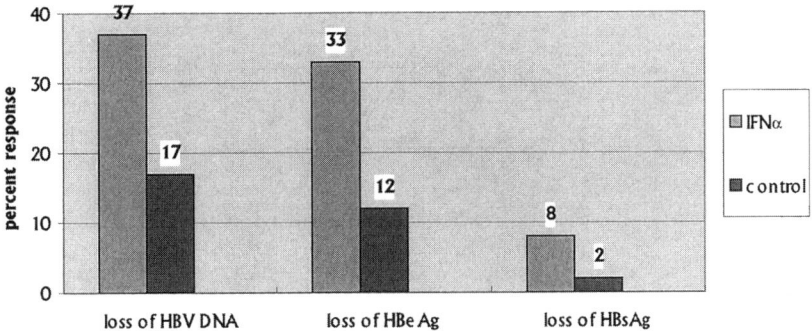

Fig 1. Treatment of chronic hepatitis B. A meta-analysis of IFN-α trials. (Adapted from ref. *2*.)

infection, and do not require antiviral treatment. Some patients are infected with HBV variants that have mutations in the pre-core region, which prevent the production of HBeAg. HBeAg-negative chronic hepatitis B (HBsAg-positive for >6 mo, HBeAg-negative, HBV-DNA-detectable in serum by nonpolymerase chain reaction [PCR]-based assays, and clinical/biochemical/histological evidence of chronic liver disease) is more commonly seen in patients from Asian and Mediterranean countries. In these patients, HBeAg seroconversion cannot be used as an end point of treatment. Response is therefore defined as loss of detectable serum HBV DNA by non-PCR assays, and normalization in ALT level. Several studies in Italy and Greece *(5–7)* found that patients with HBeAg-negative chronic hepatitis B respond during IFN-α treatment, but the posttreatment relapse rate varied from 50 to 86%, and the rate of sustained response ranged from 19 to 59%. The high relapse rate has prompted some investigators to examine longer duration of treatment. In one study, 42 patients were treated with IFN-α for 24 mo: Only 2 (25%) of the responders relapsed when treatment was stopped, but only 7 (33%) patients responded during treatment *(8)*. Thus, the rate of sustained response remained poor: 24%. In view of the costs and side effects of IFN-α, more convincing data are needed before long-term IFN-α can be recommended for these patients.

4. Asian patients with chronic HBV infection. Early trials conducted in Asian patients with HBeAg-positive chronic hepatitis B reported very low response rates *(4)*. A subsequent study *(3)* found that, although the response in patients with normal pretreatment ALT was poor (5%), the response in patients with elevated pretreatment ALT was satisfactory (39%), and comparable to that in white patients (Fig. 2). These data suggest that endogenous immune reaction to HBV is needed to optimize response to IFN-α therapy, and that Asian patients who are in the immune-clearance phase respond similarly as white patients. The efficacy of IFN-α therapy in Asian patients with HBeAg-negative chronic hepatitis B has

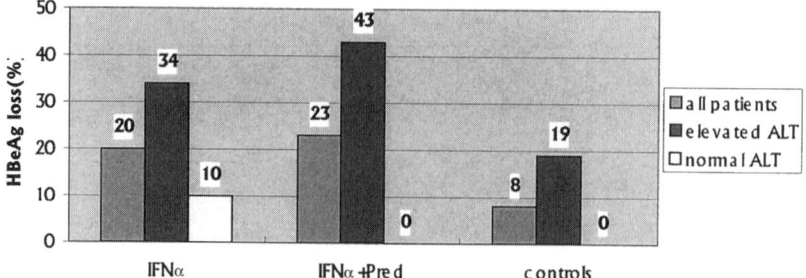

Fig 2. Response to infection treatment with or without prednisone, in patients with normal vs elevated pretreatment ALT. (Adapted ref. *3*.)

not been examined. In a recent study of 243 Chinese patients with HBeAg-negative chronic hepatitis B, only 45% had the pre-core stop codon variant *(9)*. Thus, it is unclear whether Asian patients with HBeAg-negative chronic hepatitis B respond in a way similar to patients from Mediterranean countries.

5. Children with chronic hepatitis B. The efficacy of, and tolerance to, IFN-α therapy are similar in adults and children. Trials conducted on children 2–16-yr-old, who are HBeAg- and HBV-DNA-positive, with elevated ALT, showed a HBeAg clearance rate of 26–40% *(10,11)*. Most adverse events were mild, although growth stunting was observed in very young children *(10)*. Thus, children who are HBeAg-positive, with detectable HBV DNA and elevated ALT, should be considered for IFN-α therapy. However, IFN-α therapy is associated with a very low rate of response in children who have active viral replication and normal ALT *(12)*. These children should be monitored and IFN-α therapy instituted, when they enter into the immune-clearance phase.

6. Nonresponders to IFN-α treatment. Most studies found that retreatment of IFN nonresponders, with IFN-α alone, was associated with a very low rate of response. A recent trial *(13)* reported a HBeAg clearance rate of 33% upon retreatment with IFN-α, suggesting that some patients may benefit from retreatment using IFN-α. This trial included patients who were previously treated with suboptimal doses of IFN-α and may have overestimated the benefits of IFN-α retreatment. Given the side effects of IFN, most patients would prefer to be retreated with other therapy.

7. HBV-DNA-positive, clinical cirrhosis. Approximately 20–40% of patients develop a flare in ALT during IFN-α treatment, which is believed to be a reflection of IFN-induced immune-mediated lysis of infected hepatocytes, and is considered to be a favorable sign. In most patients, the flare is asymptomatic, and not accompanied by increase in bilirubin level. In these patients, treatment can be continued. However, in patients with cir-

Table 2
Factors Associated with Favorable Response to IFN-α Therapy

High pretreatment serum ALT levels
Low pretreatment serum HBV DNA levels
Active inflammation on liver histology
HBV infection acquired during adulthood, compared to perinatal infection
Female vs male
Negative HIV serology
Negative delta virus serology

---

rhosis, the flare may precipitate hepatic decompensation. Two studies *(14,15)* evaluated the safety and efficacy of IFN-α in patients with clinical cirrhosis. In both studies, significant side effects caused by bacterial infection and exacerbation of liver disease, were reported, even with low doses of IFN-α. In one study *(14)*, all five patients with Child's A cirrhosis tolerated treatment, and responded, but response was observed in only 5/15 (33%) patients with Child's B cirrhosis, and in 0/6 patients with Child's C cirrhosis. These data indicate that patients with severe hepatic decompensation do not benefit from IFN-α treatment, and the risks are unacceptably high. With the availability of lamivudine (LAM), there is no role for IFN-α in patients with clinical cirrhosis. Nevertheless, IFN-α may be used in patients with well-compensated cirrhosis, provided that patients are carefully monitored. In a previous trial of IFN-α *(16)*, with or without prednisone priming, in patients with compensated liver disease, 65% of the patients had histological cirrhosis. Only one of the treated patients had hepatic decompensation, which was attributed to prednisone withdrawal, rather than to IFN-α.

Dose Regimen

The recommended dose of IFN-α for adults with HBeAg-positive chronic hepatitis B is 5 MU/d, or 10 MU 3×/wk, administered subcutaneously for 16 wk. The recommended dose for children is 3–6 MU/m^2 3× wk. Current data suggest that patients with HBeAg-negative chronic hep-atitis B require longer duration of treatment, but the optimal duration remains to be determined.

Factors Predictive of Response

Several factors have been associated with a favorable outcome to IFN-α therapy (Table 2). Of these, high pretreatment ALT and low pretreatment serum HBV DNA are most predictive of a response to IFN-α therapy *(17)*.

Table 3
Adverse Effects
Associated with IFN Treatment

Flu-like symptoms
Fatigue
Anorexia and weight loss
Depression and irritability
Leucopenia and thrombocytopenia
Alopecia and skin rash
Induce or aggravate autoimmune disease

Adverse Effects

IFN-α therapy is associated with a range of side effects affecting various body systems (Table 3). Of these, emotional lability is the most worrisome, because it is difficult to detect. A meta-analysis of nine randomized controlled trials, with 552 patients *(18)*, showed that 35% of the patients treated with IFN required dose reduction, and 5% required premature cessation of treatment. These figures were obtained within stringent clinical trials. Dose reductions and premature termination of treatment are probably more frequent in clinical practice.

Prednisone Priming

Prednisone can enhance HBV replication indirectly, by suppressing the immune system, or directly, by interacting with the glucocorticoid-responsive element in the HBV genome. The rationale for glucocorticoid pretreatment stems from the observation that some patients with chronic hepatitis B cleared markers of HBV replication, following tapering or discontinuing of steroid therapy *(19,20)*. These findings suggest that recovery of immune function following steroid withdrawal may be beneficial, particularly if this is timed with the initiation of IFN-α therapy. Several studies failed to demonstrate an overall benefit of prednisone priming, although patients with lower pretreatment ALT levels appeared to have a marginal benefit *(16)*. A meta-analysis of seven published studies, directly comparing IFN-α with and without prednisone priming, failed to show a significant increase in efficacy of IFN-α when steroid pretreatment was added *(21*; Table 4). However, a recent European multicenter study *(22)* involving 213 patients, found that priming with relatively low doses of prednisone for 4 wk, followed by a treatment-free period for 2 wk, increased loss of HBeAg from 28 to 44% ($P = 0.02$). Thus, prednisone priming may possibly have an added benefit in some patients, but there is a risk of fatal exacerbations in patients with underlying cirrhosis.

Table 4
Comparison of IFN-α with Prednisone Priming vs IFN-α Alone

Author/yr (ref)	Markers of response to treatment	Prednisone + IFN-α (%)	IFN-α alone (%)	p value
Cohard et al. 1994 *(21)*		n = 211	n = 259	
	Loss of HBeAg	41	35	0.37
	Loss of HBV DNA	37.5	35.7	0.78
	Loss of HBsAg	6	7	0.84
	Normalization of ALT	44.5	38	0.53
Krogsgaard et al. 1996 *(22)*		n = 101	n = 99	
	Loss of HBeAg	44	28	0.02
	HBeAg seroconversion	38	23	0.03
	Loss of HBV DNA	51	28	0.013

Durability of Response and Long-term Outcome of IFN-Treated Patients

The long-term effects of IFN-α therapy can be assessed from three perspectives.

1. Sustained suppression and/or eradication of HBV. IFN-α induced HBeAg clearance has been reported to be durable in 88–100% of patients, after a follow-up period of 4–8 yr *(23–25)*. However, HBV DNA remained detectable in the serum from most of these patients, when tested by PCR assays. Several studies found that, with time, an increasing percent of the responders cleared HBsAg. The rate of delayed HBsAg clearance among the responders was reported to be 12–65% after 5 yr, in studies from the United States and Europe *(23,24)*, but delayed HBsAg clearance was not observed in studies on Chinese patients *(25,26)*. These data suggest that white patients are more likely to have viral eradication.
2. Resolution of hepatic injury. A decrease in necroinflammation of the liver was seen in most patients, with a sustained virologic response *(2)*, but residual hepatic injury, with mild portal inflammation and fibrosis, usually persisted.
3. Increase in survival and decrease in risk of cirrhosis and HCC. Several studies found that HBeAg-positive patients, who cleared HBeAg, have improved survival, compared to patients who remained HBeAg-positive, suggesting that suppression of HBV replication can improve clinical outcome. In a long-term follow-up (median 8.2 yr) of 101 male patients who participated in a controlled trial of IFN-α therapy, Lin et al. *(25)* found that treated patients had a lower incidence of HCC, 1.5 vs 12% ($P = 0.04$), and an improved survival, 98 vs 57% ($P = 0.02$). In that study, IFN-α

treatment was also associated with a lower rate of progression to cirrhosis, but the difference did not reach statistical significance. Similar data were reported by Niederau et al. *(24)*. In their follow-up of 103 patients over a mean period of 50 mo, the length of survival, until liver transplant or death, was significantly longer in patients who had cleared HBeAg after IFN-α therapy.

LAMIVUDINE (EPIVIR™-HBV, 3TC)

This is the first orally administered antiviral agent approved for the treatment of chronic hepatitis B virus infection. It is the (−) enantiomer of 2'-3' didexoy-3'-thiacytidine. It is phosphorylated in vivo to the active triphosphate (3' thiacytidine triphosphate [3TC-TP]), which competes with deoxycytidine triphosphate for DNA synthesis. Incorporation of 3TC-TP into newly synthesized DNA results in premature chain termination during reverse transcription of the first HBV DNA strand. It has similar effect on the synthesis of the second HBV DNA strand. LAM, by decreasing the viral load, may have an added effect of reversing T-cell hyporesponsiveness to HBV antigens in patients with chronic hepatitis B virus infection *(27)*.

Efficacy

Clinical trials, using short courses (4–24 wk) of LAM, showed that, although most patients had significant decrease in serum HBV DNA levels, the antiviral effect was not sustained *(28–30)*.

Several trials have been conducted to evaluate the safety and efficacy of longer courses (≥1 yr) of LAM therapy *(31–33)*. LAM has also been examined in patients with HBeAg-positive, and in patients with HBeAg-negative, chronic hepatitis B, in treatment-naïve patients and in IFN nonresponders, as monotherapy, and in combination with IFN. These clinical trials showed that LAM is well-tolerated and effective in suppressing HBV replication in patients with HBeAg-positive, and in patients with HBeAg-negative chronic hepatitis B. Among HBeAg-positive patients, a 1-yr course of LAM therapy is associated with a HBeAg seroconversion rate similar to a 16-wk course of IFN-α therapy. As with IFN-α, LAM is most effective in patients with high pretreatment ALT. LAM is also effective in IFN nonresponders. Based on data from two studies, combination therapy of LAM and IFN-α does not seem to confer any added benefit, compared to treatment with either agent alone.

Patient Selection

1. HBeAg-positive, HBV-DNA-positive. Three clinical trials in treatment-naïve patients reported that HBeAg seroconversion (defined as loss of

Table 5
Efficacy of LAM Treatment in Patients with Chronic Hepatitis B

Author/yr (ref)	Treatment ×52 wk	n	HBeAg sero-conversion	% loss of HBeAg	% loss of HBV DNA	% with improved histology	% with normalized ALT
Lai et al. 1998 (31)	LAM 100 mg	143	16	NA	NA	56	72
	Placebo	73	4	NA	NA	25	24
Dienstag et al. 1999 (33)	LAM 100 mg	66	17	32	44	52	41
	Placebo	71	6	11	16	23	7

Table 6
Comparison of Response to LAM,
IFN, and Combination Therapy of LAM and IFN

		HBeAg seroconversion (%)			
	n	LAM	IFN-α	LAM + IFN-α	p value
Treatment-naïve patients (48)	226	18%	19%	29%	NS
IFN-α nonresponders (35)	238	18%	12%	13%	NS

HBeAg, detection of anti-HBe, and loss of serum HBV DNA, based on non-PCR assays) occurred in 16–17% of treated patients after 1 yr of LAM treatment (31,33; Tables 5 and 6). Approximately 50% of the treated patients had histological improvement (defined as decrease in Knodell score by ≥2 points). These encouraging data led to the approval of LAM as a treatment of chronic hepatitis B. However, only a small percent of patients developed HBeAg seroconversion after 1 yr of treatment. Subgroup analysis found that pretreatment ALT was the most important predictor of response. Thus, as with IFN-α therapy, HBeAg- and HBV-DNA-positive patients, with normal ALT, have poor response to LAM treatment, suggesting that successful response to LAM treatment relies on innate immune response to HBV.

2. HBeAg-negative, HBV-DNA-positive, elevated ALT. In a multicenter trial in Europe and Canada (34), 125 patients were randomized to receive LAM or placebo. Patients who had no response (defined as HBV DNA >2.5 pg/mL) after 24 wk of treatment were withdrawn. At wk 24, a significantly higher percent of LAM-treated patients responded (normal ALT and undetectable serum HBV DNA by bDNA assay): 63%, compared to

6% among the controls ($P < 0.001$). In patients who received LAM continuously for 52 wk, serum HBV DNA was undetectable by bDNA assay in 65%, and by PCR assay in 39% of the LAM-treated patients, and histological improvement was seen in 60% of patients. These data indicate that LAM is beneficial in patients with HBeAg-negative chronic hepatitis B. However, as with IFN-α therapy, posttreatment relapse is common, necessitating long-term treatment.
3. Nonresponders to IFN-α treatment. LAM was evaluated in a multicenter trial on 238 patients who previously failed to respond to a course of IFN-α monotherapy (35). In this study, patients were randomized to receive LAM monotherapy for 52 wk; LAM for 8 wk, followed by combination of LAM and IFN-α for another 16 wk; or no treatment. Patients who received LAM monotherapy had the highest HBeAg seroconversion rate; 18%, compared to 12 and 13%, respectively in the other groups (NS). Biochemical and histological improvement were also more frequent in the patients who received LAM monotherapy. These data suggest that patients who failed IFN-α treatment have similar response to LAM as treatment-naïve patients, and retreatment with combination of IFN-α and LAM did not confer any added benefit, compared to retreatment with LAM monotherapy.
4. HBV-DNA-positive liver cirrhosis. Unlike IFN-α, LAM is well-tolerated in patients with decompensated cirrhosis. In an open label study on 35 patients (36), 10 with Childs-Turcotte-Pugh (CTP) class-C and 25 CTP class-B, improvement in liver disease (defined as decrease in CTP score of ≥2) was observed in 22/23 patients, who received a minimum of 6 mo treatment (range 16–30 mo). All patients had undetectable HBV DNA, by non-PCR assay, within 6 mo of treatment. LAM-resistant mutants were detected in three patients, who were maintained on LAM, with stable CTP score, up to 30 mo after the detection of LAM-resistant mutants. These data suggest that LAM treatment is beneficial in patients with decompensated cirrhosis. However, longer follow-up is necessary, to determine the outcome of patients who developed LAM resistance. In addition, not all patients benefited from treatment. In this study, seven patients had progressive liver disease, necessitating liver transplant, and five died during the first 6 mo. Thus, further studies are needed to determine the efficacy of LAM in this patient population, the optimal timing to initiate treatment, and the subset of patients who are most likely to benefit from treatment.

Dose Regimen

LAM is administered orally at 100 mg/d. Dose-finding studies showed that 100-mg dose is more effective than 25 mg, but doses above 100 mg did not confer any added effect. Dose adjustment is needed for patients with renal failure (creatinine clearance of <50 mL/min). In patients co-infected with HIV, higher doses of LAM should be administered (150 mg bid) in conjunction with other HIV treatment. The optimum duration of LAM therapy has not been determined. LAM treatment should be administered for a minimum of 1 yr, because shorter duration of therapy is associated with lower rates of HBeAg seroconversion and less-durable response. Preliminary results from the Asian study *(37)* showed that HBeAg seroconversion increases with the duration of treatment, from 16% at 1 yr to 27% at 2 yr and 40% at 3 yr. The ease of administration and the excellent safety profile have prompted many investigators to recommend long-term or indefinite treatment. However, the incidence of LAM resistance increases with the duration of treatment, from 17% at 1 yr to 55% at 3 yr. Thus, the benefits of long-term treatment must be weighed against the potential risks of adverse outcome associated with LAM-resistant mutants.

Current recommendations are to treat patients for at least 1 yr, and to discontinue treatment in patients who have achieved HBeAg seroconversion (HBeAg loss, anti-HBe detection, and HBV-DNA-negative, by non-PCR assays, on more than one occasion). In patients who have not achieved HBeAg seroconversion, LAM may be continued, in the hope that HBeAg seroconversion will occur with longer duration of treatment. In patients with LAM-resistant mutants, treatment can be continued, as long as benefit to the patient (based on clinical assessment, ALT, and HBV DNA levels) is maintained. Continued treatment will suppress the wild-type HBV, resulting in lower HBV DNA and ALT, compared to pre-treatment values. In addition, some patients may develop HBeAg seroconversion, even after the detection of LAM-resistant mutants.

Factors Predictive of Response

In the Asian study *(38)*, pretreatment ALT level was the only independent predictor of HBeAg seroconversion. HBeAg seroconversion was observed in 64, 26, and 5% of patients with pretreatment ALT >5×, 2–5×, and <2× the upper limit of normal, respectively. Unlike IFN-α therapy, response to LAM treatment was not related to the pretreatment HBV DNA level. Similar results were obtained *(39)* when pooled data, from 406 patients in four randomized trials, involving patients from all over the world, were analyzed.

Adverse Effects

LAM does not interact with mitochondrial DNA. Common side effects associated with nucleoside analogs, such as pancreatitis and peripheral neuropathy, are rare *(40)*. In randomized, controlled trials of LAM in patients with chronic hepatitis B, various adverse events have been reported, but these events occurred with the same frequency among the controls. Mild (2–3-fold) increase in ALT has been observed more commonly during and after LAM treatment, compared to patients who received placebo. In most instances, the ALT increase was transient, and not associated with any increase in bilirubin levels. Overall, LAM appears to be a well-tolerated drug.

LAM Resistance

The selection of LAM-resistant mutants is the main limitation to LAM treatment. The most common mutation affects the tyrosine, methionine, aspartate, aspartate (YMDD) motif in the catalytic domain of the HBV DNA polymerase, resulting in a substitution from methionine to valine (M552V) or isoleucine (M552I). This mutation can occur in isolation, or in conjunction with another mutation that affects an upstream region, resulting in a substitution from leucine to methionine (L528M). These genetic changes result in a decreased capability of the virus to replicate *(41)*, which accounts for the lower HBV DNA levels observed in patients with LAM-resistant mutants.

LAM resistance is usually manifested as breakthrough infection (defined as reappearance of HBV DNA in serum after its initial disappearance). However, breakthrough infection can also be a result of noncompliance. Unlike HIV infection, LAM-resistant HBV mutants are usually not detected until patients have been on treatment for at least 6 mo. Genotypic resistance can be detected in 17% patients after 1 yr of treatment, increasing to 40% after 2 yr and 55% after 3 yr of treatment. In vitro studies *(42)* found that these mutants confer up to 10,000-fold resistance. Thus, increasing the dose cannot restore the antiviral effect of LAM on these mutants.

The clinical course of patients with LAM-resistant mutants is variable, and the long-term outcome of these patients remains to be determined. In most patients, continuation of LAM results in lower serum HBV DNA and ALT levels, compared to pretreatment. The continued benefit may be related to the suppressive effect of LAM on residual wild-type virus and the lower replication capacity of the mutants. However, some patients may develop acute exacerbations of liver disease. In a report from Taiwan *(43)*, 13/32 patients with LAM-resistant mutants were observed to have flares in ALT, during a median follow-up period of 24 wk (range 4–94 wk). Although most of the flares were asymptomatic, three (23%) patients had hepatic decompensation. Fatal exacerbations, associated with the selection of LAM-resistant mutants, have also been reported in other studies, and appear to be more common in patients with underlying cirrhosis or recurrent hepatitis B post-liver transplantation *(44,45)*. The Taiwan study *(43)* found that HBeAg seroconversion can occur after the detection of LAM-resistant mutants, and was more common in patients who had ALT flares (8/12 patients 75%), compared to no HBeAg seroconversion seen in 19 patients without ALT flares ($P < 0.001$). These findings support the continued use of LAM in patients who developed LAM-resistant mutants. However, longer follow-up of a larger cohort of patients is needed to determine if continued treatment is beneficial to all patients with LAM resistance. Clearly, there is a need to be prudent in the use of LAM, and an urgent demand to develop safe and effective therapy for patients with worsening liver disease caused by LAM-resistant HBV mutants. Several antiviral agents have been shown to be effective against LAM-resistant HBV mutants in in vitro studies, but only adefovir dipivoxil has been tested in vivo. The preliminary data are encouraging, but the long-term safety and efficacy of adefovir dipivoxil has not been determined.

Durability of Response

Data on the durability of LAM-induced response is limited. In one study *(46)*, 35 patients were treated for 1 yr, and were assessed 6 mo after cessation of treatment: 91% of the patients who had HBeAg seroconversion remained HBeAg-negative. However, recent data from Asia *(47,48)* reported lower rates of durable response, 37–73%, 1 yr after stopping treatment. In the Korean study *(48)*, the high relapse rate may be related to a shorter duration of treatment (mean 8 mo). Current data suggest that the rate of HBsAg clearance may be lower than with IFN-α therapy, but longer follow-up is needed to determine if delayed HBsAg clearance can be observed in patients with durable response after LAM treatment.

OTHER TREATMENT OPTIONS

Combination Therapy of LAM and IFN-α

LAM and IFN-α work through different mechanisms, so combination therapy of the two agents may have additive or synergistic effects. Combination therapy of LAM and IFN-α has been evaluated in two studies *(35,48*; Table 6). In both studies, LAM was administered for 8 wk prior to the initiation of IFN-α therapy. The rationale for this regimen was to optimize the response to IFN-α by decreasing the viral load with LAM pre-treatment.

In one study *(49)*, 226 treatment-naïve patients were randomized to LAM monotherapy for 52 wk, or to LAM for 8 wk, followed by LAM and IFN-α for 16 wk or IFN-α alone for 16 wk. At wk 52, the HBeAg seroconversion rates were 18, 19, and 29% in the groups that received LAM monotherapy, IFN-α monotherapy, and combination therapy, respectively (NS). Histological response was also observed in a higher percent of patients who received LAM monotherapy: 49%, compared to 37 and 46% patients who received combination therapy and IFN-α only. Subgroup analysis showed that the combination therapy appeared to have a maximum benefit in patients with moderately increased ALT (2–5× upper limit of normal) with HBeAg serconversion of almost 40%, compared to about 20% for both groups with monotherapy. These data indicate that a 1-yr course of LAM is similar to a 16-wk course of IFN-α, in antiviral efficacy. Combination of LAM and IFN-α does not seem to have any added benefit, compared to treatment with either agent alone, except in subgroup of patients with moderately elevated ALT. However, there are several flaws in the design of this study: Patients in the combination therapy group received 24 wk of LAM, but patients in the LAM monotherapy group received 52 wk of treatment; this study was underpowered; and the timing of the posttreatment liver biopsy was biased in favor of LAM monotherapy. Thus, the posttreatment liver biopsies were performed while the patients in the LAM monotherapy group were still on treatment, but the patients in the combination therapy and IFN-α monotherapy groups had completed treatment 28 wk earlier. A similar study *(35)*, in patients who previously failed to respond to IFN-α, found that retreatment with combination of LAM and IFN-α did not have any added benefit, compared to retreatment with LAM monotherapy. Although the results of these studies are discouraging, problems in their design prevent definitive conclusions on the efficacy of combination therapy. It is also possible that better results may be obtained by initiating IFN-α and LAM simultaneously.

Other Nucleoside Analogs

FAMCICLOVIR

This is the oral prodrug of penciclovir. It is a deoxyguanosine analog, and, in its triphosphate state (PCV-TP), competes with dGTP for incorporation into viral DNA. PCV-TP also competes with deoxyguanosine triphosphate (dGTP) for the priming of reverse transcription during the synthesis of the first strand of HBV DNA. Clinical studies showed that famciclovir is less potent, compared with LAM, with 1 vs 2–3 log decrease in serum HBV DNA levels. A study of 417 chronic hepatitis B patients *(50)* found that famciclovir, at 500 mg tid for 1 yr, resulted in a low rate of HBeAg seroconversion: 9 vs 3% among controls. The same study demonstrated that famciclovir, administered as a single daily dose (1.5 g), was less effective. Resistance to famciclovir has been reported. The most common mutation involves a substitution from leucine to methionine at position 528 (L528M) *(51)*. Thus, these mutants may have crossresistance with LAM *(52)*. In view of the low efficacy of famciclovir, and the need for thrice-daily administration, it is unlikely that famciclovir will have a major role in the treatment of chronic hepatitis B.

ADEFOVIR DIPIVOXIL

This is the prodrug of adefovir. It is a deoxyadenosine monophosphate analog. It inhibits HBV DNA polymerase, and is a potent inhibitor of HBV replication. Adefovir dipivoxil has been shown to decrease serum HBV DNA levels by 3–4 log in clinical studies *(53)*. In one phase-II trial *(54)*, 67 patients, treated with adefovir for 12 wk, resulted in 20% HBeAg seroconversion at 36 wk of follow-up. Adefovir at high doses is associated with nephrotoxicity. Phase-III clinical trials are ongoing, to determine the safety and efficacy of a 1-yr course of lower doses (10 and 30 mg) of adefovir. In vitro studies *(55)* showed that adefovir is effective in suppressing the replication of LAM-resistant HBV. Preliminary data *(56)* suggest that adefovir is also effective in suppressing replication of LAM-resistant HBV in vivo. These findings are encouraging because effective rescue therapy are needed for patients who develop worsening liver disease as a result of LAM-resistant mutants.

ENTECAVIR

This is a dGTP analog, which acts by inhibition of HBV DNA polymerase. In vitro and animal studies showed that it has potent antiviral activity against HBV. It is currently being evaluated in phase I/II clinical trials *(56a)*.

EMTRICITABINE (FTC)

FTC is a deoxycytidine analog, which inhibits HBV DNA polymerase, and has structural similarities to LAM. A preliminary study on 30 patients *(57)* showed that it is well-tolerated and effective in decreasing serum HBV DNA levels. As expected, FTC may select for the same mutations that are associated with LAM resistance.

IMMUNOMODULATORY THERAPIES

Patients with chronic hepatitis B virus infection exhibit impaired T-cell response to HBV Ags *(58)*. The rationale of immunomodulatory therapy is to reverse the hyporesponsive state, and to stimulate the body's innate immune system to effectively clear HBV. To date, there is little evidence that immunomodulatory therapy alone is effective in clearing HBV. The role of immunomodulatory therapy may be predominantly as an adjunct to antiviral therapy.

Thymosin

Thymosin is a thymic-derived peptide, which can stimulate T-cell response. A small pilot study on 12 patients *(59)* reported encouraging results. However, a subsequent double-blind, controlled trial, involving 97 American patients, found that the rate of HBeAg seroconversion was 25% in treated and in 13% controls ($P = 0.11$). Although thymosin was well-tolerated, its low efficacy suggests that there is no role for thymosin in the treatment of chronic hepatitis B *(60)*. Studies in Asia and Europe reported more encouraging results. In a study in Asia *(61)*, 98 patients were randomized to receive 26 or 52 wk of thymosin, or no treatment. When assessed at the end of therapy, 3, 6, and 3% of the patients who received thymosin for 26 or 52 wk, or no treatment, respectively, had lost HBeAg. When response was assessed at 18 mo after entry into the study, the corresponding rates of HBeAg loss were 41, 27, and 9% in the patients who received 26 or 52 wk of thymosin, and the control group, respectively. These data suggest that thymosin may have a role in the treatment of chronic hepatitis B, and that the antiviral effects may not be apparent until 6 mo after cessation of treatment. Because of the conflicting results, more studies are needed before thymosin can be recommended for treatment of chronic hepatitis B.

S and pre-S HBV Vaccines

The basis for peptide vaccine therapy in chronic hepatitis B is to stimulate immune response to HBV. Pre-S Ags have been shown to be more immunogenic than the S antigen (HBsAg), and may stimulate both T- and B-cell response. In one study *(62)*, 170 patients were randomized to receive GenHevac (preS2/S antigen-containing vaccine), Recombivax (S antigen-containing vaccine) or no treatment. Most patients were subsequently treated with IFN-α after completion of the vaccine schedule. The data, available only in 40 patients, showed that clearance of HBV DNA and HBeAg were seen in 5/17 patients vaccinated with GenHevac. Significant decrease in HBV DNA level was seen in 2/10 patients vaccinated with Recombivax. HBV DNA clearance was seen in 1/13 controls. Because of the design of the study, which included IFN-α treatment after the end of vaccination schedule, and the high dropout rate, it is not possible to ascertain the efficacy and durability of the response to the vaccines *per se*. Better-designed studies are needed to define the therapeutic role of HBV vaccine.

Table 7
Comparison Between LAM and IFN

LAM	IFN
Pros	
Oral administration	Finite duration of treatment
Negligible side effects	Higher rate of HBsAg clearance
Lower costs?	Resistant mutants not reported
Cons	
Long/indefinite duration of treatment	Expensive
Resistant mutants	Frequent side effects
Poor response in immune tolerant patients	Poor response in immunotolerant patients

DNA-based HBV Vaccines

Experimental DNA vaccines stimulate both T- and B-cell immune responses to HBV, and may be more effective in the treatment of chronic hepatitis B than peptide vaccines *(63)*. Trials conducted on transgenic mice that express the HBV surface gene showed that vaccination with plasmid DNA resulted in decreased production of HBsAg. The results of pilot clinical trials are eagerly awaited.

T-cell Vaccines

Cytotoxic T-cells play an important role in the clearance of intracellular virus. A vaccine incorporating a cytotoxic T-lymphocyte epitope, derived from hepatitis B core protein, was evaluated in a pilot clinical study *(64)*. Although the vaccine induced a cytotoxic T-lymphocyte response in some patients, it was not sufficient to achieve virus clearance. In addition, this vaccine appeared to be less effective in patients who are in the immune-tolerant phase of HBV infection.

MOLECULAR APPROACHES

Antisense Oligonucleotide/Ribozymes

These molecules bind to specific DNA or RNA targets, causing degradation of the DNA or RNA. Multiple or critical sites of the viral genome can be targeted, so as to render any escape mutants nonviable. However, these molecules are rapidly degraded in vivo by nucleases, limiting delivery of adequate concentrations of the active molecules to the target sites. A recent trial *(65)* conducted on ducks showed that antisense oligonucleotides, delivered in liposomes, were effective in decreasing duck HBV

Table 8
Current Recommendations for Treatment of Chronic Hepatitis B IFN

HBeAg	HBV DNA[a]	ALT	Treatment strategy
+	+	Normal	Low efficacy for both IFN-α and LAM treatment. Observe patient, consider treatment when ALT becomes elevated.
+	+	Elevated	IFN-α or LAM therapy. In IFN-α nonresponders and patients with contraindications to IFN-α, LAM is preferred.
−	+	Elevated	IFN-α or LAM. Long-term treatment required.
−	−	Normal	No treatment required.
+/−	+	Cirrhosis	Compensated: low dose IFN-α (close monitoring required) or LAM Decompensated: LAM treatment. Optimal timing and duration of therapy unknown. Transplantation.
+/−	−	Cirrhosis	Compensated: observe. Decompensated: transplantation.

[a]HBV DNA results based on non-PCR assay.

DNA levels. Further refinement of this technique is needed, before it can be used clinically.

TREATMENT STRATEGIES IN THE NEW MILLENNIUM

Current FDA-approved therapy are effective in achieving HBeAg clearance in 20–30% and HBeAg seroconversion in 15–20% of treated patients. IFN-α has the advantages of a finite duration of treatment, and no reports of drug-resistant mutants. However, side effects are common, and may be debilitating. LAM, on the other hand, has minimal side effects, but the emergence of resistant mutants, and the need for long-term treatment, limit the widespread use of LAM. Whether IFN-α or LAM should be used as the primary therapy is a decision that should be made jointly by the physician and patient, after careful discussions of the pros and cons of the two therapy (Table 7). Current recommendations for management of patients with chronic hepatitis B are summarized in Table 8.

As the armamentarium of therapeutic agents expands, combination therapy should be considered. Because of the lack of efficacy of currently available treatment on the covalently closed circular DNA, viral eradication is dependent on the turnover of infected hepatocytes and innate immune response. Although long-term treatment with a potent antiviral agent may be sufficient in some patients, it seems likely that most patients will require combination therapy, for sustained virologic response.

REFERENCES

1. World Health Organization. The World Health Report. Geneva, Switzerland, 1988.
2. Wong DK, Cheung AM, O'Rourke K, et al. Effect of alpha-interferon treatment in patients with hepatitis B e antigen-positive chronic hepatitis B. A meta-analysis. Ann Intern Med 1993; 119: 312–323.
3. Lok AS, Wu PC, Lai CL, et al. Controlled trial of interferon with or without prednisolone priming for chronic hepatitis B. Gastroenterology 1992; 102: 2091–2097.
4. Lok AS, Lai CL, Wu PC, et al. Long-term follow-up in a randomized controlled trial of recombinant alpha 2-interferon in Chinese patients with chronic hepatitis B infection. Lancet 1988; 2: 298–302.
5. Hadziyannis S, Bramou T, Makris A, et al. Interferon alfa-2b treatment of HBeAg negative/serum HBV DNA positive chronic active hepatitis type B. J Hepatol. 1990; 11(Suppl 1): S133–S136.
6. Brunetto MR, Giarin M, Saracco G, et al. Hepatitis B virus unable to secrete e antigen and response to interferon in chronic hepatitis B. Gastroenterology 1993; 105: 845–850.
7. Fattovich G, Farci P, Rugge M, et al. Randomized controlled trial of lymphoblastoid interferon-alpha in patients with chronic hepatitis B lacking HBeAg. Hepatology 1992; 15: 584–589.
8. Lampertico P, Ninno ED, Manzin A, et al. Randomized controlled trial of a 24-month course of interferon alfa 2b in patients with chronic hepatitis B who had hepatitis B virus DNA without hepatitis B e antigen in the serum. Hepatology 1997; 26: 1621–1625.
9. Chan HLY, Leung NWY, Hussain M, et al. Hepatitis B e antigen-negative chronic hepatitis B in Hong Kong. Hepatology 2000; 31: 763–768.
10. Sokal ME, Conjeevaram HS, Roberts EA, et al. Interferon alfa therapy for chronic hepatitis B in children: a multinational randomized controlled trial. Gastroenterology 1998; 114: 988–995.
11. Gregorio GV, Jara P, Hierro L, et al. Lymphoblastoid interferon alfa with or without steroid pretreatment in children with chronic hepatitis B: a multicenter controlled trial. Hepatology 1996; 23: 700–707.
12. Lai CL, Lin HJ, Lau JN, et al. Effect of recombinant alpha 2 interferon with or without prednisolone priming in Chinese HBsAg carrier children. Q J Med 1991; 78: 155.
13. Carreno V, Marcellin P, Hadziyannis S, et al. Retreatment of chronic hepatitis B e antigen-positive patients with recombinant interferon alfa-2a. Hepatology 1999; 30: 277–282.
14. Perrillo R, Tamburro C, Regenstein F, et al. Low-dose, titratable interferon alfa in decompensated LD caused by chronic infection with hepatitis B virus. Gastroenterology 1995; 109: 908–916.
15. Hoofnagle JH, Di Bisceglie AM, Waggoner JG, et al. Interferon alfa for patients with clinically apparent cirrhosis due to chronic hepatitis B. Gastroenterology 1993; 104: 1116–1121.
16. Perrillo RP, Schiff ER, Davis GL, et al. Randomized, controlled trial of interferon alfa-2b alone and after prednisolone withdrawal for the treatment of chronic hepatitis B. The Hepatitis Interventional Therapy Group. N Engl J Med 1990; 323: 295–301.

17. Lok ASF. Treatment of chronic hepatitis B. J Viral Hepatitis 1994; 1: 105–124.
18. Wong JB, Koff RS, Tine F, et al. Cost-effectiveness of interferon alfa 2b for hepatitis B e antigen-positive chronic hepatitis B. Ann Intern Med 1995; 122: 664–675.
19. Scullard GH, Robinson WS, Merigan TC, et al. Effect of immunosuppressive therapy on hepatitis B viral infection in patients with chronic hepatitis. Gastroenterology 1979; 7: A40.
20. Muller R, Vido I, Schmidt FW. Rapid withdrawal of immunosuppressive therapy in chronic active hepatitis B infection. Lancet 1981; 1: 1323–1324.
21. Cohard M, Poynard T, Mathurin P, et al. Prednisolone-interferon combination in the treatment of chronic hepatitis B: direct and indirect metaanalysis. Hepatology 1994; 20: 1390–1398.
22. Krogsgaard K, Marcellin P, Trepo C, et al. Prednisolone withdrawal therapy enhances the effect of human lymphoblastoid interferon in chronic hepatitis B. INTERPRED Trial Group. J Hepatol 1996; 25: 803–813.
23. Korenman J, Baker B, Waggoner J, et al. Long-trem remission of chronic hepatitis B after alpha-interferon therapy. Ann Intern Med 1991; 114: 629–634.
24. Niederau C, Heintges T, Lange S, et al. Long-term follow-up of HBeAg-positive patients treated with interferon alfa for chronic hepatitis B. N Engl J Med 1996; 334: 1422–1427.
25. Lin SM, Sheen IS, Chien RN, et al. Long-term beneficial effect of interferon therapy in patients with chronic hepatitis B virus infection. Hepatology 1999; 29: 971–975.
26. Lok AS, Chung HT, Liu VW, et al. Long-term follow-up of chronic hepatitis B patients treated with interferon alfa. Gastroenterology 1993; 105: 1833–1838.
27. Boni C, Bertoletti A, Penna A, et al. Lamivudine treatment can restore T-cell responsiveness in chronic hepatitis B. J Clin Invest 1998; 102: 968–975.
28. Dienstag J, Perrillo RP, Schiff ER, et al. Preliminary trial of lamivudine for chronic hepatitis B infection. N Engl J Med 1995; 333: 1657–1661.
29. Lai CL, Ching CK, Tung AK, et al. Lamivudine is effective in suppressing hepatitis B virus DNA in Chinese hepatitis B surface antigen carriers: a placebo controlled trial. Hepatology 1997; 25: 241–244.
30. Nevens F, Main J, Honkoop P, et al. Lamivudine therapy for chronic hepatitis B: a six-month randomized dose-ranging study. Gastroenterology 1997; 113: 1258–1263.
31. Lai CL, Chien RN, Leung NWY, et al. One-year trial of lamivudine for chronic hepatitis B. N Engl J Med 1998; 339: 61–68.
32. Dienstag JL, Schiff ER, Mitchell M, et al. Extended lamivudine retreatment for chronic hepatitis B: maintainance of viral suppression after discontinuation of therapy. Hepatology 1999; 30: 1082–1087.
33. Dienstag JL, Schiff ER, Wright TL, et al. Lamivudine as initial treatment for chronic hepatitis B in the United States. N Engl J Med 1999; 341: 1256–1263.
34. Tassapoulos NC, Volpes R, Pastore G, et al. Efficacy of lamivudine in patients with hepatitis B e antigen-negative/hepatitis B virus DNA-positive (precore mutant) chronic hepatitis B. Hepatology 1999; 29: 889–896.
35. Schiff E, Karayalcin S, Grimm I, et al. Placebo controlled study of lamivudine and interferon alpha 2b in patients with chronic hepatitis B who previously failed interferon therapy (abstract). Hepatology 1998; 28: 388A.
36. Villeneuve JP, Condreay LD, Willems B, et al. Lamivudine treatment for decompensated cirrhosis resulting from chronic hepatitis B. Hepatology 2000; 31: 207–210.
37. Leung NWY, Lai CL, Chang TT, et al. Three years lamivudine therapy in chronic HBV. J Hepatology 1999; 30(Suppl 1): 59.

38. Chien RN, Liaw YF, Atkins M, for the Asian Hepatitis Lamivudine Trial Group. Pretherapy alanine transaminase level as a determinant for hepatitis B e antigen seroconversion during lamivudine therapy in patients with chronic hepatitis B. Hepatology 1999; 30: 770–774.
39. Perrillo RP, Schalm, SW, Schiff, ER, et al. Predictors of HBsAg seroconversion in chronic hepatitis B patients treated with lamivudine (abstract). Hepatology 1999; 30: 317A.
40. Heylen R, Miller R. Adverse effects and drug interaction of medication commonly used in the treatment of adult HIV positive patients: part 2. Genitourin Med 1997; 73: 5–11.
41. Melagari M, Scaglioni PP, Wands JR. Hepatitis B virus mutants associated with 3TC and Famciclovir administration are replication defective. Hepatology 1998; 27: 628–633.
42. Allen MI, Deslauriers M, Andrews CW, et al. Identification and charactization of mutations in hepatitis B virus resisitant to lamivudine. Hepatology 1998; 27: 1670–1677.
43. Liaw YF, Chien RN, Yeh CT, et al. Acute exacerbation and hepatitis B virus clearance after emergence of YMDD motif mutation during lamivudine therapy. Hepatology 1999; 30: 567–572.
44. Ling R, Multimer D, Ahmed M, et al. Selection of mutations in the hepatitis B virus polymerase during therapy of transplant recipients with lamivudine. Hepatology 1996; 24: 711–713.
45. Batholomew MM, Jansen RW, Jeffers LJ, et al. Hepatitis-B-virus resistance to lamivudine given for recurrent infection after orthotopic liver transplantation. Lancet 1997; 349: 20–22.
46. Schiff E, Cianciara J, Kowdley K, et al. Durability of HBeAg seroconversion after lamivudine monotherapy in controlled phase II and III trials. Hepatology 1998; 28: 163A.
47. Chang TT, Lai CL, Liaw YF, et al. Enhanced HBeAg seroconversion rates in Chinese patients on lamivudine. Hepatology 1999; 30: 420A.
48. Song BC, Suh DJ, Lee HC, et al. Seroconversion after lamivudine treatment is not durable in chronic hepatitis B. Hepatology 1999; 30: 348A.
49. Schalm SW, Heathcote J, Cianciara J, et al. Lamivudine and alpha interferon combination treatment of patients with chronic hepatitis B infection: a randomized trial. Gut 2000; 46: 562–568.
50. De Man RA, Habal E, Marcellin P, et al. A randomized placebo-controlled study on the efficacy of 12 months famciclovir treatment in patients with chronic HBeAg positive hepatitis (abstract). J Hepatol 1999; 30(Suppl 1): GS5/27.
51. Aye TT, Bartholomuesz A, Shaw T, et al. Hepatitis B virus polymerase mutations during antiviral therapy in a patient following liver transplant. J Hepatol 1997; 26: 1148–1153.
52. Xiong X, Yang H, Westland CE, et al. In vitro evaluation of hepatitis B virus polymerase mutations associated with famciclovir resistance. Hepatology 2000; 31: 219–224.
53. Tsiang M, Rooney JF, Toole JJ, et al. Biphasic clearance kinetics of hepatitis B virus from patients during Adefovir Dipivoxil therapy. Hepatology 1999; 29: 1863–1869.
54. Heathcote EJ, Jeffers L, Wright T, et al. Loss of serum HBV DNA and HBeAg seroconversion following short-term (12 weeks) of adefovir dipivoxil therapy in chronic hepatitis B: Two placebo controlled phase II studies (abstract). Hepatology 1998; 28: 317A.

55. Xiong X, Flores C, Yang H, et al. Mutations in hepatitis B DNA polymerase associated with lamivudine do not confer resistance to adefovir in vitro. Hepatology 1998; 28: 1669–1673.
56. Perrillo R, Schiff E, Magill A, et al. In vivo demonstration of sensitivity of YMDD variants to adefovir (abstract). Gastroenterology 1999; 116: A1261.
56a. deMan R, Wolters L, Nevens F, et al. A study of oral entecevir given for 28 days in both treatment-naive and pre-treated subjects with chronic hepatitis (abstract). Hepatology 2000; 322: 376A.
57. Gish RG, Leung NWY, Wright TL, et al. Anti-hepatitis B virus (HBV) activity and pharmacokinetics of FTC in a 2 month trial in HBV infected patients (abstract). Gastroenterology 1999; 116: A1216.
58. Chisari FV. Heaptitis B virus immunopathogenesis. Annu Rev Immunol 1995; 13: 29–60.
59. Mutchnick MG, Appelman HD, Chung HT, et al. Thymosin treatment of chronic hepatitis B: a placebo-controlled double blind study (abstract). Hepatology 1991; 14: 409–415.
60. Mutchnick MG, Lindsay KL, Schiff ER, et al. Thymosin $\alpha 1$ treatment of chronic hepatitis B: a multicenter randomized placebo-controlled double blind study. J Viral Hepatitis 1999; 6(5): 397–403.
61. Chien RN, Liaw YF, Chen TC, et al. Efficacy of thymosin $\alpha 1$ in patients with chronic hepatitis B: a randomized, controlled trial. Hepatology 1998; 27: 1383–1387.
62. Couillin I, Pol S, Mancini M, et al. Specific vaccine therapy in chronic hepatitis B: induction of T cell proliferative responses specific for envelope antigens. J Infect Dis 1999; 180: 12–26.
63. Davis HL. DNA vaccines for prophylactic or therapeutic immunization against hepatitis B virus. Mt Sinai J Med 1999; 66: 84–90.
64. Heathcote J, McHutchison, Lee S, et al. Pilot study of the CY-1899 T-cell vaccine in subjects chronically infected with hepatitis B virus. Hepatology 1999; 30: 531–536.
65. Soni PN, Brown D, Saffie R, et al. Biodistribution stability, and antiviral efficacy of liposome-entrapped phosphorothioate antisense oligodeoxynucleotides in ducks for the treatment of chronic duck hepatitis B virus infection. Hepatology 1998; 28: 1402–1410.

8 Treatment of Chronic Hepatitis C Infection

Manal F. Abdelmalek, MD
and Gary L. Davis, MD

CONTENTS
INTRODUCTION
TREATMENT OF CHRONIC HEPATITIS C
PROSPECTS FOR NEW TREATMENT OPTIONS
SUMMARY
REFERENCES

INTRODUCTION

Hepatitis C virus (HCV) infection often causes insidious and progressive liver injury in infected individuals. Acute infection is typically mild and subclinical, yet there is a high rate of chronicity after infection. As many as 55–85% of individuals who contract HCV infection will develop chronic infection and hepatitis. Of these, at least 20% will progress to cirrhosis after a 10–30 yr period, and are at risk to develop hepatocellular carcinoma *(1)*. The estimated worldwide prevalence of chronic HCV infection is over 170 million *(2–4)*, and 2.7–3.9 million are infected in the United States *(5,6)*. Cirrhosis caused by HCV infection is currently the leading indication for liver transplantation in the United States *(7)*.

The high prevalence of infection, progressive nature of the resulting liver disease, and the burden that complications of cirrhosis place on the health care system, justify an aggressive approach to prevention and treatment. Acute infections have been dramatically reduced by limiting risk factors, especially infection among blood donors *(2)*. Other preventive measures, such as immune globulin prophylaxis or vaccines, are not

From: *Clinical Gastroenterology: Diagnosis and Therapeutics*
Edited by: R. S. Koff and G. Y. Wu © Humana Press Inc., Totowa, NJ

currently available. In those patients with chronic infection, goals of treatment may include eradication of the virus, prolonged suppression of viral replication, and reduction of hepatic inflammation. However, the ultimate goal of any treatment of hepatitis C is to prevent the development of cirrhosis because the complications of HCV infection, and its impact on survival, occur almost exclusively in these patients *(8)*.

Treatment regimens have evolved significantly over the past decade. Initially, short courses of type I interferons (IFNs) were shown to decrease alanine aminotransferase (ALT) and HCV levels, and to reduce hepatic inflammation *(9–14)*. However, eradication of virus was unusual, and most patients who did respond during treatment promptly relapsed when the therapy was stopped. Longer courses of IFN were more likely to clear virus, and were also shown to reduce inflammation and fibrosis in patients in whom virus levels were suppressed *(14–18)*. Current treatment regimens that combine IFN with oral ribavirin, a nucleoside analog, are able to eradicate infection in nearly 40% of patients. Although successful treatment of HCV infection is durable and associated with reduction of hepatic inflammation, with long-term reversion of liver biopsies to normal in most cases *(19–22)*, longitudinal studies have not yet enrolled enough subjects, or been continued long enough, to demonstrate improved survival.

This chapter discusses the current approach for treatment of patients with chronic hepatitis C infection. Despite impressive improvements in the efficacy of IFN-based regimens, the majority of treated patients still do not achieve lasting benefit, and therefore the search continues for additional approaches to treatment. This search, of course, requires some understanding of the pathogenesis on HCV-induced liver disease, and how different therapeutic agents may interrupt these mechanisms *(23,24)*. Future options discussed include antiviral agents directed at the replicative and assembly machinery of the virus, cytoprotective agents that either prevent infection or cell injury, anti-inflammatory drugs that block or alter host responses to infection, or antifibrotic agents that inhibit fibrogenesis and remodeling of extracellular matrix.

TREATMENT OF CHRONIC HEPATITIS C

Who to Consider for Treatment

All patients with HCV-induced liver disease should be considered for treatment with IFN and ribavirin. A liver biopsy provides considerable information for patient management, and is highly desirable. Serum liver aminotransferases, symptoms, physical findings, and HCV RNA level do not correlate closely with histologic activity, and cannot be used as surrogates for liver biopsy *(25,26)*. Liver biopsy confirms the cause of liver disease, and documents the degree of inflammation activity and fibrosis. The latter, specifically the presence or absence of cirrhosis, is essential in counseling the patient regarding long-term prognosis, and establishing a management plan to monitor for hepatic decompensation and development of hepatocellular carcinoma. Liver biopsy also provides a sense of the urgency of treatment and an estimation of the likelihood of response to treatment. The National Institutes of Health Consensus Development Conference on Hepatitis C *(27)*, and the more recent European Consensus Conference *(28)*, concluded that the need for treatment in patients with moderate or severe histologic inflammation activity, with or without fibrosis, was essential. Patients with mild inflammation on histology, or those with advanced cirrhosis, need to be considered for treatment on an individual basis, after weighing the clinical factors. However, there is no compelling evidence to exclude these patients altogether, and the good results with recent treatment regimens makes therapy more attractive in these cases.

Other factors that need to be considered include patient's age, estimated prognosis with and without therapy, co-morbid medical illnesses, pre-existing cytopenias, and patient tolerability to potential side effects of therapy. Currently recommendations say that patients with persistently normal serum ALT levels and minimal histologic disease activity should not be treated, since their rate of disease progression is slow and their long-term prognosis is excellent. However, this recommendation may well change as treatment responses continue to improve. On the other hand, the presence of hepatic fibrosis, despite normal ALT values, although unusual, should compel consideration for treatment. Patients with decompensated cirrhosis (specifically, diminished liver synthetic function, encephalopathy, or ascites) do not tolerate treatment well, because of side effects and cytopenia. This group should be considered for liver transplantation. Treatment requires vigilant monitoring, and should only be undertaken by experienced hepatologists or gastroenterologists.

IFN Monotherapy for CHC

Type I IFNs are natural glycoproteins produced by cells in response to viral infections. IFNs can be commercially manufactured by cell culture techniques, or with recombinant technology, and have been commercially available for the treatment of chronic hepatitis for a decade. Although type I IFN include both α and β species, the IFN-αs have been most extensively studied, and are the only agents approved for the treatment of

HCV infection in the United States *(9,10)*. IFNs inhibit the replication of many viruses, including hepatitis viruses, through a variety of mechanisms, including direct antiviral mechanisms (inhibition of virus attachment and uncoating, induction of intracellular proteins and ribonucleases), and by amplification of specific (cytotoxic T-lymphocyte [CTL]) and nonspecific (natural killer cell) immune responses *(29)*. Direct antiviral mechanisms probably account for their effectiveness in HCV infection.

In 1986, Hoofnagle et al. *(11)* showed that short-term, low-dose treatment with recombinant IFN-α2b reduced serum ALT levels and hepatic inflammation in some patients with non-A, non-B hepatitis. These initial observations were subsequently borne out in large, randomized controlled studies using IFN-α monotherapy for 6 mo, at a dose of 3 million units administered subcutaneously 3× weekly (3 MU tiw). Although initial biochemical and virologic responses were seen in 40–50% of patients, the treatment effect was transient, and sustained responses were disappointingly low, generally averaging less than 10% *(12–17)*. Treatment also reduced hepatic inflammation. This effect was most pronounced in sustained treatment responders, but was also seen in other treated patients *(12)*.

Efforts to increase the IFN-α treatment response included use of higher doses or a longer duration of therapy. Most studies with doses higher than 3 MU usually showed little-to-no increase in treatment response, and patients were more likely to require discontinuation of therapy because of side effects *(30)*. Treatment induction with high doses of IFN caused an earlier and more pronounced drop in viral levels, but did not improve sustained response rates (SRRs) *(31)*. Although initial studies *(32)* also seemed to show a lack of benefit with longer courses of treatment, treatment for at least 12 mo clearly reduces relapse, compared to a 6-mo course. A longer course of treatment is particularly beneficial in those patients with viral genotype 1 *(33)*.

There are currently few indications for IFN monotherapy, since the introduction of combination therapy with IFN and ribavirin. Monotherapy is still preferred in patients with anemia, renal insufficiency *(34)*, or sensitivity to ribavirin. IFN should be used with extreme caution, or not at all, in patients with certain pre-existing condition that may significantly worsen with IFN use *(35)*. These include significant cytopenias, severe depression or other psychiatric conditions, severe congestive or ischemic cardiac diseases, poorly controlled diabetes, seizure disorders, inflammation bowel disease, neuropathies, and autoimmune or potentially immune-mediated diseases, such as rheumatoid arthritis or systemic lupus erythematosis. For a more detailed discussion of therapy in patients with immunological disorders, *see* Chapter 10.

Combination Therapy with IFN Plus Ribavirin

Ribarivin is an orally active synthetic guanosine analog that has recently been approved for use in combination with IFN for the treatment of chronic hepatitis C. Ribavirin has in vitro activity against several DNA and RNA viruses, including the flaviviridae such as HCV *(36,37)*. The mechanism of action of HCV infection, particularly the mechanism(s) that account for the increased efficacy of IFN, when it is used in combination, is not clear *(38,39)*. Ribavirin appears to increase the antiviral effects of IFN in the infected cell, since it results in a longer suppression of replication after the dose *(40,41)*. Ribavirin may augment virus-specific CTL, as well as nonspecific immune response, by inhibiting interleukin-4, an inhibitor of CTL activity, while preserving interleukin-2 and IFN-γ activity *(42,43)*. Finally, anecdotal observations of flu-like side effects that were more severe with combination therapy, than with IFN alone, suggests that ribavirin may somehow increase the end-organ effects of IFN itself. This is supported by the observation that ribavirin increases intracellular 2'5'-oligoadenylate synthetase activity in IFN-incubated peripheral blood mononuclear cells *(43)*. Ribavirin has a half-life of 44–49 h, after a single dose, and there is up to a sixfold accumulation with chronic dosing *(34,38)*. Thus, drug elimination can take several weeks, after discontinuation of dosing. Ribavirin elimination is markedly reduced in patients with renal dysfunction; therefore, ribavirin should not be used in patients with creatinine clearances of <50 mL/min *(34)*.

Ribavirin alone is well-tolerated, and decreases serum aminotransferase levels, often into the normal range, but has no effect on HCV RNA levels *(25)*. However, early studies *(44)* showed that combination of ribavirin with a standard IFN regimen significantly reduced relapse, after treatment was stopped. Many studies *(45)* have now confirmed this effect, and have also demonstrated higher end-of-treatment response rates. Thus, in comparison to IFN monotherapy, the combination of IFN and ribavirin results in significantly higher rates of both end-of-treatment and sustained biochemical, virological, and histologic responses. This benefit has now been confirmed *(45–50)*, both in treatment-naïve patients and those who have relapsed after an end-of-treatment response to IFN monotherapy. The benefit of this regimen in nonresponders to IFN monotherapy is controversial, and still unproven.

TREATMENT-NAÏVE PATIENTS

Three small, randomized, controlled trials, conducted in previously untreated patients with CHC, clearly demonstrated that the addition of ribavirin to a standard IFN regimen resulted in significant improvement in the sustained virologic response, from approx 16% (IFN monotherapy) to 42% *(44,46,47)*. Biochemical (serum ALT) and histologic benefit were also seen in those patients who achieved a virologic response. The results of these and other European trials were reviewed by Schalm et al. *(48)*. Among the 60 patients who had not received previous treatment, 40% achieved an end-of-treatment virologic response with combination therapy, compared to only 30% with IFN monotherapy. Sustained virologic response was noted in 30% of patients after combination therapy, compared to only 5% with monotherapy *(48)*.

The encouraging results of these early studies with combination therapy led to two large multicenter trials, one conducted in the United States *(45)*, and the other conducted internationally, primarily in Europe *(33)*. In the U.S. trial, 912 previously untreated patients were randomized 1:1:1:1 to receive either combination therapy (IFN 3 MU 3×/wk subcutaneously with ribavirin [1000 mg for weight <75 kg, or 1200 mg for weight ≥75 kg] in a divided daily dose) or IFN monotherapy plus placebo, for a duration of either 24 or 48 wk. The international trial randomized 840 treatment-naïve subjects, and was similar in design, except there was no 24-wk IFN monotherapy arm. In both studies, subjects were stratified according to HCV genotype (1 or non-1), viral load (above or below 2×10^6 copies/mL), and the presence or absence of cirrhosis. Study end points, for assessing treatment outcome, were similar in the studies, and involved biochemical, virologic, and histologic findings. The combined results of these studies were recently reported *(49)*. Combination therapy enhanced the end-of-treatment response rates and reduced relapse following cessation of therapy, compared to IFN monotherapy. This benefit was observed for virologic and biochemical responses (*see* Table 1 for virologic results). Histologic improvement in inflammation, as measured by the Knodell hepatic activity index score, was also greater in patients receiving combination therapy than in those receiving IFN monotherapy (Table 2). The most impressive histologic improvement was observed in durable virologic responders, regardless of treatment regimen, and this explains the greater mean improvement among recipients of combination therapy.

Several viral and host factors, including viral genotype, HCV RNA level, and the presence of fibrosis, have been associated with the response to IFN-based therapy *(50)*. These factors are also related to the responsiveness to combination therapy (Table 3; *33,45,49*). However, combination therapy is more effective than IFN monotherapy in all groups, irrespective of HCV genotype, viral load, or fibrosis stage. Genotype is the most important factor in determining the response to IFN or combination therapy. Genotypes 2 and 3 respond better than genotype 1. Only 6 mo of combination treatment is required to achieve the optimal response

Table 1
Sustained Response Rate to IFN Monotherapy and Combination Therapy

Treatment group[a]	Duration (wk)	US trial	International trial	Combined
Sustained virologic response rate				
IFN	24	6%	–	6%
IFN	48	13%	19%	16%
IFN + ribavirin	24	31%	35%	33%
IFN + ribavirin	48	38%	43%	40.5%
Sustained biochemical (ALT) response rate				
IFN	24	11%	**	11%
IFN	48	16%	24%	20%
IFN + ribavirin	24	32%	39%	36%
IFN + ribavirin	48	36%	50%	43%

[a] IFN, recombinant IFN-α2b; ALT, alanine aminotransferase.
**This study did not contain a 24-wk monotherapy treatment arm.
Data adapted from refs. 33 and 50.

Table 2
Histologic Response to IFN Monotherapy and Combination Therapy[a]

Histologic HAI[b]	IFN + placebo 24 wk (n = 176)	IFN + placebo 48 wk (n = 158)	IFN + ribavirin 24 wk (n = 179)	IFN + ribavirin 48 wk (n = 157)
% patients improved >2 points	44%	41%	57%	61%
Mean change from baseline (all treated patients)	–0.6	–1.0	–1.8[c]	–2.4[d]
Mean change from baseline (sustained responders)	3.8	–5.2	–4.4	–4.5

[a] Includes results of U.S. trial only.
[b] Includes Knodell I + II + III components.
[c] $p = .005$ for comparison with 48 wk treatment with IFN alone.
[d] $p < .001$ for comparison with 48 wk treatment with IFN alone.
HAI, hepatic activity index; IFN, recombinant interferon α-2b.
Data from ref. 50.

rate for genotype 2 or 3, regardless of HCV RNA level; 12 mo is required for genotype 1, particularly in those with high viral levels or fibrosis. Patients with bridging fibrosis or cirrhosis require 12 mo of therapy, to have the best chance to respond, regardless of genotype.

The optimal treatment for most patients with CHC is the combination of IFN plus ribavirin, and this should be considered the standard of care.

Table 3
Impact of Virologic
and Histologic Factors on Sustained Virologic Response Rates[a]

Variable	IFN + placebo 24 wk (%)	IFN + placebo 48 wk (%)	IFN + ribavirin 24 wk (%)	IFN + ribavirin 48 wk (%)
HCV genotype 1	2	9	17	29
viral load				
>2 × 10^6 copies/mL	0.8	3	10	27
≤2 × 10^6 copies/mL	4	25	32	33
HCV genotype 2 or 3	15	31	66	65
viral load				
>2 × 10^6 copies/mL	11	26	62	60
≤2 × 10^6 copies/mL	25	36	61	64
Fibrosis stage				
3 or 4	5	12	23	36
0 or 1	5	18	36	43

[a]Combined results from both U.S. and international studies.
IFN, recombinant interferon α-2b; HCV, hepatitis C virus.
Adapted from refs. 33 and 50.

This combination increases both the end-of-treatment and sustained virologic responses, compared to IFN monotherapy, and is also associated with normalization of serum ALT and a reduction in hepatic inflammation. Determination of viral genotype, HCV RNA levels, and histologic stage before initiation of treatment are essential for choosing the best duration of therapy in individual patients. Overall, approx 40% of patients achieve a sustained virologic response when given the optimal treatment regimen (49). Sustained responses in these clinical trials is usually defined by an undetectable HCV RNA level, by polymerase chain reaction (PCR), 6 mo after discontinuation of treatment. In support of this definition, several reports (20,21,51,52) have now documented that this is a reliable end point, and late relapses are rare.

Algorithm for Approach
to Previously Untreated (Naïve) Patients

A proposed treatment algorithm is outlined in Fig. 1. Patients who are good candidates for combination therapy should generally be offered treatment, irrespective of liver histology, if there are no contraindications to treatment. Prior to the initiation of IFN and ribavirin therapy, all patients should have viral genotype and HCV RNA level measured. Liver biopsy is highly desirable. Patients should be instructed on self-injection and use of sterile technique. In addition, counseling regarding avoidance of alcohol, and anticipated side effects of therapy, should be discussed. Use of contraception for all patients of child-bearing potential, for the

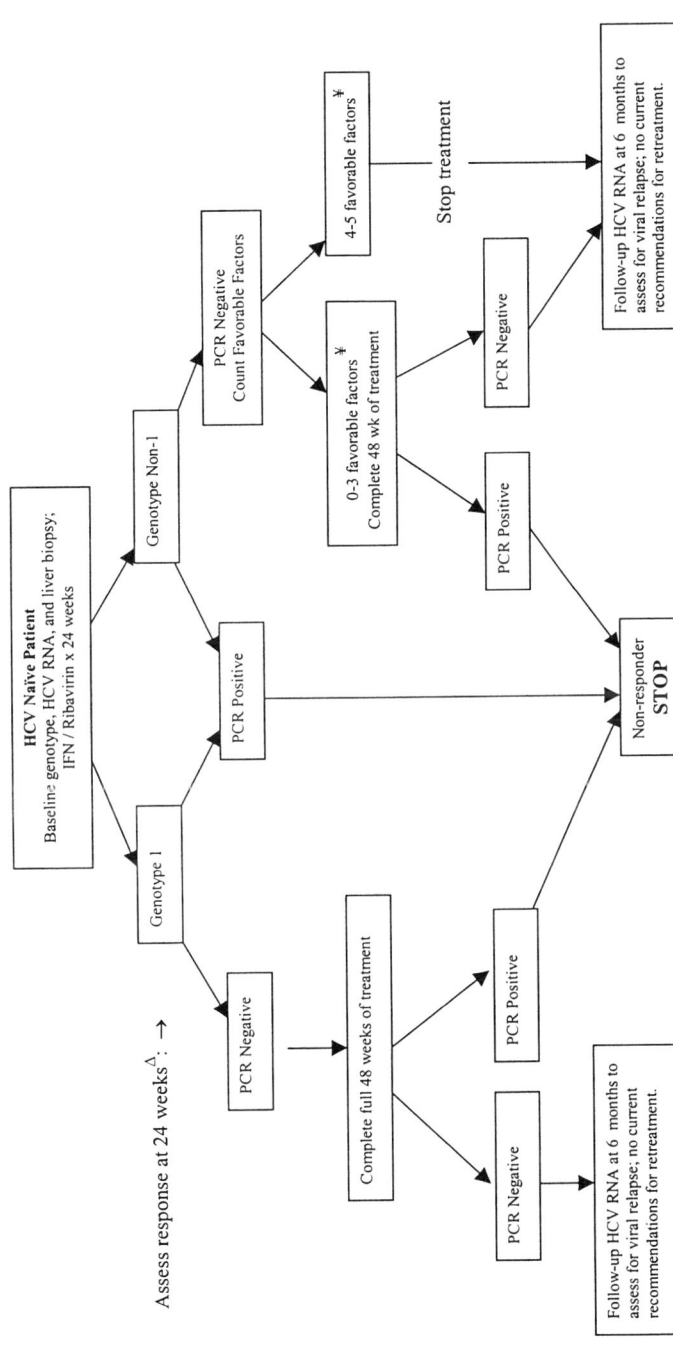

Fig. 1. Algorithm for treatment of naïve HCV infection.

* Viral genotype determination requires the presence of detectable HCV RNA and should be obtained before treatment is begun.
Δ Recent studies suggest that assessment of antiviral response can be made within the first few weeks of treatment (see text).
¥ See reference 54.

duration of therapy and an additional 6 months thereafter, to allow for clearance of tissue stores of ribavirin, should be emphasized. Baseline thyroid function panel, pregnancy test, and clinical assessment of cardiovascular and psychological risk factors are advised.

The simple treatment strategy, suggested by the results of the initial trials with combination therapy, considered only viral genotype. This strategy called for 24 wk in those with genotype 2 or 3, but a full year in others *(27)*. However, a simple algorithm like this, which utilizes only one of the several predictive factors, can lead to suboptimal treatment of some patients. Therefore, the choice of 24 or 48 wk for combination therapy is dependent on genotype, HCV RNA level, and histology (Table 3). Currently, it is recommended that all patients receive at least 24 wk of therapy. Treatment should be stopped if HCV RNA is still detectable by PCR, although some recent data *(53)* suggests that failure to respond can be accurately predicted much earlier in the treatment course. Treatment should also be stopped after 6 mo if the patient had genotype 2 or 3 before treatment, and had no fibrosis on the pretreatment liver biopsy. Therapy should be continued for an additional 24 wk in others, i.e., patients with fibrosis/cirrhosis or genotype 1.

A recent paper *(54)* has suggested that treatment can be further refined and tailored to the individual patient. Such "á la carte" treatment would consider five different factors, including genotype 2 or 3, viral level less than 3.5×10^6 copies/mL, absence of fibrosis, female gender, and age less than 40 yr. The authors proposed that there was a significant response advantage with a total of 48 wk of treatment, in any patient who was HCV RNA negative at 24 wk, and had fewer than four of these favorable factors (74 vs 50%, with only 24 wk of treatment) *(54)*.

Retreatment of IFN Monotherapy Relapsers

End-of-treatment response (normal ALT level and undetectable serum HCV RNA) is achieved in 35–40% of patients treated with the 6-mo course of IFN monotherapy *(12,14)*. However, about 80% of these patients relapse after treatment is discontinued. A longer duration of therapy, lasting 12–24 mo, decreases relapse *(14,16)*. However, overall, only 6–16% of patients treated for 6–12 mo maintain a virologic response; most relapse within 6 mo of stopping treatment *(14,45,55)*. Relapse is more common in patients with fibrosis on liver biopsy, high pretreatment levels of HCV RNA, or genotype 1 *(56–59)*. Relapse after IFN monotherapy remains a major issue in the long-term management of the disease.

Several studies examining the efficacy of retreating IFN relapsers have now been published. Retreatment with the same dose and duration of IFN is rarely effective *(60–63)*. Retreatment with higher doses, or for a longer duration of treatment, may achieve a sustained response in a portion of relapsers *(60)*. One study found that a year of high-dose consensus IFN achieved sustained response in 58%, a rate similar to combination therapy *(64)*. However, these findings were not confirmed in another study *(63)*, which did a head-to-head comparison of treatment with high doses or a standard dose of IFN. A meta-analysis of 549 patients *(65)*, who relapsed following IFN monotherapy, found that sustained virologic response occurred in only 3.4% of those retreated with standard doses, but in 12.8–28.7% of those retreated with higher doses and/or longer period of time. Thus, retreatment with a long course of high-dose IFN monotherapy remains an option in some patients who relapse after IFN, and cannot be retreated with combination therapy.

The first large controlled trial *(44)* of the combination of IFN and ribavirin, in previously untreated patients with CHC, suggested that combination therapy achieved a higher SRR, chiefly by reducing relapse, rather than by increasing the initial response rate. Thus, it was likely that many of the patients who relapsed, after an initial end-of-treatment response to IFN monotherapy, would have a sustained response, if retreated with combination therapy. This has indeed proven to be the case *(48,50,66–68)*. The results of recent randomized controlled trials of combination therapy, in IFN relapsers, have been reviewed elsewhere *(69)*. Taken together, these studies show that retreatment of IFN relapsers with IFN alone, or in combination therapy, results in end-of-treatment response in 47 and 80%, and sustained virologic response in 7 and 48%, respectively. To date, no published, controlled studies have compared high-dose IFN to combination therapy for retreatment of IFN relapsers.

As with treatment-naïve patients, genotype is the most important factor affecting response to retreatment of relapsers with combination therapy. Patients with genotypes 2 or 3 have a sustained virologic response rate of 73%, compared to only 30% of patients with genotype 1 *(50)*. A recent report *(70)* found that retreatment with 12 mo of combination therapy increased sustained response from 24 to 61% in relapsers with genotype 1. The HCV RNA level before retreatment also affects outcome: Only 42% of patients with an HCV RNA level greater than 2 million copies/mL developed sustained virologic response, compared to 67% of those with lower levels *(50)*. The combination of these two factors, HCV genotype and viral load, acted together to increase sustained response. The best SRR rate was in those with HCV genotype 2 or 3 and a low HCV RNA level (100%); the worst rate was in those with geno-type 1 and a high viral level (25%) *(50)*.

Combination of IFN and oral ribavirin is the best current regimen for the retreat-ment of patients who relapse after initially responding to IFN monotherapy. Retreatment with dual therapy offers a striking advantage, compared to IFN monotherapy, resulting in more than a 2–10-fold increase in the SRR. Retreatment with high-dose IFN, especially high-dose consensus IFN, remains an option.

ALGORITHM FOR APPROACH TO RETREATMENT OF IFN RELAPSERS

A proposed treatment algorithm is outlined in Fig. 2. All IFN responders who relapse should be retreated with combination therapy, if possible. Viral genotype should be determined, if it was not performed prior to the initial course of IFN treatment. All patients should be instructed again on self-injection and use of sterile technique. All should be counseled about the need to avoid alcohol. Potential adverse effects of IFN should be reviewed, and the additional possible side effects of ribavirin therapy should be discussed. The need for careful monitoring of hematocrit, during the first weeks of treatment, should be stressed. Finally, the potential teratogenic and embryotoxic effects of ribavirin must be discussed. Use of contraception is essential for all patients (both men and women) of childbearing potential, for the duration of therapy and an additional 6 mo thereafter.

HCV RNA level should be measured by a PCR method after the first 12 wk of treatment. Current data suggest that there is no advantage to continuing treatment in those who remain HCV-RNA-positive. Treatment should continue for an additional 12 wk in patients who have genotype 2 or 3 *(50)*, and for an additional 36 wk (12 mo total) in those with genotype 1 *(70)*. Patients should be monitored for an additional 6 mo after treatment is stopped. If the HCV RNA level remains undetectable by PCR, a sustained and durable response is anticipated *(52)*. There are currently no recommendations for patients who relapse after combination therapy.

RETREATMENT OF PATIENTS WHO FAIL TO RESPOND TO IFN

Patients who do not lose detectable serum HCV RNA or normalize serum liver aminotransferases by the end of treatment, are called nonresponders. Although nonresponders were originally defined on the basis of an abnormal end-of-treatment ALT level, current practice is to define the absence of response by detectable HCV RNA.

Retreatment of IFN monotherapy nonresponders with another course of IFN is effective in some, only if higher doses, longer treatment period, or both, are used *(60,71–73)*. Although some studies *(74)* have implied that changing to another form of IFN may be beneficial, this does not appear to be supported by larger experiences *(60,71,72)*.

Preliminary results from several studies *(48,51,75–77)* have suggested that IFN-α nonresponders may have up to a 20% SRR with combination

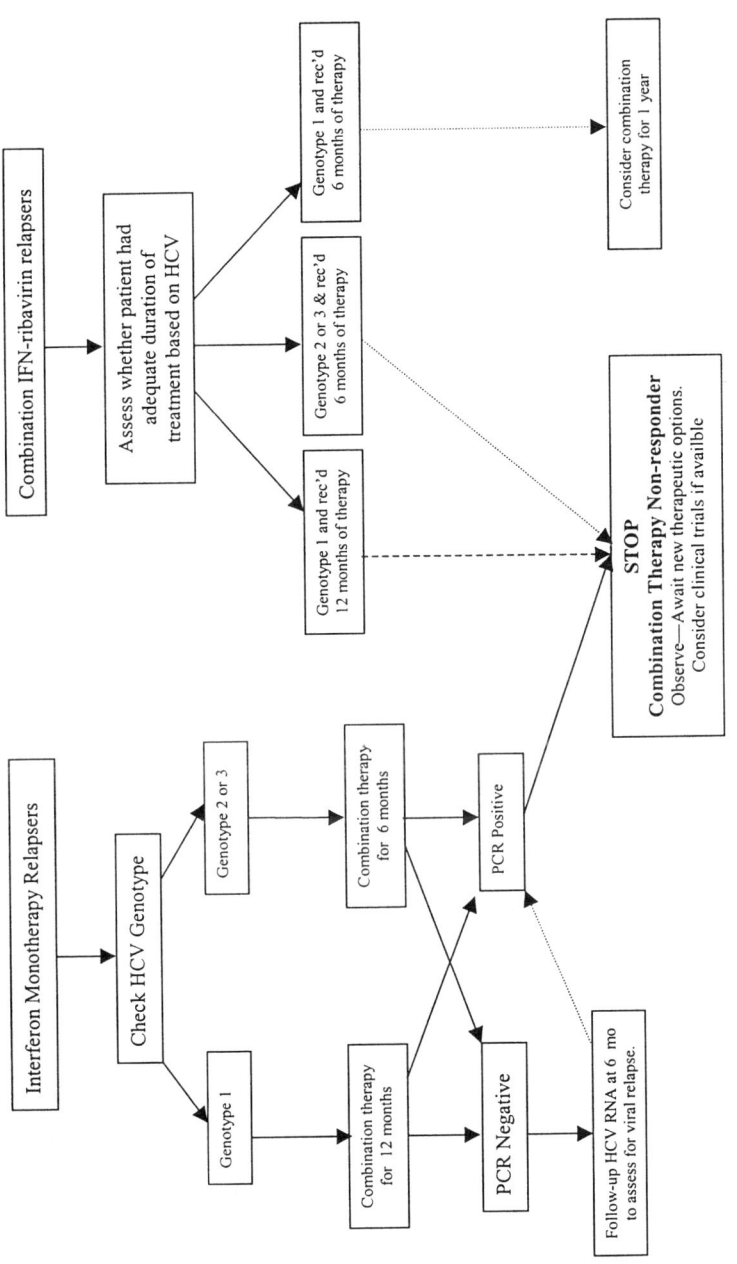

Fig. 2. Algorithm for treatment of HCV relapse.

therapy of IFN plus ribavirin. A recent review found that 36% of IFN nonresponders achieved an end-of-treatment virologic response, but the durability of virologic response appears to be much less, and remains to be clearly established *(78,79)*. In general, sustained virologic response rates have been low, averaging less than 10%, and ranging from 0 to 20%. Furthermore, recent data *(80)* suggest that retreatment of IFN nonresponders with high-dose IFN is far more likely to achieve a sustained response in patients who had a substantial drop in HCV RNA during the initial course of IFN, but did not clear virus.

Overall, retreatment probably offers little long-term benefit in this subgroup of patients, and cannot be generally recommended. Considering the expense of combination therapy, added to that of the previous course(s) of IFN, cost-effectiveness of a treatment strategy targeting all nonresponders must be questioned. It may be more cost-effective to identify subgroups that are more likely to have a sustained response with retreatment. Such subgroups may include those with favorable genotypes for retreatment (genotype 2 or 3) or a partial virologic response to the initial course of treatment. Finally, the recent approval of IFN and ribavirin as initial therapy of CHC has made the issue of retreatment of IFN nonresponders less relevant. There are currently no data on therapy alternatives for nonresponse to combination therapy.

Safety and Tolerance of Combination Therapy

The safety and tolerability of combination therapy have recently been reviewed in detail by Maddrey *(81)*. The safety and tolerance of the combination of IFN and ribavirin is similar to those treated with IFN alone.

Ribavirin predictably causes hemolysis at currently recommended doses. The mean fall in hemoglobin (Hb) is 2–3 gm/dL, and this occurs during the first 4 wk of treatment, remains relatively stable thereafter, and returns to baseline within 4 wk of stopping treatment *(33,45,50)*. Although only about 5% of patients develop Hb levels less than 9.6 gm/dL, rapid and significant drops may occur in a short period of time, and therefore careful monitoring is required during the first few weeks of combination therapy. The fall in Hb is accompanied by a reticulocytosis. Recombinant erythropoietin has been shown to increase Hb levels back to near baseline, despite continuation of treatment, and may be useful in selected patients who become profoundly or symptomatically anemic *(82)*. Decreases in white blood cell and neutrophil are similar to those with the decline with IFN alone. Likewise, platelet counts decline, whether or not ribavirin is added to the regimen, but the decrease is less in those receiving ribavirin, which is probably the result of a relative reactive thrombocytosis resulting from anemia.

Most clinical trials have shown that the addition of ribavirin to the treatment regimen of chronic hepatitis does not increase clinically perceived side effects of treatment *(33,45,50)*. However, many patients complain of more intense flu-like side effects when receiving combination treatment. Discontinuation of treatment is more common in those receiving both drugs than with IFN alone (9 vs 5%). The most common reason for dose reduction or interruption is anemia and resulting fatigue *(33,45,50)*.

Clearly, from the side effect profile of ribavirin, that combination therapy is not indicated for every patient. It should be used with great caution, or not at all, in patients with pre-existing anemia or hemolytic disorders, coronary artery disease, or hypoxia. Careful consideration should be given to the potential effects of an acute anemia in each patient in whom combination treatment is considered. Because of the potential for teratogenic and embryotoxic effects in animals, it should not be used in patients of child-bearing potential, unless adequate contraception is assured. Trial and postmarketing surveillance data suggests that most patients or spouses of patients who become pregnant during or within 6 mo after treatment will spontaneously abort, if the pregnancy is not otherwise terminated, but one fetal anomaly has been observed (Davis, unpublished data).

Issues in Assessing Treatment Response

The development of accurate molecular assays for assessing HCV genotype and level of viremia has resulted in significant progress in the clinical assessment of the treatment responses in patients with HCV infection. HCV RNA testing can be either qualitative (present or not) or quantitative. The former are typically PCR-based methods; the latter are performed with either a PCR-based or signal-amplification method. Qualitative measurement of HCV RNA by PCR confirms active infection. It is a useful diagnostic tool in clinical situations in which the presence of infection requires documentation, e.g., during the early weeks of acute infection, in immunosuppressed patients in whom antibodies to HCV may be undetectable *(83)*, and in the anti-HCV-positive patient with persistently normal ALT values. Documentation of viremia by either method is important prior to consideration of therapy. Quantitative HCV RNA methods are helpful in monitoring the response to treatment. Failure of the HCV RNA level to drop, by at least 2 logs in the first 4–12 wk, reliably predicts a low likelihood of later response to therapy *(84)*. Persistence of HCV viremia by a qualitative test (PCR), after 24 wk of combination therapy, is also associated with a lack of response to further therapy.

The optimal HCV RNA assay should be standardized, reproducible, sensitive to PCR range (<1000 copies/mL), and quantitative throughout a wide dynamic range. Few assays that meet these criteria are currently available. A major clinical problem related to HCV RNA testing is the high variability between different assays, so that results from different laboratories or assays are not comparable. In addition, numerous factors, such as specimen storage conditions, design of amplification primers, variability of biochemical reactions, DNA contamination products, and efficiency of postamplification detection systems, may impact results *(85–88)*.

Quantitative assessment of HCV RNA levels via signal amplification and quantitative PCR are valuable tools in the clinical management of patients before, during, and after IFN therapy. The Roche Monitor assay (Amplicor HCV Monitor, Roche Molecular Systems, Nutley, NJ) is highly sensitive in detecting levels as low as 1000 RNA copies/mL *(89)*, but its dynamic range is narrow, and samples with levels greater than 1 million copies/mL (at least 80% of samples) require dilution, for the result to be considered reliable. The HCV Superquant™ assay (National Genetics Institute, Culver City, CA) has a limit of detection of 100 copies/mL, and is a linear assay, with detection up to 5×10^6 copies/mL. Higher HCV RNA levels can be quantified after sample dilution. There are several "home brew" quantitative PCR methods available in reference lab, but these are usually not standardized, and values by these methods should not be considered to be comparable to the abovementioned methods. The bDNA assay (Bayer Diagnostics, Emeryville, CA) is a signal-amplification technique, rather than a nucleic acid amplification method. It is standardized and highly reproducible throughout a wide dynamic range, but its usefulness has been limited, in some situations, by a lower limit of sensitivity of 2×10^5. A new version of the bDNA assay, with a lower limit of sensitivity of 5000 copies per mL, should be released soon.

Whichever method is chosen, the same assay must be used for each determination in the same patient. Although the Bayer, NGI, and Roche assays give comparable results within the range of 200,000–1 million copies, they are not necessarily comparable outside of this limited range. Other assays should not be considered to be comparable, at this time.

Genetic variation may determine the success of therapy in patients infected with the HCV. Hepatitis C genotypes, specific subtypes of the virus, are distributed differently, depending on geography and etiology. Several screening tests, including the reverse-hybridization line-probe assay (INNOLIPA™ HCV II, Innogenetics, Zwiunaarge, Belgium), restriction fragment-length polymorphism (RFLP) of the PCR amplicons, and nested PCR with sequencing (genotype-specific parameters to the core region) have been developed to identify HCV genotype. The results of all of these methods are comparable. The line-probe assay is a reliable assay applicable to routine typing and subtyping of HCV specimens *(89,90)*. RFLP uses universal primers to amplify a single PCR fragment from a particular region of the HCV genome. Restriction enzyme recognition sites, present in the DNA fragment, show type- or subtype-specific distribution. The electrophoretic separation of the PCR fragments allows for the approximate length of the restricted fragments, thereby identifying the genotype, to be determined. At the present time, the identification of viral genotype is critical for choosing the appropriate duration of antiviral therapy.

PROSPECTS FOR NEW TREATMENT OPTIONS

Current therapy for hepatitis C infection is believed to be based mostly on the ability of IFNs to directly inhibit intracellular HCV replication and prevent infection in uninfected hepatocytes. However, the exact mechanism of action, by which IFN and ribavirin exert their action remains unclear. On average, the currently available therapy regimens for CHC infection appears capable of eradicating HCV in up to 40% of treated patients. However, the majority of patients treated do not achieve an initial response, or never respond to these therapy regimens.

Conjugation of currently available IFNs to polyethylene glycol (PEG), so-called pegylation, decreases clearance, and results in sustained exposure to higher drug levels. This allows 1/wk dosing. Results of the initial trials with PEG-IFN monotherapy have been encouraging, with sustained viral response rates of 36–39% *(91,92)*. The results with PEG-IFN may be nearly as good as with combination therapy, and this treatment may have fewer side effects. Trials of pegylated IFNs plus ribavirin are underway. One could speculate that SRRs of 50% may be achievable.

The current treatments available for HCV are far from ideal, and new cost-effective, safe, and well-tolerated agents are needed. There are several other potential avenues open to the development of new antiviral treatment strategies for HCV infection. Virus could be neutralized outside of the hepatocyte, by neutralizing antibodies *(93)* or receptor inhibition, thereby preventing viral binding, uptake, and uncoating. Intracellular replication of HCV could be blocked in a variety of ways, including inhibition of host or viral enzymes *(94)*, or interruption of replication by anti-sense oligonucleotides or ribozyme peptides *(95)*. Elimination of infected cells could be facilitated by enhancing the host immune response to HCV by passive or adaptive immune transfer *(24)*. Finally, direct inhibition of hepatic inflammation may be accomplished by blocking proinflammatory cytokines, such as tumor necrosis factor or IFN-γ, with agents such as interleukin-10 *(96)*. Anti-fibrotic agents may prove useful in advanced disease, particularly if virus inhibiton could not be achieved.

SUMMARY

The combination of IFN and ribavirin is better first-line treatment, compared to IFN monotherapy, in the treatment of previously untreated (naïve) patients with HCV *(33,50)*. Patients who are good candidates for combination therapy should be offered treatment, irrespective of liver histology, unless there are absolute clinical or lab contraindications. Clinical studies to date suggest that the majority of patients benefit most from 48 wk of treatment *(33,45,54)*. The exception would be the patient with genotype 2 or 3, who has neither fibrosis nor other unfavorable predictive factors *(54)*. For this patient, 24 wk of treatment should prove effective. The treatment strategies outlined in the algorithms in this paper should result in an overall sustained virological response rate of ~40%.

REFERENCES

1. Kiyosawa K, Sodeyama T, Tanaka E, et al. Interrelationship of blood transfusion, non-A, non-B hepatitis and hepatocellular carcinoma: analysis by detection of antibody to hepatitis C virus. Hepatology 1990; 12: 671–675.
2. Alter MJ. Epidemiology of hepatitis C in the West. Semin Liver Dis 1995; 15: 5–14.
3. Alter MJ, Sampliner RE. Hepatitis C and miles to go before we sleep. N Engl J Med 1989; 321: 1538–1540.
4. Kuo G, Choo QL, Alter HJ, et al. Assay for circulating antibodies to a major etiologic virus of human non-A, non-B hepatitis. Science 1989; 244: 362–364.
5. Alter MJ. Epidemiology of hepatitis C. Hepatology 1997; 26(Suppl 1): 62S–65S.
6. Alter MJ, Kruszon-Moran D, Nainan OV, et al. Prevalence of hepatitis C infection in the United States, 1988-1994. N Engl J Med 1999; 341: 556–562.
7. Harper AM, Rosendale JD, McBride MA, et al. UNOS OPTN waiting list and donor registry. Clin Transplant 1998; 73–90.
8. Fattovich G, Giustina G, Degos F, et al. Morbidity and mortality in compensated cirrhosis type C: a retrospective follow-up study of 384 patients. Gastroenterology 1997; 112: 463–472.
9. Davis GL. Recombinant alpha interferon treatment of non-A, non-B (type C) hepatitis: review of studies and recommendations for treatment. J Hepatol 1990; 11(Suppl 1): S72–S75.
10. Davis GL, Hoofnagle JH. Interferon in viral hepatitis: role in pathogenesis and treatment. Hepatology 1986; 6: 1038–1041.
11. Hoofnagle JH, Mullen KD, Jones DB, et al. Treatment of chronic non-A, non-B hepatitis with recombinant human alpha interferon: a preliminary report. N Engl J Med 1986; 315: 1575–1578.
12. Davis GL, Balart LA, Schiff ER, et al. Treatment of chronic hepatitis C with recombinant interferon alfa. A multicenter randomized, controlled trial. N Engl J Med 1989; 321: 1501–1506.
13. Causse X, Godinot H, Chevallier M, et al. Comparison of 1 or 3 MU of interferon alfa-2b and placebo in patients with chronic non-A, non-B hepatitis. Gastroenterology 1991; 101: 497–502.
14. Poynard T, Leroy V, Cohard M, et al. Meta-analysis of interferon randomized trials in the treatment of viral hepatitis C: effects of dose and duration. Hepatology 1996; 24: 778–789.

15. Lin R, Roach E, Zimmerman M, et al. Interferon alfa-2b for chronic hepatitis C: effects of dose increment and duration of treatment on response rates. Results of the first multicentre Australian trial. Australia Hepatitis C Study Group. J Hepatol 1995; 23: 487–496.
16. Poynard T, Bedossa P, Chevallier MA, et al. Comparison of three interferon alfa-2b regimens for the long-term treatment of chronic non-A, non-B hepatitis. N Engl J Med 1995; 322: 1457–1462.
17. Saracco G, Rosina F, Abate ML, et al. Long-term follow-up of patients with chronic hepatitis C treated with different doses of interferon α-2b. Hepatology 1993; 18: 1300–1305.
18. Shiffman ML, Hofmann CM, Thompson EB, et al. Relationship between biochemical, virological, and histological response during interferon treatment of chronic hepatitis C. Hepatology 1997; 26: 780–785.
19. Castilla A. Prieto J, Fausto N. Transforming growth factors beta 1 and alpha in chronic liver disease. Effects of interferon alfa therapy. N Engl J Med 1991; 324: 933–940.
20. Marcellin P, Boyer N, Gervais A, et al. Long-term histologic improvement and loss of detectable intrahepatic HCV RNA in patients with chronic hepatitis C and sustained response to interferon-alpha therapy. Ann Intern Med 1997; 127: 875–881.
21. Reichard O, Glaumann H, Fryden A, et al. Long-term follow-up of chronic hepatitis C patients with sustained virological response to alpha-interferon. J Hepatol 1999; 30: 783–787.
22. Schvarcz R, Glaumann H, Weiland O, et al. Histological outcome in interferon alpha-2b treated patients with chronic posttransfusion non-A, non-B hepatitis. Liver 1991; 11: 30–38.
23. Nelson DR, Lau JYN. Pathogenesis of chronic hepatitis C virus infection. In: *Therapies for Viral Hepatitis* (Schinazi RF, Sommadossi J-P, Thomas HC, eds.), London: International Medical, 1998; 8: 65–76.
24. Davis GL, Nelson DR, Reyes GR. Future options in the management of hepatitis C. Semin Liver Dis 1999; 19(Suppl 1): 103–112.
25. Bodenheimer HC, Lefkowitch J, Lindsay K, et al. Histological and clinical correlation in chronic hepatitis C. Hepatology 1990; 12: 844A.
26. Schoeman MN, Liddle C, Bilous M, et al. Chronic non-A, non-B hepatitis: lack of correlation between biochemical and morphological activity, and effects of immunosuppressive therapy on disease pregression. Aust NZ J Med 1990; 20: 56–62.
27. Ahmed A, Keeffe EB. Treatment strategies for chronic hepatitis C: update since the 1997 National Institutes of Health Consensus Development Conference. J Gastroenerol Hepatol 1999; 14(Suppl): S14–S18.
28. EASL International Consensus Conference on Hepatitis C. Paris, 26–28, February 1999, Consensus Statement. European Association for the Study of the Liver. J Hepatol 1999; 30: 956–961.
29. Peters M, Davis GL, Dooley JS, et al. Interferon system in acute and chronic viral hepatitis. In: *Progress in Liver Diseases* (Popper H, Schaffner F, eds.), Grune and Stratton, New York, NY, 1996; 8: 453–467.
30. Lindsay KL, Davis GL, Schiff ER, et al. Response to higher doses of interferon alfa-2b in patients with chronic hepatitis C: a randomized multicenter trial. Hepatitis Interventional Therapy Group. Hepatology 1996; 24: 1034–1040.
31. Gross JB, Brandhagen DJ, Poterucha JJ, et al. Daily high dose interferon suppresses viremia in patients with chronic hepatitis C without a previous sustained response. Gastroenterology 1998; 114: 1248A.

32. Métreau JM, Calmus Y, Poupon R, et al. Twelve month treatment compared to 6-month treatment does not improve the efficacy of alpha-interferon in NANB chronic active hepatitis. Hepatology 1991; 14: 72A.
33. Poynard T, Marcellin P, Lee SS, et al. Randomized trial of interferon alfa-2b plus ribavirin for 48 weeks or for 24 weeks versus interferon alpha2b plus placebo for 48 weeks for treatment of chronic infection with hepatitis C virus. Lancet 1998; 352: 1426–1432.
34. Glue P. Clinical pharmacology of ribavirin. Semin Liver Dis. 1999; 19(Suppl 1): 17–24
35. Dusheiko G. Side effects of interferon alpha in viral hepatitis C. Hepatology 1997; 26(Suppl 1): 112S–121S.
36. Crumpacker CS. Overview of ribavirin treatment of infection caused by RNA viruses. In: *Clinical Applications of Ribavirin* (Smith RA, Knight V, Smith JAD, eds.), Orlando, Academic, 1984, pp. 33–38.
37. Patterson JL, Fernandez-Larson R. Molecular action of ribavirin. Rev Infect Dis 1990; 12: 1132–1346.
38. Khakoo S, Glue P, Grellier L, et al. Ribavirin and interferon alfa-2b in chronic hepatitis C: assessment of possible pharmacokinetic and pharmacodynamic interactions. Br J Clin Pharmacol 1998; 46: 563–570.
39. Davis GL. Combination therapy with interferon alfa and ribavirin as retreatment of interferon relapse in chronic hepatitis C. Semin Liver Dis 1999; 19(Suppl 1): 49–55.
40. Ning Q, Brown D, Parodo J, et al. Ribavirin inhibits viral induced macrophage production of tumor necrosis factor, interleukin 1, and procoagulant activity and preserves TH1 cytokine production, but inhibits TH2 cytokine response. J Immunol 1998; 160: 3487–3493.
41. Pawlotsky JM, Dahari H, Conrad A, et al. Effect of intermittent interferon (IFN), daily IFN and IFN plus ribavirin induction therapy on hepatitis C virus genotype 1b replication kinetics and clearance. Hepatology 1998; 28: 288A.
42. Ilyin GP, Langouet S, Rissel M, et al. Ribavirin inhibits protein synthesis and cell proliferation induced by mitogenic factors in primary human and rat hepatocytes. Hepatology 1998; 27: 1687–1694.
43. Martin J, Navas S, Quiroga JA, et al. Effects of the ribavirin-interferon alpha combination on cultured peripheral blood mononuclear cells from chronic hepatitis C patients. Cytokine 1998; 10: 635–644.
44. Reichard O, Norkrans G, Fryden A, et al. Randomised, double-blind, placebo-controlled trial of interferon alpha-2b with and without ribavirin for chronic hepatitis C. The Swedish Study Group. Lancet 1998; 352: 83–87.
45. McHutchison JG, Gordon SC, Schiff ER, et al. Interferon alfa-2b alone or in combination with ribavirin as initial treatment for chronic hepatitis C. N Engl J Med 1998; 339: 1485–1492.
46. Lai MY, Kao JH, Yang PM, et al. Long-term efficacy of ribavirin plus interferon alfa in treatment of chronic hepatitis C. Gastroenterology 1996; 111: 1307–1312.
47. Chemello L, Cavalletto L, Bernardinello E, et al. Effect of interferon alfa and ribavirin combination therapy in naive patients wtih chronic hepatitis C. J Hepatol 1995; 23(Suppl 2): 8–12.
48. Schalm SW, Hansen BE, Chemello L, et al. Ribavirin enhances the efficacy but not the adverse effects of interferon in chronic hepatitis C. Meta-analysis of individual patient data from European centers. J Hepatol 1997; 26: 961–966.
49. McHutchison JG, Poynard T. Combination therapy with interferon plus ribavirin for the initial treatment of chronic hepatitis C. Semin Liver Dis 1999; 19(Suppl 1): 57–65.

50. Davis GL, Esteban-Mur R, Rustgi V, et al. Interferon alpha-2b alone or in combination with ribavirin for the treatment of relapse of chronic hepatitis C. N Engl J Med 1998; 339: 1493–1499.
51. Lau DTY, Kleiner DE, Ghany MG, et al. 10-year follow-up after interferon-alpha therapy for chronic hepatitis C. Hepatology 1998; 28: 1121–1127.
52. Davis GL, McHutchison J, Poynard T, Esteban-Mur R, for the International Hepatitis Interventional Therapy Group. Durability of viral response to interferon alone or in combination with oral ribavirin in patients with chronic hepatitis C. Hepatology 1999; 30: 303A.
53. Neumann AU, Dahari H, Conrad A, et al. Early prediction and mechanism of the ribavirin/IFN-α dual therapy effect on chronic hepatitis C virus (HCV) infection. Hepatology 1999; 30: 309A.
54. Poynard T, McHutchinson J, Goodman Z, et al. Is an "á la carte" combination interferonal alfa-2b plus ribavirin regimen possible for the first line treatment in patients with chronic hepatitis C? The ALGOVIRC Project Group. Hepatology 2000; 31: 211–218.
55. Cammà C, Giunta M, Pinzello G, et al. Chronic hepatitis C and interferon alpha: conventional and cumulative meta-analysis of randomized controlled trials. Am J Gastroenterology 1999; 94: 581–595.
56. Davis GL, Lindsay K, Albrecht J, et al. Clinical predictors of response to recombinant alpha interferon treatment in patients with chronic non-A, non-B hepatitis (hepatitis C). The Hepatitis Interventional Therapy Group. J Viral Hepatol 1994; 1: 55–63.
57. Lau JYN, Davis GL, Kniffen J, et al. Significance of serum hepatitis C virus RNA levels in chronic hepatitis. Lancet 1993; 341: 1501–1504.
58. Martinot-Peignoux M, Marcellin P, Pouteau M, et al. Pretreatment serum hepatitis C virus RNA levels and hepatitis C virus genotype are the main and independent prognostic factors of sustained response to interferon alfa therapy in chronic hepatitis C. Hepatology 1995; 22: 1050–1056.
59. Davis GL. Treatment of acute and chronic hepatitis C. Clin Liver Dis 1997; 1: 615–630.
60. Alberti A, Chemello L, Noventa F, et al. Therapy of hepatitis C: retreatment with alpha interferon. Hepatology 1997; 26(Suppl 1): 137S–142S.
61. Picciotti A, Brizzolara R, Campo N, et al. Two year interferon retreatment may induce a sustained response in relapsing patients with chronic hepatitis (abstract). Hepatology 1996; 24: 273A.
62. Le X, Zhou X, Dai X, et al. Evaluation of interferon-2b for the treatment of relapsed hepatitis C. Hepatology 1996; 24: 536.
63. Craxi A, Almasio P, Fuschi P, et al. Should patients with chronic hepatitis C who relapse after interferon be retreated? J Hepatol 1997; 26: 192A.
64. Heathcote EJ, Keeffe EB, Lee SS, et al. Retreatment of chronic hepatitis C with consensus interferon. Hepatology 1998; 27: 1136–1143.
65. Cammà C, Giunta M, Chemello L, et al. Chronic hepatitis C: interferon retreatment of relapsers. A meta-analysis of individual patient data. Hepatology 1999; 30: 801–807.
66. Bellobuono A, Mondazzi L, Tempini S, et al. Ribavirin and interferon-alpha combination therapy vs interferon-alpha alone in the retreatment of chronic hepatitis C: a randomized clinical trial. J Viral Hepatol 1997; 4: 185–191.
67. Brillanti S, Garson J, Foli M, et al. Pilot study of combination therapy with ribavirin plus interferon alfa for interferon alfa-resistant chronic hepatitis C. Gastroenterology 1994; 107: 812–817.

68. Pol S, Couzigou P, Bourliere M, et al. A randomized trial of ribavirin and interferon-alpha vs interferon alpha alone in patients with chronic hepatitis C who were nonresponders to a previous treatment. J Hepatol 1999; 31: 1–7.
69. Davis GL. Combination treatment with interferon alfa and ribavirin as retreatment of interferon relapse in chronic hepatitis C. Clin Liver Dis 1999; 19(Suppl 1): 49–55.
70. Di Marco V, Almasio P, Vaccaro A, et al. Combined treatment of relapse of chronic hepatitis C with high dose α-2B interferon plus ribavirin for 6 or 12 months. Hepatology 1999; 30: 303A.
71. Keeffe EB, Hollinger FB. Therapy of hepatitis C: consensus interferon trials. Hepatology 1997; 26(Suppl 1): 101S–107S.
72. Lindsay KL. Therapy of hepatitis C: overview. Hepatology 1997; 26(Suppl 1): 71S–77S.
73. Bacon BR. Available options for treatment of interferon nonresponders. Am J Med 1999; 107: 67S–70S.
74. Montalto G, Tripi S, Cartabellotta A, et al. Intravenous natural beta-interferon in white patients with chronic hepatitis C who are nonresponders to alpha-interferon. Am J Gastroenterology 1998; 93: 950–953.
75. Schalm SW, Brouwer JT, Chemello L, et al. Interferon-ribavirin combination therapy for chronic hepatitis C. Dig Dis Sci 1996; 41(Suppl 12): 131S–134S.
76. Schalm SW, Brouwer JT. Antiviral therapy of hepatitis C. Scand J Gastroenterol 1997; 223(Suppl): 46–49.
77. Davis GL. Current therapy for chronic hepatitis C. Gastroenterology 2000; 118 (Suppl 1): S104–S114.
78. Brass CA. Efficacy of interferon monotherapy in the treatment of relapsers and nonresponders with chronic hepatitis C infection. Clin Ther 1998; 20: 388–397.
79. Sjogren MH, Holzmuller K, Kadakia S, et al. High response rate to interferon/ribavirin treatment in HCV relapsers but not in non-responders. Hepatology 1998; 28: 287A.
80. Heathcote EJ, James S, Mullen K, et al. Chronic hepatitis C virus patients with breakthroughs during interferon treatment can successfully be retreated with consensus interferon. Hepatology 1999; 30: 562–566.
81. Maddrey WC. Safety of combination interferon alfa-2b/ribavirin therapy in chronic hepatitis C: relapsed and treatment-naïve patients. Semin Liver Dis 1999; 19: 67–75.
82. Weisz CK, Kreiswirth S, McMeeking M, et al. Erythropoietin use for ribavirin/interferon induced anemia in patients with hepatitis (abstract). Hepatology 1998; 28: 288A.
83. Lau JYN, Davis GL, Brunson ME, et al. Hepatitis C in kidney transplant recipients. Hepatology. 1993; 18: 1027–1031.
84. Neumann AU, Conrad A, Pianco S, McHutchison J. Early prediction and mechanism of the ribavirin/IFN dual therapy effect on chronic hepatitis C virus infection. Hepatology 1999; 30: 309A.
85. Bukh J, Purcell R, Miller R. Importance of primer selection for the detection of hepatitis C virus RNA with the polymerase chain reaction assay. Proc Natl Acad Sci USA 1992; 89: 187–191.
86. Busch MP, Wiber JC, Johnson P, et al. Impact of specimen handling and storage on detection of hepatitis C virus RNA. Transfusion 1992; 32: 420–425.
87. Cristiano K, Di Bisceglie A, Hoofnagle J, et al. Hepatitis C RNA in serum of patients with chronic non-A, non-B hepatitis: detection by the polymerase chain reaction using multiple primer sets. Hepatology 1991; 14: 51–55.

88. Wang JT, Wang TH, Sheu JC, et al. Effects of anticoagulants and storage of blood samples on efficacy of the polymerase chain reaction assay for hepatitis C virus. J Clin Microbiol 1992; 30: 750–753.
89. Schiff ER, DeMedina M, Kahn RS. New perspectives in the diagnosis of hepatitis C. Semin Liver Dis 1999; 19(Suppl 1): 3–15.
90. Stuyver L, Rossau R, Maertens G, et al. Line probe assays for the deduction of hepatitis B and C virus genotypes. Antiviral Ther 1996; 124(Suppl 3): 868–876.
91. Shiffman M, Pockros P, Reddy RK, et al. Controlled, randomized, multicenter descending dose phase II trial of pegylated interferon alfa-2A vs standard interferon alfa-2A for treatment of chronic hepatitis C. Gastroenterology 1999; 116: A1275.
92. Heathcote EJ, Shiffman M, Cooksley G, et al. Multinational evaluation of the efficacy and safety of once weekly PEG-interferon α-2A in patients with chronic hepatitis C with compenstaed cirrhosis. Hepatology 1999; 30: 316A.
93. Krawczynski K, Fattom A, Spelbring J, et al. Early termination of HCV infection by passive anti-HCV transfer in experimentally infected chimpanzees. Hepatology 1998; 28: 398A.
94. Dimasi N, Martin F, Volpari C, et al. Characterization of engineered hepatitis C virus NS3 protease inhibitors affinity-selected from human pacreatic secretory trypsin inhibitor and minibody repertoires. J Virol 1997; 71: 7461–7469.
95. Blatt LM, Macejak DG, Lee Pa, et al. Antiviral activity and liver localization of nuclease resistant ribozymes directed against hepatitis C virus RNA. Antiviral Ther 2000; 5(Suppl 1): 50.
96. Nelson DR, Lauwers GY, Lau JY, et al. Interleukin 10 treatment reduces fibrosis in patients with chronic hepatitisi C: a pilot trial in interferon nonresponders. Gastroenterology 2000; 118; 655–660.

9 Treatment of Chronic Viral Hepatitis in Patients with Autoimmune Diseases

Gehad Ghaith, MD
and Stuart C. Gordon, MD

CONTENTS

INTRODUCTION
AUTOIMMUNE MANIFESTATIONS OF VIRAL HEPATITIS
AUTOIMMUNE EFFECTS OF IFN-α
TREATMENT OF CHRONIC VIRAL HEPATITIS IN PATIENTS
  WITH PRE-EXISTING AUTOIMMUNE DISORDERS
CONCLUSION
REFERENCES

INTRODUCTION

There exists an intricate relationship between chronic viral hepatitis, its treatment, and autoimmunity. A vast array of extrahepatic manifestations is associated with hepatitis C *(1)* and, to a lesser extent, hepatitis B *(2)*; many of these conditions are mediated through autoimmune mechanisms. Shortly after the release of interferon α-2b (IFN-α2b) for the treatment of these viral infections came reports of autoimmune disorders that were either caused or unmasked by the use of this agent. Because patients with known autoimmune diseases were routinely excluded from IFN treatment trials, literature regarding the use of this agent in this important patient group is scant. Anecdotal reports and a review of the available literature, however, provide valuable clinical information, and shed light on this intriguing, but poorly documented subject.

From: *Clinical Gastroenterology: Diagnosis and Therapeutics*
Edited by: R. S. Koff and G. Y. Wu © Humana Press Inc., Totowa, NJ

The treatment of chronic viral hepatitis in patients with autoimmune disorders involves an analysis of complex interactions of multiple factors, with many confounding variables. Thus, there exists autoimmune manifestations of viral hepatitis in the absence of IFN therapy; autoimmune adverse effects of IFN itself in the patient with chronic hepatitis C virus without underlying autoimmunity; and the effect of IFN on the patient with viral hepatitis, who also has an underlying autoimmune disease.

AUTOIMMUNE MANIFESTATIONS OF VIRAL HEPATITIS

Chronic viral hepatitis, both type B *(3)* and type C, has been associated with a spectrum of autoimmune phenomena. McMurray and Elbourne *(4)* summarized many of the reported autoimmune complications of HCV hepatitis (Table 1). Some of these HCV-related entities, such as membranous glomerulonephritis (GN) *(5)*, cryoglobulinemia, and associated vasculitis *(6–9)*, tend to improve following successful treatment and viral eradication. Among HBV-associated autoimmune phenomena, the HBV-related proteinuria *(10)* and polyarteritis nodosa *(11–16)* usually improve, following successful IFN antiviral therapy. Nevertheless, the opposite may also occur: Worsening of cryoglobulinemic neuropathy and fatal bleeding secondary to vasculitic gastritis occurred when IFN-α was given to a hepatitis C patient with highly symptomatic cryoglobulinemia *(17)*, in whom steroids had not been tried before IFN. It is not clear whether corticosteroids should be started before, or along with, IFN in the patient with symptomatic cryoglobulinemia. In addition, HCV-associated thyroid disease *(18–20)* and lichen planus *(21–23)* may worsen or flare during IFN therapy. Thus, it would appear that autoimmune complications of chronic viral hepatitis pursue a variable course during IFN therapy, and that clinicians must approach each case individually.

AUTOIMMUNE EFFECTS OF IFN-α

Infections are cytokines with both antiviral and antiproliferative properties. IFN-α increases the expression of human lymphocyte antigen (HLA) class I and II, which results in a magnified activity of both helper and cytotoxic lymphocytes, and subsequent upregulation of the immune system. This, in turn, can lead to the induction of a new autoimmune disease, or to the exacerbation of an existing autoimmune disease. Shortly after IFN-α2b was Food and Drug Administration-approved for the therapy of hepatitis C, came reports that showed a worsening of aminotransferase levels in HCV patients during therapy, with an autoimmune

Table 1
Autoimmune Manifestations of HCV Infection

Serological
   ANA positivity
   Anticardiolipins antibodies
   Antithyroid antibodies
   Antismooth muscles antibodies
   Rheumatic factor
Cryoglobulins-related
   Vasculitis
   Neuropathy
Lymphoproliferative diseases
   Monoclonal gammopathy
   Low-grade lymphoma
Musculoskeletal manifestations
   Polyarthralgia
   RA
   SLE
Glandular manifestations
   Thyroiditis
   Sialoadenitis
   Sjögren's syndrome
Autoimmune liver disease
   Autoimmune hepatitis
Antiphospholipid syndrome and thrombotic disorders
Renal manifestation
   Membranoproliferative GN
   Membranous GN
   Acute proliferative GN

hepatitis-like picture *(24–27)*. Over the past 10 yr, numerous reports have described *de novo* autoimmune conditions that appeared to be hastened by IFN therapy (Table 2). Most of these manifestations appear to improve after the cessation of interferon (IFN).

Okanoue et al. *(28)* studied the IFN-related autoimmune complications of 677 patients with chronic HCV who underwent antiviral therapy. These conditions included autoimmune thyroiditis (18 patients); hemolytic anemia (two patients); rheumatoid arthritis (RA) (two patients); immune-mediated thrombocytopenia (ITP), psoriasis, and systemic lupus erythematosus (SLE)-like syndrome (one patient each). In that retrospective study, the autoimmune complications generally occurred from 12 to 20 wk after starting IFN. After cessation of therapy, most of these entities completely resolved.

Table 2
Autoimmune Effects
of IFN in Chronic Viral Hepatitis Patients

Endocrine
    Thyroid autoantibodies
    Graves' disease
    De novo insulin-dependent diabetes mellitus
Dermatologic
    Alopecia
    Vitiligo
Hematologic
    Hemolytic anemia
    Autoimmune thrombocytopenia
    Factor VIII inhibitors
Rheumatologic
    ANA positivity
    Systemic lupus-like syndrome
    Immune-complex vasculitis
Renal
    Membranous GN
    Nephrotic syndrome
Pulmonary
    De novo sarcoidosis
    Interstitial pneumonitis
Neuromuscular
    Peripheral neuropathy
    Myelopathy
Gastrointestinal and Hepatic
    De novo biliary cirrhosis
    De novo celiac disease
    Ischemic colitis

Data adapted from refs. 76–79.

TREATMENT OF CHRONIC VIRAL HEPATITIS IN PATIENTS WITH PRE-EXISTING AUTOIMMUNE DISORDERS

The role of IFN therapy in patients with chronic viral hepatitis and a pre-existing autoimmune disorder raises separate issues: What is the course of the autoimmune disorders during IFN therapy? What is the virologic response to IFN in such patients? In addition, does the mere presence of circulating autoantibodies define the existence of an autoimmune disorder, and does the presence of such antibodies affect the response to IFN? The following discussion, therefore, focuses on both the role of IFN in the patient with autoantibodies, but without autoimmune disorders, and the effect of IFN in the patient with a well-defined autoimmune disease.

Positive Autoantibodies, but Without Symptoms of Autoimmune Disorders

The presence of serum autoantibodies is essential for the diagnosis of an autoimmune disorder, but no one marker is pathognomonic for a certain autoimmune condition. In addition, many healthy persons carry "silent" autoantibodies, and they remain asymptomatic throughout their lives. These autoantibodies may represent a subclinical autoimmune dysregulation state, which may become manifest when a trigger, such as HCV or IFN, affects the subject. The presence of these autoantibodies ultimately does not compromise the host's immunologic response to pathogens, compared to the general population, and the literature suggests that these individuals have an acceptable response to IFN therapy. Nevertheless, these patients appear to be at a higher risk for the development of autoimmune complications during IFN therapy.

The report by Okanoue et al. *(28)*, which followed 677 patients with chronic hepatitis C virus during therapy, found that autoimmune side effects were more frequent among those individuals who had pre-existing autoantibodies. Of 24 patients with pretreatment antimicrosomal antibodies, for example, four individuals (16%) developed hypothyroidism during therapy, compared to 2/653 (0.32%) without antimicrosomal antibodies, who developed this problem. Likewise, Custro et al. *(29)* found that HCV patients with pretreatment thyroid autoantibodies (antimicrosomal thyroid peroxidase and antithyroglobulin antibodies) were 3× more likely to develop hypothyroidism during therapy than HCV patients who were seronegative. Bell et al. *(30)* studied a group of patients with HCV hepatitis, including 20 patients who had one or more pre-existing autoantibody, and 20 patients without any pre-existing autoantibodies. During treatment with IFN-α, 6/20 patients (30%) with autoantibodies developed new immune-mediated disorders (hypothyroidism in two patients, hyperthyroidism in one patient, arthropathy in one patient, and psoriasis in one patient). In 20 patients without pretreatment autoantibodies, treatment with IFN did not result in any autoimmune complications. These authors concluded that patients with no detectable autoantibodies have a low risk for developing autoimmune complications during treatment of IFN-α, but patients with circulating antibodies are at significant risk for the development of such complications.

Patients with circulating autoantibodies appear to have an adequate viral response to IFN therapy, which is comparable to the response of the general population. Clifford et al. *(31)*, in a retrospective review of 244 patients with HCV hepatitis, compared the viral response of patients who were positive for autoimmune markers (antinuclear antibody [ANA] antismooth muscle antibody, rheumatoid factor, and anti-liver-kidney microsome [LKM] antibodies), and the response of patients who were seronegative. The two groups of patients were similar in age, gender, and severity of disease, and had no significant differences in their response to IFN therapy (as defined by normalization of aminotransferase) during the therapy. Similarly, Bayraktar et al. *(32)* found no significant differences in the response to IFN, as defined by both HCV RNA negativity and normalization of serum alanine aminotransferase levels, between patients who were positive for autoantibodies and those who were not. A report by Van Thiel et al. *(33)* found similar results. In a well-designed prospective study, those investigators used IFN-α to treat chronic hepatitis C virus hepatitis patients with positive autoimmune "dysregulation" markers. The antiviral response rate was not affected by the presence of these autoantibodies. Likewise, Wada et al. *(34)* suggested that the presence of autoimmune markers in HCV patients does not necessarily predict a poor response to IFN-α therapy.

Two studies evaluated the antiviral response among patients with HCV, who were positive for the anti-LKM antibody. Todros et al. *(35)*, from Italy, in 1995, treated 92 HCV patients with IFN-α2b, including 12 patients who were anti-LKM positive. Those investigators found that the virologic response to the therapy, and the side effects, were similar in the two groups. Similarly, Duclos-Vallee et al. *(36)* studied 5 HCV patients who were positive for anti-LKM, and each was treated with IFN-α2b. Side effects and viral response were similar to the autoantibody-seronegative population.

The above studies indicate that HCV patients with underlying anti-LKM autoantibody may be successfully treated with IFN-α2b; in most cases, the virologic response is not affected by the presence of underlying autoantibodies. Should IFN induce a clinical autoimmune syndrome in an asymptomatic carrier of autoantibodies, this phenomenon appears to be reversible after the cessation of IFN. Based on reported experience, asymptomatic patients with autoantibodies should not be excluded from treatment programs.

Antiviral Therapy in Patients with Autoimmune Diseases

INFLAMMATORY BOWEL DISEASE

Available information suggests that an immune mechanism may be involved in the pathogenesis of inflammatory bowel disease (IBD), including ulcerative colitis (UC) and Crohn's disease. This theory is partially based on the observation that the extraintestinal manifestations that may accompany these disorders (i.e., arthritis, pericholangitis) may represent autoimmune phenomena. In addition, it is believed that therapy agents, including glucocorticoids and azathioprine, may exert their effects via immunosuppressive mechanisms. Several reports describe IFN therapy for chronic viral hepatitis in patients with IBD, but the unpredictable course of IBD itself makes it difficult to predict the risks associated with the use of IFN in these patients.

IFN has been evaluated as an immunomodulator to treat IBD in patients who did not have chronic viral hepatitis, with inconclusive results. Summer et al. *(37)*, in a prospective open-label study, treated 28 UC patients, including two with underlying hepatitis B, but none of the 28 patients had hepatitis C: 23 patients (83%) responded well to the therapy, with prompt improvement within 15 d, and these patients were in complete clinical and endoscopic remission after 6 mo. Boerr et al. *(38)* reported conflicting results, however, and found a much lower (10%) response rate, with a 30% rate of colitis exacerbation in response to IFN therapy.

Specifically addressing the issue of IFN treatment in patients with chronic viral hepatitis and underlying UC, Mitoro et al. *(39)* described a 34-yr-old man with UC and chronic hepatitis C virus hepatitis, treated with IFN-α2b. Within 3 wk of the therapy, he developed melena. IFN was stopped, and treatment with sulfasalazine allowed the reinstitution of IFN therapy, with improvement of aminotransferase, and no worsening of UC. Yosumori et al. *(40)* likewise described a patient with HBV hepatitis and UC. Shortly after initiating IFN therapy, he had worsening of both hepatitis and colitis; discontinuation of IFN resulted in clinical improvement. Subsequent administration of sulfasalazine then allowed the patient to receive IFN without flare-up of his colitis, and he finished the course with good response. The course of these two cases suggests that UC may initially worsen during IFN therapy for chronic viral hepatitis, perhaps because of immunomodulation. The disease exacerbation appears to be reversible, however, with temporary discontinuation of IFN and the addition of conventional medical therapy for the underlying colitis, thus allowing IFN therapy to be completed.

Several authors have also described cases of hepatitis and IBD, which had a favorable course during IFN therapy. De Diego et al. *(41)* reported on a 32-yr-old man with UC and hepatitis C, who was treated with IFN-α2b therapy. Before IFN therapy, the patient was experiencing an exacerbation of his UC. Antiviral therapy achieved normalization of the aminotransferases, negativity of HCV RNA by polymerase chain reaction, and complete control of the colitis. Legaz et al. *(42)* also described good virologic response to IFN-α2b in a patient with HBV and UC. With IFN therapy, the patient became hepatitis-seronegative, and the course of the

IBD remained unchanged during treatment and the posttreatment follow-up period.

A retrospective study done by Cottone et al. *(43)* discussed the clinical course of 14 patients with chronic viral hepatitis (2 with hepatitis B, 12 with hepatitis C) and associated IBD. Seven patients with UC and seven patients with Crohn's disease received IFN as treatment for chronic viral hepatitis. During IFN therapy, 11/14 patients had no change in their disease activity; one patient experienced mild relapse during the treatment with IFN; one patient, with active ileal Crohn's disease, experienced marked improvement in his disease during the treatment; and another patient with similar disease before treatment had no modification of his clinical course.

Therefore, the literature regarding the antiviral therapy of chronic viral hepatitis patients with underlying IBD is conflicting. A careful examination of such cases should be undertaken when considering IFN therapy for patients with IBD. Although worsening of IBD may occur, appropriate modification in the treatment of IBD may allow successful completion of antiviral therapy.

PRIMARY BILIARY CIRRHOSIS

An interesting body of literature discusses the interaction of primary biliary cirrhosis (PBC) and hepatitis C. Treatment of HCV with IFN-α2b was reported, by D'Amico et al. *(44)*, to induce *de novo* PBC. Those investigators treated a 55-yr-old woman, who was HCV-positive and antimitochondrial antibody (AMA)-negative. A pretreatment liver biopsy was compatible with chronic hepatitis, and there were no features of PBC. The patient responded to the treatment, but, after cessation, cholestasis developed, along with positive AMA (titer, 1:256), and a liver biopsy showed features of both PBC and chronic hepatitis.

Garrido et al. *(45)* investigated the role of pretreatment AMAs in patients with HCV hepatitis. These investigators used IFN to treat three women (age range, 21–51 yr), who were both HCV-RNA-positive and AMA-positive. Two of these three women experienced a marked rise in serum alkaline phosphatase during therapy. Gimbert et al. *(46)* also studied the presence and the significance of AMA positivity among HCV patients. Those investigators used IFN to treat seven patients who were AMA-positive. None of the seven patients had clinical or histologic evidence of PBC, and all seven patients received IFN without any worsening of their liver disease. The authors of that report suggested that the presence of AMA positivity might only be an immunologic reaction to the presence of HCV, and not a marker of PBC in these patients. One patient who cleared HCV virus, in that study, also became negative for AMA during IFN therapy. In another report, by Madea et al. *(47)*, one patient, with biopsy-proven PBC, received IFN-α for HCV hepatitis. Significant worsening of cholestasis occurred during IFN treatment.

These reports generate conflicting data regarding IFN treatment in the presence of positive mitochondrial antibodies in patients with hepatitis C. Although additional data are needed, preliminary literature suggests that incidental mitochondrial antibody positivity may be seen in patients with hepatitis C, and that patients with more classic PBC may experience disease exacerbation in response to IFN.

Psoriasis

Psoriasis is a chronic inflammatory skin disorder characterized by erythematous papules and plaques, covered by silvery scale, as well as by hyperactivity of certain populations of T-helper1 cells, which are directly activated by IFN-α. Wolfer et al. *(48)* described three of their own patients and 17 other cases selected from the literature, in which psoriasis was induced or made worse after IFN therapy for chronic viral hepatitis B and hepatitis C, and other indications, such as renal cell carcinoma, malignant melanoma, and hairy cell leukemia. A number of carefully documented cases *(49–51)* have convincingly shown that underlying psoriasis is clearly exacerbated when IFN is used for the treatment of hepatitis C. In one case report by Lombardini et al. *(51)*, IFN therapy for HCV in a psoriasis patient led to worsening of skin lesions, oligoarthritis and sacroiliitis. These case reports also note that disease exacerbations improve following the discontinuation of IFN. Thus, psoriasis is among the few AIDs that were consistently made worse with IFN therapy. Risk vs benefit discussion must be carefully weighed, before deciding to commence antiviral treatment in individuals with underlying psoriasis.

Immune Thrombocytopenia

ITP is a form of thrombocytopenia in which there is peripheral destruction of platelets via an immune-complex mechanism. Prednisone therapy is beneficial. Although many reports illustrated the thrombocytopenic effect of IFN-α *(52)*, the course of pretreatment thrombocytopenia has been described in some anecdotal reports. Bacq et al. *(53)* reported a 40-yr-old woman with chronic hepatitis C virus hepatitis and stable ITP, who developed profound thrombocytopenia during IFN therapy, which prompted the discontinuation of IFN and the use of oral corticosteroid. However, lower doses of IFN-α may be better-tolerated, with less thrombocytopenic effect *(54)*. Tappero et al. *(55)* tried IFN-β as an alternative for IFN-α, for the treatment of a patient with chronic hepatitis C virus, who had developed severe thrombocytopenia following IFN-α2b therapy.

The patient's platelet count remained above 140,000/mL during treatment, but there was no sustained viral response.

IFN, known to cause thrombocytopenia, even in the absence of ITP, may exacerbate a pre-existing ITP. Although overt ITP is clearly a contraindication for IFN therapy, HCV patients, with history of latent and stable ITP, may also be at higher risk for profound thrombocytopenia on IFN, and should be monitored closely.

Myasthenia Gravis

Myasthenia gravis (MG) is a neuromuscular disorder characterized by weakness and fatigability of skeletal muscles. An autoimmune response, mediated by specific antiacetylcholine receptor antibodies, is believed to be responsible for the underlying pathophysiology of the disease. Immunosuppressive agents, such as prednisone, azathioprine, and cyclosporine are highly effective in the treatment of MG.

Multiple case reports have demonstrated significant neuromuscular deterioration in MG patients with chronic viral hepatitis, when given IFN. Gurtubay et al. *(56)* described a case of MG that presumably developed *de novo* after the start of IFN therapy for HCV. Konishi et al. *(57)* described the case of a patient with HCV and MG, who received IFN for HCV treatment. Before therapy, his disease had been stable for many years, and he had only mild ocular symptoms. Three mo after starting IFN, however, he developed generalized weakness, dysarthria, and dysphagia. IFN was stopped at that point, but his condition became worse, and he required artificial ventilation for 2 wk. Harada et al. *(58)* also describe a case of MG that was made worse by IFN therapy, albeit IFN-β, rather than IFN-α. These anecdotal cases, therefore, repeatedly show that a significant morbidity occurs when IFN is given to chronic viral hepatitis patients with either clinical or subclinical evidence of MG.

An interesting perspective on the subject of HCV and MG was provided by Shenoy et al. *(59)*, who showed that IFN-α was beneficial in suppressing the development of experimental MG in mice. Bolay et al. *(60)* applied these results in human studies, and treated seven MG patients (but no underlying viral hepatitis) with IFN-α. Those investigators showed that the underlying neuromuscular status actually improved in four patients, remained unchanged in two patients, and worsened in only one individual. Those authors concluded that IFN, when given to patients with HCV, may have different immunological mechanisms as they relate to the underlying MG; they also speculated that the immunologic effects of HCV infection were perhaps more important than IFN itself in inducing or worsening MG.

IFN therapy when given in the standard dose needed for chronic viral hepatitis, therefore, appears to be unsafe in the patient with MG.

Although screening for this rare disease with antiacetylcholine antibodies is not cost-effective, a history of diplopia and dysphagia should be further investigated before starting IFN therapy.

MULTIPLE SCLEROSIS

Multiple sclerosis (MS) is a disease characterized by recurrent attacks of focal or multifocal neurologic dysfunction that results from demyelinating lesions in the central nervous system. Autoimmune factors play a role in the pathogenesis of MS, and T-lymphocytes sensitized to specific myelin antigen may be responsible for the attack on the myelin. Glucocorticosteroids are widely used in the treatments of the flare-ups, and some immunosuppressive agents have been used, with variable results.

There is only one report *(69)* that described severe neurologic complications resulting from IFN, when given to a chronic viral hepatitis patient with underlying MS. This 38-yr-man was affected by MS, which was stable for 5 yr. He was given IFN to treat "non-A, non-B" hepatitis. A few hours after the injection of the first IFN dose, he developed high fever, hypertonia, and severe impairment of the sensory and motor functions of his four extremities. Based on this one case report, therefore, it seems reasonable to suspect that IFN should be avoided in MS patients until further data are available. The biologic effects of IFNs are not fully understood, and, although it is believed that both IFN-α and -β increase the expression of major histocompatability complex class II, with upregulation of the immune system, there are still unclear differences in their functions. These poorly understood differences may explain why IFN-β is actually useful in treating MS *(70)*, but IFN-α was reported to exacerbate the same disease.

SARCOIDOSIS

Sarcoidosis is a multisystem disorder that is characterized by an accumulation of T-lymphocytes and mononuclear phagocytes, forming noncaseating granulomas. The disease is associated with exaggerated helper T-lymphocyte immune response, and oral glucocorticosteroids are the treatment of choice. Worsening or unmasking of sarcoidosis during IFN therapy has been reported frequently, but there are also anecdotal reports that sarcoidosis actually improves when IFN is given for the treatment of chronic viral hepatitis.

In a report by Hoffman et al. *(61)*, three patients with HCV received IFN-α2b, two of them in combination with ribavirin. None of these patients had clinical evidence of sarcoidosis before the IFN therapy, but, at treatment wk 12, 20, and 21, respectively, each showed symptoms of pulmonary sarcoidosis. IFN was stopped, and spontaneous remission was observed in all three cases. Similarly, Teragawa et al. *(62)* described a previously healthy 62-yr-old woman, who developed complete atrioventricular block and noncaseating pulmonary granulomas, 24 wk into IFN therapy for HCV.

Among patients with a previous history of sarcoidosis, Nakajima et al. *(63)* reported the case of a 67-yr-old man, whose disease had been in remission for 15 yr. He received IFN-α2b for the treatment of chronic hepatitis C virus hepatitis, and 5 mo into the treatment, he developed bilateral swelling of the parotid glands, and bilateral diffuse reticulonodular pulmonary parenchymal opacities on chest X-ray. IFN therapy was discontinued, and oral prednisone was started. Clinical, radiologic, and biochemical status resolved after the administration of oral prednisone.

Only one case of sarcoidosis was reported to improve with IFN therapy. Lures et al. *(64)* described a 35-yr-old patient with chronic hepatitis B virus hepatitis and a 6-yr history of documented sarcoidosis, who received treatment with IFN. The treatment resulted in not only a complete virologic response, but also a complete clinical and radiographic response of his sarcoidosis.

Thus, these anecdotal case reports do not provide an answer regarding the role of IFN in the presence of sarcoidosis. Whether patients with underlying HBV may pursue a different course than those with HCV is also unclear. Although instances of flare have been reported following IFN therapy, so too has a case of sarcoidosis remission.

Addison's Disease

Addison's disease is a form of primary adrenocortical deficiency that is characterized by skin and mucosal membrane pigmentation, weight loss, nausea and vomiting, and weight loss. The disorder results from the destruction of the adrenal cortex, with autoimmune-mediated idiopathic atrophy being responsible for most cases of the disease.

Because of the autoimmune nature of this disease, one might anticipate some modification of its course when IFN therapy is given. A case report by Oshimoto et al. *(65)* described a 47-yr-old man with Addison's and HCV hepatitis, who developed somnolence, fatigue, and significant hyponatremia 4 wk into the IFN therapy. This one case, therefore, suggests that Addison's patients are at risk of adrenal decompensation when IFN-α is given.

Asthma

Asthma is a disease of the airways, in which there is increased responsiveness of the tracheobronchial tree to a multiplicity of stimuli, including allergens and medications. Autoimmune mechanisms may play a role in the pathogenesis of asthma, given the fact that steroids are used to treat refractory cases of asthma, and recently immunosuppressive agents, including methotrexate, were used in the treatment of asthma.

Bini and Weinshel *(66)* described two patients with mild asthma, in whom treatment with IFN-α for CHC resulted in exacerbation of the underlying asthma. The severe asthmatic symptoms resolved promptly after IFN was discontinued and corticosteroid therapy was initiated. A repeat attempt at treatment with IFN-α several months later resulted in a rapid, more severe exacerbation of asthma in both patients. This report suggests that allergic asthma may be a relative contraindication for IFN therapy.

ATOPIC DERMATITIS

Atopic dermatitis (AD) is a type of dermatitis that occurs in patients who have an atopic state. The majority of these patients have a family history of asthma, hay fever, or dermatitis. An autoimmune mechanism may play a role in the pathogenesis of the disease, and glucocorticosteroids are used in refractory cases. The effect of IFN on this disease may vary, depending on the age of the patient. Mackie et al. *(67)* reported a beneficial effect of IFN-α when used for the treatment of AD in children, but not adults. Based on this observation, Kimata et al. *(68)* suggested that AD is not a contraindication for the use of IFN for treating chronic viral hepatitis and other conditions, in children who have underlying AD. They studied five children who had both AD and another disease potentially treatable with IFN-α: one child with chronic myelogenous leukemia, two children with hepatitis B, and two children with HCV. All four children with viral hepatitis achieved viral clearance, and there was no worsening of their AD. Although it appears that IFN-α may be safely used for the treatment of chronic viral hepatitis in children with AD, data are lacking regarding the role of IFN therapy in adults with the same condition.

RHEUMATOLOGIC DISEASES: SLE, RA, AND OTHERS

The rheumatologic diseases are the most common forms of autoimmune disorders. In addition, the estimated prevalence of RA in the U.S. population is 1%. Unfortunately, the literature does not provide useful data to evaluate the role of IFN therapy in viral hepatitis patients who are affected by these rheumatologic diseases. It is known that the onset of *de novo* rheumatologic diseases, or their unmasking, may complicate IFN therapy in HCV patients. These observations, therefore, lead to reluctance among clinicians to treat chronic viral hepatitis patients who have overt rheumatologic diseases. Reports of HCV patients with rheumatologic diseases in general, and RA in particular, who were treated with IFN, are limited. Anecdotal cases from the author's clinical practice, and those of other hepatologists, suggest that underlying RA is not worsened by the use of IFN-α for the treatment of hepatitis C (J. McHutchison, K. Sherman, personal communications).

Kimura et al. *(71)* reported a 34-yr-old woman with both HCV and inactive SLE, who was given IFN-α to treat HCV hepatitis. She subsequently developed pancytopenia, and required platelet transfusions and oral prednisone. Likewise, Kurihara et al. *(72)* described a patient with both chronic hepatitis C virus hepatitis and RA, who received IFN-β, with good viral response and no worsening of his rheumatologic complaints. Again, the poorly understood differences in the biologic effects between IFN-α and IFN-β may account for these different outcomes. IFN-β was studied by Tak et al. *(73)* as an option for treating RA, not necessarily associated with chronic viral hepatitis, and found a moderate improvement in 20% of these patients. The treatment of viral hepatitis co-existing with other rheumatologic diseases, such as polymyositis, scleroderma, spondyloarthritis, polymyalgia rheumatica, and giant-cell arteritis, has not been well-described in the literature.

CONCLUSION

The widespread use of IFN-α for the treatment of chronic viral hepatitis has created a poorly understood interrelationship between hepatitis and autoimmunity and autoimmune disorders. This relationship is complex, and involves several co-factors and confounding variables. The autoimmune adverse effects of IFN itself appear to be transient and reversible, and the patient with asymptomatic autoantibodies may experience an unmasking of autoimmune disease while on IFN therapy. Nevertheless, viral eradication may be achieved, and risk–benefit considerations must be evaluated. The presence of an underlying autoimmune disease among chronic viral hepatitis patients is particularly problematic, and the literature suggests that patients with MG, Addison's disease, MS, ITP, allergic asthma, psoriasis, or sarcoidosis may experience disease worsening on IFN therapy (*see* Table 3). Individuals with IBD may experience transient flares on IFN, but its presence is not an absolute contraindication for therapy.

Literature on rheumatologic diseases is, unfortunately, limited. In the United States, there are an estimated 2.1 million patients with RA *(74)*, and even more with other RDs. An estimated 3 million Americans are infected with hepatitis C *(75)*. It is not unusual, therefore, for autoimmune disorders to co-exist with chronic viral hepatitis, and the treatment of such patients is a major health problem. Newer antiviral agents are awaited, and clinicians are encouraged to share their clinical experiences, and to report anecdotal accounts; such reporting should lead to better insight into this arena, and improved patient care.

Table 3
IFN-α in Patients with Underlying Autoimmune Disorders

Autoimmune	Treatment with IFN-α	Comments
Autoantibodies without autoimmune disease	Safe	An autoimmune disease may be unmasked by IFN, but it is reversible when IFN-α2b is stopped (30). Response to IFN-α2b is same as autoantibody seronegative (31–34). HCV patients with anti-LKM antibody have good response to IFN-α2b, without worsening of hepatitis (35–36).
Inflammatory bowel disease (IBD)	Generally safe (41–43), but worsening of IBD has been reported (39,40).	If worsening occurs, hold IFN, adjust IBD treatment, and restart antiviral therapy (39,40).
Primary biliary cirrhosis (PBC)	Possible disease-worsening	Biopsy-proven PBC may worsen with IFN-α2b (47). Role of IFN in patients with positive AMA, but without cholestasis or biopsy-proven PBC is not clear, but probably safe (45,46).
Psoriasis	Possible disease-worsening	Most reports document severe exacerbation of psoriasis with IFN-α2b (48–51).
Lichen planus	Possible disease-worsening (21–23)	
Idiopathic autoimmune thrombocytopenia (ITP)	Contraindicated	IFN-β (55), or a lower dose of IFN-α (54), may be better-tolerated.

(continued)

Myasthenia gravis (MG)	Contraindicated	Severe and prolonged myasthenic attacks were induced by IFN-α (57) or IFN-β2b (58), when given to HCV patients. Lower-dose IFN-α2b therapy was used safely in MG patients with no viral hepatitis (60).
Sarcoidosis	Possible disease-worsening	Features of sarcoidosis that emerge *de novo* during IFN therapy are reversed when IFN-α2b is stopped (61). One case of heart block (62). One patient with sarcoidosis was treated with IFN-α2b for chronic HBV, and symptoms of sarcoidosis improved (64).
Addison's disease	Possible disease-worsening (65)	
Allergic asthma	Possible disease-worsening	Asthmatic attacks were induced shortly after IFN-α2b administration (66).
Atopic dermatitis	Relatively safe in children (68)	Data limited in adults.
Multiple sclerosis (MS)	Contraindicated	Severe exacerbation of MS was observed hours after IFN-α2b administration (69).
Rheumatoid arthritis (RA)	Probably safe (72)	Data limited.
Systemic lupus erythematosus (SLE)	Insufficient data	One case of HCV and lupus, treated with IFN-α, resulted in severe pancytopenia (71). Patients with ANA, but without evidence of systemic lupus, were safely treated with IFN-α2b for chronic hepatitis C virus (26–28).

REFERENCES

1. Gordon SC. Extrahepatic manifestations of hepatitis C. Dig Dis 1996; 14: 157–168.
2. Hartman H. Extra hepatic manifestations of HBV and HCV infection. Schweiz Rundsch Med Prax 1997; 86: 1163–1166.
3. Zurn A, Schmied E, Saurat JH. Cutaneous manifestations of infection due to hepatitis B virus. Schweiz Rundsch Med Prax 1990; 79: 1254–1257.
4. McMurray RW, Elbourne K. Hepatitis C virus infection and autoimmunity. Semin Arthritis Rheum 1997; 26: 689–701.
5. Jefferson J, Johnson R. Treatment of hepatitis C-associated glomerular disease. Semin Nephrol 2000; 20: 286–292.
6. Adinolfi LE, Utili R, Zampino R, et al. Effects of long-term course of alpha-interferon in patients with chronic hepatitis C associated to mixed cryoglobulinemia. Eur J Gastroenterol Hepatol 1997; 9: 1067–1072.
7. Calleja JL, Albillos A, Moreno-Otero R, et al. Sustained response to interferon-alpha or interferon-alpha plus ribavirin in hepatitis C virus-associated symptomatic mixed cryoglobulinemia. Aliment Pharmacol Ther 1999; 13: 1179–1186.
8. Polzien F, Schott P, Mihm S, et al. Interferon-alpha treatment of hepatitis C virus-associated mixed cryoglobulinemia. J Hepatol 1997; 27: 63–71.
9. Sepp NT, Umlauft F, Illersperger B, et al. Necrotizing vasculitis associated with hepatitis C virus infection: successful treatment of vasculitis with interferon-alpha despite persistence of mixed cryoglobulinemia. Dermatology 1995; 191: 43–45.
10. Shapiro RJ, Steinbrecher UP, Magil A. Remission of nephrotic syndrome of HBV-associated membranous glomerulopathy following treatment with interferon. Am J Nephrol 1995; 15: 343–347.
11. Avsar E, Savas B, Tozun N, et al. Successful treatment of polyarteritis nodosa related to hepatitis B virus with interferon alpha as first-line therapy. J Hepatol 1998; 28: 525–526.
12. Simsek H, Telatar H. Successful treatment of hepatitis B virus-associated polyarteritis nodosa by interferon alpha alone. J Clin Gastroenterol 1995; 20: 263–265.
13. Wicki J, Olivieri J, Pizzolato G, et al. Successful treatment of polyarteritis nodosa related to hepatitis B virus with a combination of lamivudine and interferon alpha. Rheumatology 1999; 38: 183–185.
14. Kruger M, Boker KH, Zeidler H, et al. Treatment of hepatitis B-related polyarteritis nodosa with famciclovir and interferon alfa-2b. J Hepatol 1997; 26: 935–939.
15. Guillevin L, Deblois P, Trepo C. Treatment of polyarteritis nodosa related to hepatitis B virus with interferon alpha and plasma exchanges. Ann Rheum Dis 1994; 53: 334–337.
16. Molloy PJ, Friedlander L, Van thiel DH, et al. Combined interferon, famciclovir and GM-csf treatment of HBV infection in an individual with periarteritis nodosa. Hepatogastroenterology 1999; 46: 2529–2531.
17. Frieman G, Metha S, Sherker AH. Fatal exacerbation of hepatitis C-related cryoglobulinemia with interferon-alpha therapy. Dig Dis Sci 1999; 44: 1364–1365.
18. Deutsh M, Dourakis S, Manesis EK, et al. Thyroid abnormalities in chronic viral hepatitis and their relationship to interferon therapy. Hepatology 1997; 26: 206–210.
19. Benelhadj S, Marcellin P, Castelnau, et al. Incidence of hypothyroidism during interferon therapy in chronic hepatitis C. Horm Res 1997; 48: 209–214.
20. Mmenomori M, Mori T, Fukuda Y, et al. Incidence and characteristics of thyroid dysfunction following interferon therapy in patients with chronic hepatitis C. Intern Med 1998; 37: 246–252.

21. Areias J, Velho GC, Cerqueira R, et al. Lichen planus and chronic hepatitis C: exacerbation of the lichen under interferon-alpha-2a therapy. Eur J Gastroenterol Hepatol 1996; 8: 825–828.
22. Protzer U, Ochsendorf FR, Leopolder-Ochsendorf A, et al. Exacerbation of lichen planus during interferon alfa-2b therapy for chronic active hepatitis C. Gastroenterology 1993; 104: 903–905.
23. Rongioletti F, Rebora A. Worsening of lichen myxedematosus during interferon alfa-2a therapy for chronic active hepatitis C. J Am Acad Dermatol 1998; 38: 760–761.
24. Ohta M, Ishii Y, Takami S, et al. Case of autoimmune hepatitis developed by the treatment with interferon. Nippon Shokakibyo Gakkai Zasshi 1991; 88: 209–212.
25. Tran A, Beusnel C, Montoya ML, et al. Autoimmune hepatitis type 1 revealed during treatment with interferon. Gastroenterol Clin Biol 1992; 16: 722–723.
26. Shindo M, Di Bisceglie AM, Hoofnagle JH. Acute exacerbation of liver disease during interferon alfa therapy for chronic hepatitis C. Gastroenterology 1992; 102: 1406–1408.
27. Garcia-Buey L, Garcia-Monzon C, Rodriguez S, et al. Latent autoimmune hepatitis triggered during interferon therapy in patients with chronic hepatitis C. Gastroenterology 1995; 8: 1770–1777.
28. Okanoue T, Shakamoto S, Itoh Y, et al. Side effects of high-dose interferon therapy for chornic hepatitis C. J Hepatol 1996; 25: 283–291.
29. Custro N, Montalto G, Scafidi V, et al. Prospective study on thyroid autoimmunity and dysfunction related to chronic hepatitis C and interferon therapy. J Endocrinol Invest 1997; 20: 374–380.
30. Bell TM, Bansal AS, Shorthouse C, et al. Low-titre auto-antibodies predict autoimmune disease during interferon-α treatment of chronic hepatitis C. J Gastroenterol Hepatol 1999; 14: 419–422.
31. Clifford BD, Donahue D, Smith L, et al. High prevalence of serological markers of autoimmunity in patients with chronic hepatitis C. Hepatology 1995; 21: 613–619.
32. Bayraktar Y, Bayraktar M, Gurakar A, et al. Comparison of the prevalence of autoantibodies in individuals with chronic hepatitis C and those with autoimmune hepatitis: the role of interferon in the development of autoimmune diseases. Hepatogastroenterology 1997; 44: 417–425.
33. Van Thiel DH, Molloy PJ, Friedlander L, et al. Interferon alpha treatment of chronic hepatitis C in patients with evidence for co-existent autoimmune dysregulation. Hepatogastroenterology 1995; 42: 900–906.
34. Wada M, Kang KB, Kinugasa A, et al. Does the presence of serum autoantibodies influence the responsiveness to interferon-alpha 2a treatment ic chronic hepatitis C? Intern Med 1997; 36: 248–254.
35. Todros L, Touscoz G, D'Urso N, et al. Hepatitis C virus-related chronic liver disease with autoantibodies to liver-kidney microsomes (LKM). Clinical characterization from idiopathic LKM-positive disorders. J Hepatol 1991; 13: 128–131.
36. Duclos-Vallée J-C, Nishioka M, Hosomi N, et al. Interferon therapy in LKM-1 positive patients with chronic hepatitis C: follow-up by a quantitative radioligand assay for CYP2D6 antibody detection. J Hepatol 1998; 28: 965–970.
37. Sümer N, Palabiyikoglu M. Induction of remission by interferon in patients with chronic active ulcerative colitis. Eur J Gastroenterol Hepatol 1995; 7: 597–602.
38. Boerr LAR, Sambuelli A, Gil A, et al. Alpha-interferon was not effective treatment of patients with ulcerative colitis. Gastroenterology 1996; 110: A868.
39. Mitoro A, Yoshikawa M, Yamamoto K, et al. Exacerbation of ulcerative colitis during alpha-interferon therapy for chronic hepatitis C. Intern Med 1993; 32: 327–331.
40. Yasumori K, Aramaki T, Mizuta Y, et al. Exacerbation of ulcerative colitis and chronic hepatitis by the treatment with interferon for chronic hepatitis B. Nippon Shokakibyo Gakkai Zasshi 1995; 92: 1066–1070.

Chapter 9 / Treatment of Chronic Viral Hepatitis in AIDs Patients

41. De Diego LA, Kashoob M, Romero M, et al. Recombinant alpha-2b-interferon treatment in a patient with chronic C concomitant hepatitis and outbreak of ulcerative colitis. Rev Esp Enferm Dig 1997; 89: 399–401.
42. Legaz H, Aztra VT, Alcantara TM, et al. Recombinant alfa-2 interferon treatment of a patient with chronic hepatitis B and ulcerative colitis. Gastroenterol Hepatol 1996; 19: 55–57.
43. Cottone M, Magliocco A, Trallori G, et al. Clinical course of inflammatory bowel disease during treatment with interferon for associated chronic active hepatitis. Ital J Gastroenterol 1995; 27: 3–4.
44. D'Amico E, Paroli M, Fratelli V, et al. Primary biliary cirrhosis induced by interferon-alpha therapy for hepatitis C virus infection. Dig Dis Sci 1995; 40: 2113–2116.
45. Garrido PG, Sánchez CJM, Olaso V, et al. Response to treatment with interferon in patients with chronic hepatitis C and high titers of –M2, –M4, and –M8 antimitochondrial antibodies. Rev Esp Enferm Dig 1999; 91: 175–181.
46. Grimbert S, Johanel C, Benjaballah F, et al. Antimitochondrial antibodies in patients with chronic hepatitis C. Lancet 1996; 16: 161–165.
47. Madea T, Onishi S, Miura T, et al. Exacerbation of primary biliary cirrhosis during interferon alfa-2b therapy for chronic hepatitis C. Dig Dis Sci 1995; 40: 1226–1230.
48. Wolfer LU, Goerdt S, Schroder K, et al. Interferon-alpha-induced psoriasis vulgaris. Hautarzt 1996; 47: 124–128.
49. Georgetson MJ, Yarze JC, Lalos AT, et al. Exacerbation of psoriasis due to interferon-alpha treatment of chronic active hepatitis. Am J Gastroenterol 1993; 88: 1756–1758.
50. Pauluzzi P, Kokelj F, Perkan V, et al. Psoriasis exacerbation induced by interferon-alpha. Report of two cases. Acta Derm Venereol 1993; 73: 395.
51. Lombardini F, Taglione E, Riente L, et al. Psoriatic arthritis with spinal involvement in a patient receiving alpha-interferon for chronic hepatitis C. Scan J Rheumatol 1997; 26: 58–60.
52. Shresta R, McKinley C, Everson GT, et al. Possible idiopathic thrombocytopenic purpura associated with natural alpha interferon therapy for chronic hepatitis C infection. Am J Gastroenterol 1995; 90: 1146–1147.
53. Bacq Y, Sapey T, Gruel Y, et al. Exacerbation of an autoimmune thrombocytopenic purpura during treatment with interferon alpha in a woman with chronic viral hepatitis C. Gastroenterol Clin Biol 1996; 20: 303–306.
54. Yoshida E, Rock N, Zeng L, et al. Use of interferon-alfa 2b in the treatment of chronic viral hepatitis in patients with preexisting idiopathic thrombocytopenia purpura. Am J Gastroenterol 1995; 90: 853–854.
55. Tappero G, Negro F, Gallo M, et al. Safe switch to beta interferon treatment of chronic hepatitis C after interferon induced autoimmune thrombocytopenia. J Hepatol 1996; 25: 270–271.
56. Gurtubay IG, Morales G, Arechaga O, et al. Development of myasthenia gravis after interferon alpha therapy. Electromyogr Clin Neurophysiol 1999; 39: 75–78.
57. Konishi T. Case of myasthenia gravis which developed myasthenic crisis after alpha-interferon therapy for chronic hepatitis C. Rinsho Shinkeigaku 1996; 36: 980–985.
58. Harada H, Tamaoka A, Kohno Y, et al. Exacerbation of myasthenia gravis in a patient after interferon-beta treatment for chronic active hepatitis C. J Neurol Sci 1999; 165: 182–183.
59. Shenoy M, Baron S, Wu B, et al. INF-alpha treatment suppresses the development of experimental autoimmune myasthenia gravis. J Immunol 1995; 154: 6203–6208.
60. Bolay H, Karabudak R, Varli K, et al. Low dose interferon-alpha is safe in patients with myasthenia gravis. J Neurol Neurosurg Psychiatry 1997; 62: 302–303.

61. Hoffman RM, Jung MC, Motz R, et al. Sarcoidosis associated with interferon-alpha therapy for chronic hepatitis C. J Hepatol 1998; 28: 1058–1063.
62. Teragawa H, Hondo T, Takahashi K, et al. Sarcoidosis after interferon therapy for chronic active hepatitis C. Intern Med 1996; 35: 19–23.
63. Nakajima M, Kubota Y, Miyashita N, et al. Recurrence of sarcoidosis following interferon alpha therapy for chronic hepatitis C. Intern Med 1996; 35: 376–379.
64. Luers C, Sudhop T, Spengler U, et al. Improvement of sarcoidosis under therapy with interferon-alpha 2b for chronic hepatitis B virus infection. J Hepatol 1999; 30: 347.
65. Oshimoto K, Shimizu H, Sato N, et al. Case of Addison's disease which became worse during interferon therapy: insulin secretion under hyperosmolarity. Nippon Naibunpi Gakkai Zasshi 1994; 70: 511–516.
66. Bini EJ, Weinshel EH. Severe exacerbation of asthma: a new side effect of interferon-alpha in patients with asthma and chronic hepatitis C. Mayo Clin Proc 1999; 74: 367–370.
67. Mackie RM. Interferon-alpha for atopic dermatitis. Lancet 1990; 335: 1282–1283.
68. Kimata H, Akiyama Y, Kubota M, et al. Interferon-alpha treatment for severe atopic dermatitis. Allergy 1995; 50: 837–840.
69. Larrey D, Marcellin P, Freneaux E, et al. Exacerbation of multiple sclerosis after the administration of recombinant human interferon alfa. JAMA 1989; 261: 2065.
70. Arnason BG. Treatment of multiple sclerosis with interferon beta. Biomed Pharmacother 1999; 53: 344–350.
71. Kimura Y, Kajiama K, Nomura H, et al. Severe thrombocytopenia during interferon-alpha therapy for chronic active hepatitis C associated with systemic lupus erythematous. Fukuoka Igaku Zassi 1994; 85: 329–333.
72. Kurihara T, Abe K, Ishirguro H, et al. Effect of interferon therapy in a patient with chronic active hepatitis type C associated with interstitial pneumonia and rheumatoid arthritis: a case report. Clin Ther 1994; 16: 1028–1035.
73. Tak PP, Hart BA, Kraan MC, et al. Effects of interferon beta on arthritis. Rheumatology 1999; 38: 362–369.
74. Lawrence R, Helmick C, Arnett F, et al. Estimate of the prevalence of arthritis and selected musculoskeletal disorders in the United States. Arthritis Rheum 1998; 41: 778–799.
75. Alter MJ. Hepatitis C virus infection in the United States. J Hepatol 1999; 31(Suppl 1): 88–91.
76. Dumoulin FL, Leifeid L, Sauerbruch T, et al. Autoimmunity induced by interferon alfa therapy for chronic viral hepatitis. Biomed Pharmacother 1999; 53: 242–254.
77. Dusheiko G. Side effects of alfa interferon in chronic hepatitis C. Hepatology 1997; 26: 1125–1195.
78. Bardella MT, Marino R, Meroni PL. Celiac disease during interferon treatment. Ann Intern Med 1999; 131: 157–158.
79. Tada H, Saitoh S, Nakagawa Y, et al. Ischemic colitis during interferon-alpha treatment for chronic active hepatitis C. J Gastroenterol 1996; 31: 582–584.

10 Developing Therapeutic Plans for Patients with Chronic Hepatitis B or C
A Practical Approach

Robert Reindollar, MD

CONTENTS

INTRODUCTION
INITIAL EVALUATION
EDUCATING THE PATIENT
SUITABILITY AND CONTRAINDICATIONS FOR TREATMENT
SPECIAL POPULATIONS: DEVELOPING THERAPY PLANS
SUMMARY
REFERENCES

INTRODUCTION

Each patient with chronic viral hepatitis has a unique medical and psychosocial history. Developing the therapeutic plan and effectively managing the patient with chronic viral hepatitis involves taking care of the entire patient, anticipating the needs and potential problems for each patient, and educating the patient regarding their disease and its management. Developing the therapeutic plan and initiating treatment for the patient with chronic viral hepatitis is best achieved with a team approach, with the patient clearly in the center of the team.

For the patient with chronic hepatitis B, there are currently two licensed therapies, including interferon (IFN) or lamivudine (LAM). Each drug regimen has distinct advantages and disadvantages. For the patient with chronic hepatitis C (CHC), the current standard treatment is IFN in com-

From: *Clinical Gastroenterology: Diagnosis and Therapeutics*
Edited by: R. S. Koff and G. Y. Wu © Humana Press Inc., Totowa, NJ

bination with ribavirin. Favorable virologic and host factors have been identified that allow the clinician to begin to tailor treatment for the individual patient *(1–4)*. There are well-known potential side effects of all of the drug regimens for both chronic hepatitis B and C, with distinct indications and contraindications.

The success of any prescribed course of treatment for either chronic hepatitis B or C depends on establishing an accurate diagnosis, establishing patient co-factors and co-morbidities that would represent contraindications to treatment, and obtaining complete virologic, biochemical, and histologic data. Finally, educating the patient regarding every aspect of their disease and, most importantly, the potential side effects of treatment will also help achieve treatment success.

INITIAL EVALUATION
History and Physical Examination

A detailed history and physical examination on the initial patient-physician encounter, will provide the most important early information leading to the therapeutic plan, and ultimately aid in managing the potential side effects of treatment. Taking a detailed history from the patient with chronic viral hepatitis will provide the approximate time and source of infection in many cases, symptoms of liver disease, if present, and disease co-factors, such as alcoholism and drug addiction. Furthermore, significant co-morbidities, such as uncontrolled depression or heart disease, which would be contraindications to treatment, will also be identified by the initial patient history (*see* Table 1).

A careful physical examination at the time of the initial evaluation will identify with reasonable certainty the patient with advanced liver disease, and additional medical conditions that might be contraindications to treatment. Important skin diseases, such as psoriasis and lichen planus, which are immune-mediated diseases that may worsen with IFN therapy, should be documented. A baseline retinal examination, at the time of the initial physical examination, should be done; IFN-associated retinopathy has rarely been reported to occur during treatment *(5,6)*.

Initial Laboratory Evaluation

Establishing an accurate serologic and virologic diagnosis of either chronic hepatitis B or C is necessary, as well as testing for other, possibly concomitant, causes of chronic liver disease. Lab studies are also necessary for establishing a pretreatment baseline, identifying advanced liver disease, or contraindications to treatment.

SEROLOGIC DIAGNOSIS OF CHRONIC HEPATITIS B

The diagnosis of chronic hepatitis B requires evidence of viral infection with the hepatitis B surface antigen (HBsAg), which that persists for greater than 6 mo. The patient with chronic hepatitis B virus infection may be a healthy carrier with no evidence of viral replication, normal serum aminotransferase (AT) levels, and no evidence of chronic hepatitis on liver biopsy. Only those patients with chronic hepatitis B, elevated ATs, and active viral replication require consideration for treatment. The markers of ongoing viral replication that are most important to the clinician considering the patient with chronic hepatitis B include hepatitis B e antigen (HBeAg) and HBV DNA.

Most patients encountered, with chronic hepatitis B with ongoing viral replication, will be both HBeAg- and HBV-DNA-positive. There is a small group of patients with chronic hepatitis B, who have developed a pre-core mutant strain of the virus that does not produce HBeAg, and is only diagnosed by the presence of HBV DNA *(7)*.

Occasionally, while evaluating a patient, evidence of prior hepatitis B infection will be identified by the isolated presence of the hepatitis B core antibody in the absence of HBsAg. In some instances, low-level HBV replication can be demonstrated by highly sensitive techniques, and HBsAg is present, but below the level of detectability of current assays. Management of such cases is problematic. Fortunately, this appears to be an uncommon event.

SEROLOGIC DIAGNOSIS OF HEPATITIS C

For the patient with risk factors for HCV, who not infrequently has an elevated alanine aminotransferase (ALT), the screening HCV antibody test (enzyme-linked immunosorbent assay or enzyme immunoassay [EIA]) is adequate in making the serologic diagnosis of hepatitis C. The second-generation EIA blood test, developed in 1992, is 97% sensitive, inexpensive, and generally used as the screening antibody test for making the diagnosis of HCV *(8)*. A positive EIA does not distinguish acute, chronic, or resolved hepatitis C infection, and does not indicate viremia. False-negatives can occur in immunosuppressed patients, such as the patient with chronic renal failure, or the transplant patient. Much more frequently, the clinician is faced with a false-positive EIA, which typically occurs in an individual with no risk factors and normal serum ATs. A false-positive EIA may occur in individuals with autoimmune disease or hypergammaglobulinemia of any cause.

Not infrequently, the clinician is faced with a patient identified to be HCV-positive upon blood donation, or on an insurance physical exami-

Table 1
Important Information from Initial Evaluation for Developing Therapeutic Plan in Patients with Chronic Viral Hepatitis

History of present illness
  Date and circumstance of HCV diagnosis
  Initial history and date of elevated ALT
  Date and place of diagnosis of HCV
Risk factors for bloodborne pathogens
  Blood transfusions prior to 1992
  Injection drug use
  High-risk sexual practices
  Contact with jaundiced persons
  Occupational exposure
  Tattoos and body piercing
  Intranasal cocaine use
  Household members with hepatitis or risk factors
Symptoms of hepatitis
  Fatigue
  Right upper quadrant pain
  Joint pain
  Pruritus
  History of jaundice
  Nausea and anorexia
Symptoms/history of advanced liver disease
  Jaundice
  Ascites or edema
  GI bleeding from varices or portal hypertensive gastropy

Review of systems
  HEENT: History of retinopathy
  Pulmonary: History of asthma or severe COPD
  Cardiac: History of severe or uncontrolled coronary artery disease
  GI: Concomitant liver disease
  GU: History of renal insufficiency; document birth control
  MS/Rheumatology: Uncontrolled RA or severe unspecified arthritis
  Neurologic: History of carpel tunnel, peripheral neuropathy, or uncontrolled seizure disorder
  Psychiatric: History of depression, anxiety, and other psychiatric diagnoses, prior hospitalizations, prior or ongoing treatments, history of suicide attempt(s), family history of depression or suicide attempt(s)
  Skin: Psoriasis, lichen planus, porphyria cutanea tarda
  Hematalogic/lymphatic: History of bone marrow suppression, anemia or cytopenia
  Immunologic: Autoimmune diseases, document HIV testing
  Endocrine: History of diabetes mellitus or thyroid disease
Physical exam
  General inspection
  Scleral icterus
  Pallor
  Needle tracks
  Evidence of skin excoriations
  Ecchymoses or petechiae

Encephalopathy
Past medical history
   Identify history of serious illnesses including, but not limited to, severe or uncontrolled cardiopulmonary, thyroid, autoimmune, or renal disease, diabetes, or active malignancy.
   Complete list of current medications, including over-the-counter medications or complementary therapies
Family history
   Family history of liver disease, hepatitis, alco, psychiatric disease, or autoimmune disease
Social history
   Identify psychosocial problems at home or at work
   Alcoholism and drug abuse
   Detailed history of previous and current alcoholism and drug use with quantification
   Family history of alcoholism and/or drug abuse
   History of withdrawal, blackouts or driving while intoxicated CAGE criteria for alcoholism

Muscle wasting, tenderness, or weakness
Fetor hepaticus
Asterixis
Peripheral stigmata of liver disease
   Spider angiomata
   Palmar erythema
   Gynecomastia
   Dupuytren's contracture
   Paratoid enlargement
   Testicular atrophy
   Paucity of axillary and pubic hair
Abdominal examination
   Hepatomegaly
   Splenomegaly
   Ascites
   Prominent abdominal collateral veins

nation, but who has no risk factors for HCV, and usually normal serum ATs. Confirmation of an HCV infection, identified by a positive screening EIA, is obtained by testing for HCV RNA, which indicates viremia and active infection.

Prior to the availability of the HCV RNA, the supplemental test used for confirmation of an HCV infection was the HCV recombinant immunoblot assay (RIBA), which contains the same basic HCV antigens as the EIA, but is an IBA. It can confirm or refute a positive EIA in a low-prevalence population *(9)*. The utility of the RIBA is limited, since it has been mostly replaced by the HCV RNA, when used for confirmation. However, for the patient who is identified with HCV by a positive EIA, but who has a negative HCV RNA, the RIBA is helpful in distinguishing a resolved HCV infection from a false-positive EIA.

Qualitative and quantitative polymerase chain reaction (PCR) tests are available. For HCV RNA quantification, both PCR and bDNA tests are available. The bDNA test is less sensitive than PCR, and cannot detect levels below 200,000 copies/mL blood *(10)*. Currently, most clinicians use the quantitative PCR, rather than the qualitative PCR, for confirming diagnosis, because the viral load gives additional information when developing the therapeutic plan. The viral load has been established as a prognostic indicator for treatment outcome *(1–4)*. A patient with a high viral load is less likely to respond to treatment, but should not be denied treatment.

Serial HCV RNA determinations are only helpful at specific time intervals during treatment, to assess response to treatment, and to make a therapeutic decision to continue or discontinue treatment *(2,3)*. Serial HCV RNA determinations are not helpful in monitoring an untreated patient, because they are generally static over time, and do not correlate with disease progression.

There are at least six known genotypes of the HCV *(11,12)*. Obtaining the HCV genotype is done after PCR confirmation, and prior to developing the therapeutic plan. The importance of genotyping the HCV patient became apparent in the recent U.S. and international combination trials, in which it was found that non-1 genotype patients require only 24 wk of combination therapy. In contrast, genotype-1 patients require a full 48 wk of combination therapy *(2,3)*. The majority of patients in the United States are infected with the genotype-1 infection, and less frequently with genotype 2 and 3, which have a much greater sustained response rate, when treated with IFN alone, or in combination with ribavirin *(2,3,13)*. The remaining non-1-genotype patients, including genotypes 4, 5, and 6, are rarely found in the United States.

Serum ATs

Not infrequently, the original diagnosis of chronic hepatitis B or C came as a result of finding an elevated serum AT at the time of a routine physical examination, as a result of blood donation, or by an insurance physical examination.

Patients with chronic hepatitis B can have a wide range of serum AT levels, from normal to markedly elevated during exacerbations. Most patients will have mild-to-moderate elevations *(7)*. If the patient with persistently normal serum ATs is a healthy carrier of the HBV, no serologic evidence of viral replication will be present. In patients with viral replication and liver biopsy evidence of chronic hepatitis B, the level of the ALT has direct implications when developing the therapeutic plan. Patients with an ALT that is less than 2× elevated are less likely to respond to treatment with IFN *(14–16)*.

For the patient with CHC, since the National Institutes of Health (NIH) consensus statement, the ALT has become the primary serum AT that is followed when considering for treatment *(17)*. Patients with CHC can also have a wide range of ALT elevations, although most patients have a mildly elevated ALT, generally not more than twice the upper limits of normal. Hoofnagle *(18)* has estimated that approx 30% of patients with CHC will have a persistently normal ALT.

There is little correlation between the ALT level and disease severity, for the hepatitis C patient, although the patient with the persistently normal ALT generally has milder histologic evidence of chronic liver disease *(18,19)*. A normal ALT associated with HCV should be repeated, to determine whether it is persistently normal (on several occasions over a period of 1 yr). This becomes important in developing the therapeutic plan, because it has been recommended that patients with persistently normal liver enzymes should not be treated outside of a clinical trial *(17,20)*.

Baseline Lab Studies

There are a number of lab studies that are necessary for developing the therapeutic plan, which include complete blood count (CBC) renal, and liver function tests, and a baseline thyroid-stimulating hormone. The CBC and the liver function tests may be the first indication that the patient has advanced liver disease, and may not be appropriate for IFN. In addition, the finding of baseline anemia or renal insufficiency may preclude the use of ribavirin. Given that IFN is an immunomodulatory drug, it is necessary to rule out underlying autoimmune disease. In addition, other causes of chronic liver disease should be ruled out, as well (Table 2). Routine pregnancy testing prior to treatment is mandatory for

Table 2
Baseline Laboratory Testing

Autoimmune disease screening
  Immunoglobulins (IgG, IgM, IgA)
  Antinuclear Antibody (ANA)
  Antimitochondrial Antibody (AMA)
  Antismooth muscle Antibody (ASMA)
Liver function and chronic liver disease screening
  Prothrombin time (PT)
  Albumin
  Total bilirubin
  Ferritin/iron studies
  $\alpha 1$ antitrypsin
  Ceruloplasmin
Routine laboratory testing
  WBC
  Hemoglobin/hematocrit
  Platelet count
  Thyroid-stimulating hormone (TSH)
  Creatinine
  Glucose

patients or partners of childbearing potential, because of the teratogenicity of ribarivin.

LIVER BIOPSY

In the United States, liver biopsy is generally recommended prior to initiating treatment for the patient with chronic viral hepatitis, unless an absolute contraindication is present. In developing the therapeutic plan, a liver biopsy serves as baseline, and helps to determine the natural history of a patient with chronic viral hepatitis. Second, it also helps to determine the sense of urgency for treatment (Fig. 1; *21*). Third, the biopsy may identify cirrhosis, which may be a contraindication for the use of IFN, especially for the chronic hepatitis B patient, and also should initiate screening for hepatocellular carcinoma. Infrequently, a liver biopsy will identify other concomitant liver diseases, such as granulomatous hepatitis, alcoholic liver disease, or non-alcoholic steatohepatitis.

EDUCATING THE PATIENT

The patient must be included in the development of the therapeutic plan. All patients should be educated regarding the transmission of viral hepatitis, the natural history of the disease, the treatment, and the potential side effects of treatment. Each patient has a unique medical history

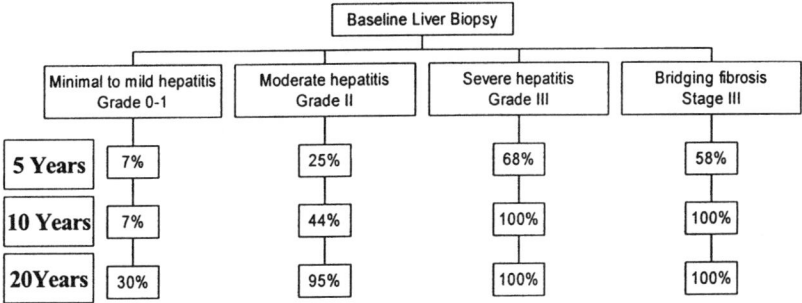

Fig. 1. Likelihood of histologic progression to cirrhosis. Adapted with permission from ref. *21*.

and psychosocial background, and therefore has distinctly different needs. Careful listening to each patient, beginning with the initial encounter, will identify specific questions, concerns, needs, and preferences, and potential problems for treatment. Problematic psychosocial issues, and the patient's sense of urgency and willingness for treatment, may alter both specific treatment plans and timing of treatment. Ultimately, education of the patient will help ensure the success of the treatment plan.

SUITABILITY AND CONTRAINDICATIONS FOR TREATMENT

Patient Data Analysis

Once all of the patient information from the history, physical examination, and diagnostic studies has been gathered, and psychosocial issues and medical co-morbidities are identified, the clinician can determine the patient's suitability for treatment, and begin to formulate the specific therapeutic plan, including the timing of treatment. In addition, the patient for whom treatment is contraindicated is identified (Table 3).

Chronic Hepatitis B: Developing the Therapeutic Plan

PATIENTS SUITABLE FOR TREATMENT

The clinician is faced with the decision of which of two licensed therapists is appropriate for treating the patient with chronic hepatitis B. In 1992, IFN-α2b was first approved in the United States for the treatment of patient with chronic hepatitis B. In December 1998, the Food and Drug Administration (FDA) approved the nucleoside analog, LAM, for the treatment of chronic hepatitis B.

Table 3
Contraindications to Treatment

Absolute contraindications to therapy
   Decompensated cirrhosis (IFN only)
   Active alcoholism or active drug use
   Noncompliance
   Significant psychosocial issues at home or at work
Contraindications to IFN
   Unstable or severe psychiatric disease
   Unstable autoimmune disease, e.g., rheumatoid arthritis, autoimmune hepatitis, severe psoriasis
   Hyperthyroidism
   Renal transplant
   Pregnancy
   Uncontrollable seizures
   Bone marrow suppression; thrombocytopenia ($<50,000/\mu L$)
   Neutropenia (ANC $<750/\mu L$)
   Uncontrolled diabetes mellitus
Contraindications to ribavirin
   Significant coronary artery or cerebrovascular disease
   Severe or intractable anemia
   Pregnancy
   Inability to practice birth control
   Significant renal insufficiency (creatinine clearance <50 mL/min)

There are two reasons to consider IFN as the first-line treatment of choice for the appropriate patient. In those patients who achieve seroconversion, the response is sustained in most. Furthermore, the development of a HBV mutant strain during IFN therapy is uncommon.

For the appropriate patient treated with IFN, loss of HBV DNA and HBeAg, with seroconversion to HBeAb, will occur in 33–37% of patients *(22)*. Patients most likely to respond are those with a low pretreatment HBV DNA (<200 pg/mL) and a high serum AT (>100 U/L), and histologic evidence of active necroinflammation found on liver biopsy *(14, 15)*. Other factors for a favorable response include absence of immunosuppression, female gender, short duration of hepatitis, wild-type virus (HBeAg$^+$), and horizontal, rather than perinatal, transmission of the virus.

The downside of IFN treatment is the fact that it is given by injection, and that its well-known potential side effects make this therapy difficult for many patients, and contraindicated in some. IFN is contraindicated in the unstable or severely disturbed psychiatric patient, in addition to the other contraindications listed on Table 3. In addition, the cirrhotic patient treated with IFN is at risk for decompensation. Two-thirds of patients who achieve a sustained response will have an AT flare, either during or following cessation of IFN *(23)*. A potential flare of hepatitis associated with IFN treatment could be deleterious to the cirrhotic patient.

LAM is an ideal therapy for those patients with chronic hepatitis B, for whom IFN is ineffective or contraindicated. It is an effective alternative for those patients who have a low ALT (100 U/L), or a high HBV DNA (>200 pg/mL), and therefore would not likely respond to IFN. It is also effective for those patients for whom IFN is contraindicated, or is likely to be ineffective, such as the decompensated cirrhotic patient, the immunosuppressed patient *(24)*, the patient infected with pre-core mutant strains *(25)*, or the patient with severe psychological problems.

LAM, which is given orally in a dose of 100 mg/d for 52 wk, is effective in suppressing viral replication in 93–100% of patients, with histologic improvement in half of the patients, a loss of HBeAg in 16–33% of patients by wk 52, and seroconversion to HBeAb in 16–18% of patients *(26,27)*.

It is tempting to use LAM as a first-line drug for most chronic hepatitis B patients: Up to 90% of patients who seroconvert have a sustained response; the drug is given orally; and it does not have the IFN side effects *(25)*.

However, there are several important considerations prior to making this the first-line treatment. First, following cessation of LAM treatment at 52 wk, patients who achieved viral suppression, as evidenced by loss of HBV DNA without HBeAg seroconversion or loss of HBeAg, will have a return of HBV DNA, and should be considered for prolonged therapy to suppress viral replication, or until HBeAg seroconversion is documented *(25,26)*. In addition, LAM therapy has been associated with the development of tyrosine-methionine-aspartate-aspartate (YMDD) mutations during treatment, which generally start to appear after 6 mo of viral suppression. By 1 yr, mutations have occurred in 14–32% of patients *(26,27)*. The development of this mutation is generally associated with a rise in HBV DNA and ALT while on LAM therapy. The YMDD mutant strain has been associated with a less-aggressive course, but the original wild-type virus usually remains suppressed, suggesting that LAM should be continued *(25)*.

Finally, prior to the use of LAM, all patients must be screened for HIV. LAM is not appropriate as monotherapy for HIV, and could initiate drug resistance. Periodic screening for HIV is also appropriate while treating the chronic hepatitis B patient with LAM.

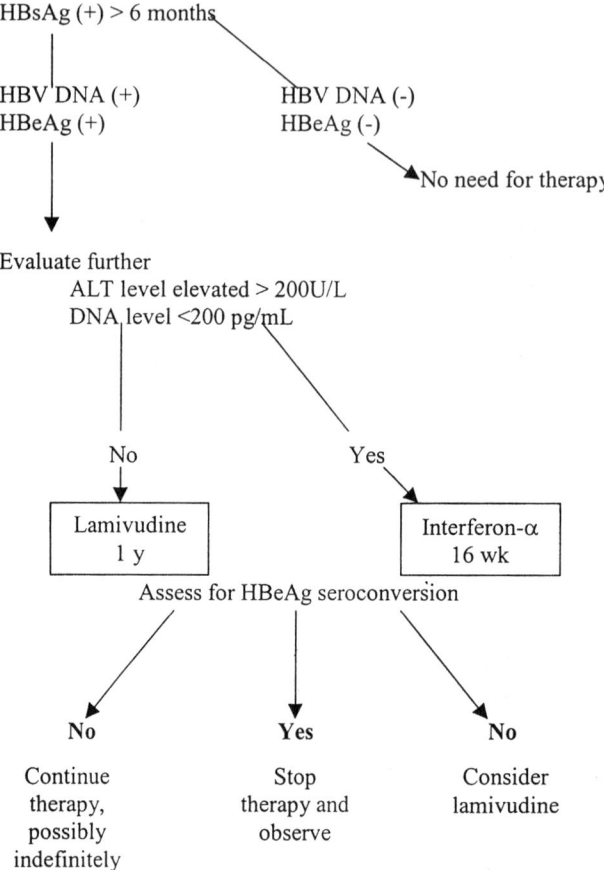

Fig. 2. Proposed algorithm for treatment of chronic hepatitis B virus infection. Adapted with permission from ref. *25*.

Although all patients with chronic hepatitis B are candidates for treatment with LAM, the development of the YMDD mutation, which occurs in a significant number of patients with prolonged treatment, makes LAM a cautious first line drug. Malik and Lee *(25)* have suggested an algorithm for the treatment of the patient with chronic hepatitis B, which considers all of the pros and cons of both therapies (Fig. 2).

CHC: Developing the Therapeutic Plan

PATIENTS SUITABLE FOR TREATMENT

Currently, patients with hepatitis C, who have been confirmed to be HCV RNA-positive, have elevated serum alanine AT levels, and a biopsy consistent with CHC, and who have no contraindications to treatment,

Chapter 10 / Therapy Plans for Chronic Hepatitis B or C

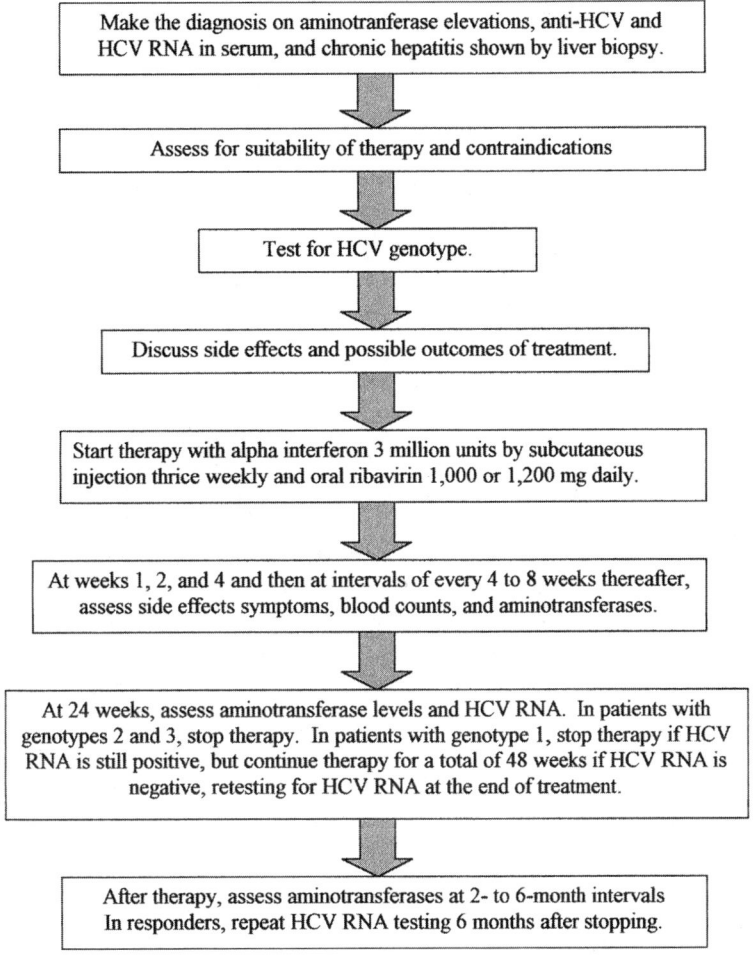

Fig. 3. NIH/NIDDK HVC treatment algorithm. Adapted with permission from ref. *20*.

should be considered for combination treatment (Fig. 3; *20*). It was initially recommended in 1997, at the NIH Consensus Conference, and updated in 1999, with the more recent (NIDDK) recommendations that those patients with fibrosis or moderate-to-severe inflammation, on liver biopsy, be the primary patients targeted for treatment *(17,20)*. Patients who have mild histologic disease should be treated on an individual basis *(20)*. However, it may be now appropriate to offer treatment to any suitable patient, regardless of the degree of inflammation or fibrosis. Certainly, there are many patients who, regardless of biopsy findings, want to be treated to clear the virus.

Since treatment was first initiated with IFN as monotherapy, a number of prognostic indicators of a sustained response to treatment have been reported, including short duration of disease, younger age, female gender, absence of cirrhosis, low HCV RNA pretreatment levels, and genotype 2 or 3, and the early disappearance of HCV RNA *(1)*. Over time, the most important of these predictors have been the presence of non-1 genotype; low viral load and absence of fibrosis or cirrhosis have been less-powerful predictors. Selection for treatment should not be based on the presence or absence of any of these factors, but they should be used for counseling in the total context of each HCV-infected patient being considered for treatment.

More recently, because of the findings of the large combination trials, the clinician can begin to tailor treatment, based on the genotype. Genotype-2 and -3 patients were found to have no significant difference in the sustained response rate, when comparing 24 to 48 wk of combination treatment with IFN and ribavirin *(2,3)*. As a result, it is now recommended that these non-1-genotype patients be treated with only 24 wk of combination therapy. In addition, essentially all patients who achieved a sustained virologic response became HCV RNA-negative prior to 24 wk of treatment *(2,3)*. As a result, the previous "3-month stop rule" of monotherapy has been replaced. It is now recommended that, after initiating combination treatment, the HCV RNA level only be re-evaluated at 24 wk of treatment, and, if virus is present, treatment should be terminated and considered for newer therapy *(2)*. A recent comprehensive review of the combination data, by Poynard et al. *(4)* suggests that, with the finding of five favorable factors for a sustained virologic response, treatment can now begin to be tailored even further, and an algorithm has been proposed (Fig. 4).

Patients Not Suitable for Treatment:
Developing the Therapeutic Plan

There are many patients infected with HBV or HCV, who, at the time of initial evaluation, are not considered suitable for treatment. These patients include the alcoholic who is actively drinking, the active drug user, the patient with a significant psychiatric history, and those patients with significant psychosocial issues. These patients should have a well-formulated plan centered on those factors.

ALCOHOLIC PATIENT

The HCV-infected alcoholic patient is at increased risk for the development of cirrhosis *(28)*. In addition, the response rate to treatment has been shown to be significantly lower in these patients *(29,30)*. Cessation

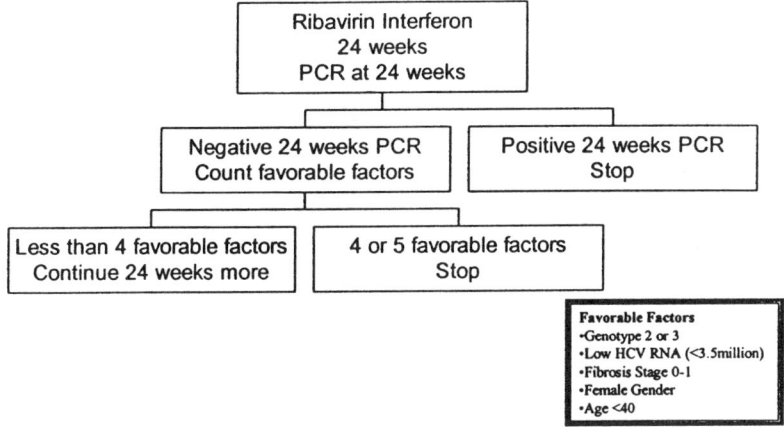

Fig. 4. Proposed treatment algorithm. Adapted with permission from ref. 4.

of drinking, and treating the alcoholic, should be the first line of therapy. Abstinence for at least 6 mo is necessary, prior to considering further treatment. In fact, alcohol use should be condemned for all HCV-infected patients. One of the few positive outcomes of the HCV epidemic has been the cessation of drinking in many HCV-infected patients, including alcoholics.

Active Drug User

The active drug user may represent an even greater challenge for treatment. Aggressive drug rehabilitation, and cessation of drug use for an extended period of time, will be necessary before any consideration for the treatment of chronic viral hepatitis. It is widely known that these individuals are a high risk for relapse during treatment, and for experiencing the potential neuropsychiatric side effects of IFN.

Psychiatric Disorders

The potential neuropsychiatric side effects of IFN may represent the greatest challenge to treating the patient with chronic viral hepatitis. It has been estimated that as high as 37% of patients who present to the practitioner for evaluation of HCV will be found to have psychiatric disorders prior to treatment *(31)*.

The mechanism of IFN-induced neuropsychiatric side effects remains mostly unknown, although there is increasing evidence that IFN alters certain neurotransmitter functions in the brain. Increasing evidence points to the serotonin pathway as one of the most important targets of IFN in the development of the neuropsychiatric side effects *(31)*, which occur in more than 20% of patients treated for CHC with this drug *(2,32,32)*.

Patients with a history of psychiatric disorders are particularly at risk for the development of the neuropsychiatric side effects of IFN.

A history of significant or severe psychiatric disease is a contraindication to the use of IFN. Since the serotonin pathway may be at the center of the potential neuropsychiatric side effects, it is not surprising that the selective serotonin reuptake inhibitors have been found to be helpful in managing the patients who are at risk, and those who experience these troublesome side effects. However, each drug has a different profile of effects and specific uses for the patient with psychiatric disorders, which requires the practitioner to become knowledgable about the use of these drugs, and makes trial and error inappropriate.

In a recent concise review *(31)*, an algorithm for assessing the risk of the hepatitis patient for developing neuropsychiatric side effects of IFN, and for managing the side effects when they occur, has been proposed. In developing the therapeutic plan for the patient with chronic viral hepatitis, this approach recommends identifying the patient who has underlying psychiatric disease, or who is at risk for developing psychiatric disease during IFN therapy. Prior to initiating therapy, a psychiatric evaluation should be obtained for patients who have a significant past or present history of depression, and, most notably, those with a history of hospitalization, or of a suicide attempt. A psychiatric evaluation should also be considered for those patients at risk, including a family history of depression or suicide attempts, a personal history of alcoholism or substance abuse, or a history of other chronic medical conditions. For the patient with active depression, and those particularly at risk for these side effects, treat first with the appropriate psychotropic drug, before initiating IFN therapy *(31)*.

Patients with Psychosocial Issues

Patients with significant psychosocial issues are not suitable for treatment until resolution of these issues. The importance of obtaining a thorough social history can never be underscored enough, to identify problems or demands at home or at work, which would make treatment not only challenging but invariably worsen the issue at hand. This emphasizes the importance of the timing of treatment. The psychosocially challenged patient is unlikely to be able to complete a successful course of treatment, and it is rarely so urgent that treatment could not be delayed until a later time, when the patient's problem has been stabilized or resolved. Successfully completing a course of therapy is much more likely to occur for the HBV- or HCV-infected patient who does not have any concurrent psychosocial issues.

SPECIAL POPULATIONS: DEVELOPING THERAPEUTIC PLANS

Cirrhotic Patient

For the chronic hepatitis B patient with cirrhosis and liver failure, IFN is inappropriate. However, LAM can be safely used in the cirrhotic patient with chronic hepatitis B, including those with liver failure awaiting liver transplantation and may help to slow the progression of disease. Posttransplantation, LAM, in conjunction with other therapy, may decrease the recurrence rate of hepatitis B.

The patient with cirrhosis deserves special consideration. Hepatitis C is the number one reason for liver transplantation in most centers in the United States. As of June 2000, 14,707 patients were listed for liver transplantation in the United States. For the year 1999, there were only 5843 donor livers available, and this number is not expected to significantly increase over time *(34)*. However, with nearly 4 million HCV-infected people in the United States, and a yearly increase of approx 4%, a recent model suggested that the disease burden will substantially increase by the year 2008, at which time there well may be a 528% increase in the need for liver transplantation *(35)*. Therefore, by the year 2008, it can be expected that the liver transplantation waiting list will have increased to approx 77,652 patients with end-stage liver disease, with only about 6000 available donors. This fact underscores the need to consider treatment of the HCV-infected cirrhotic patient, when appropriate.

The recent combination of IFN and ribavirin has significantly improved the sustained virologic response for the cirrhotic patient with HCV, and in fact was not much different than the sustained response for the noncirrhotic patient *(2,3)*. In addition, a significantly improved, sustained virologic response, from 6 to 29%, was achieved in the cirrhotic patient treated with polyethylene glycol–IFN-α2a, compared to standard treatment with IFN-α2a *(36)*. While waiting for better therapy, there may be a place for maintenance IFN in the virologic nonresponders to combination therapy, who have advanced fibrosis or stable cirrhosis. The utility of maintenance therapy for the virologic nonresponders recently has been demonstrated to result in histologic improvement *(37)*. IFN for the cirrhotic patients with CHC has been found to decrease the rate of decompensation and development of hepatocellular carcinoma *(38)*. Maintenance therapy may be useful in a select group of compensated cirrhotic patients, to avert progressive disease while awaiting better therapy. As recently reported *(39)*, the anti-inflammatory and antifibrotic potential of interleukin-10 may prove a new approach to treating those HCV-infected patients with advanced fibrosis or cirrhosis, unresponsive to standard antiviral drugs.

Children/Elderly Patient

Currently, IFN is not licensed for the use in children under the age of 18 yr. However, there is a substantial population of virally infected children. There is increasing successful experience nationwide treating the child with CHC, reported at national meetings by a relatively small number of qualified pediatric gastroenterologists and hepatologists. There are now studies in progress, which may identify the appropriate children for treatment with CHC, and may result in FDA approval.

The elderly patient with CHC may be a challenge for treatment. The primary question to answer before treating the elderly patient is whether the HCV infection is going to impact longevity or quality of life. Knowing the approximate time of infection, and the severity of liver disease on liver biopsy, may suggest that treatment is unnecessary in the patient with advanced age. In addition, the elderly patient may have other co-morbidities that make treatment of the CHC inappropriate. However, the decision to treat the elderly HCV-infected patient should be individualized, and not be denied because of age.

HBV–HCV and HCV–HIV Co-infected Patients

These co-infected patients have been thoroughly discussed in prior chapters in this text. For the HCV–HBV co-infected patient, generally only one virus is active, usually HCV. The active virus dictates treatment. There is increasing evidence of the benefit of treating the HCV, in HIV-infected patients, with IFN. They seem to achieve ALT and virologic responses similar to those in non-HIV-infected patients, and, furthermore, have been shown to result in decreased fibrosis and a decreased incidence of hepatocellular carcinoma. There has been some reluctance to use ribavirin in these patients concomitantly with other nucleoside analogs, such as zidovudine. Initial data, however, suggests that combination therapy can be safely used, with an increased response rate. It has been recommended, however, that further clinical trials need to resolve these concerns, before widespread use *(40)*.

Persistently Normal ALT Patients

The current NIH/NIDDK recommendation for HCV-infected patients, with persistently normal ATs, is not to treat outside of a controlled clinical trial *(20)*. This issue is becoming increasingly controversial. The current controversies are over the need for liver biopsy and the response to treatment. The ongoing clinical trials will likely help in answering these questions. The HCV-infected patient should not be denied treatment based solely on a persistently normal ALT.

SUMMARY

The success of treatment is dependent on the early recognition of the unique medical and psychosocial issues of each patient. Developing the therapeutic plan requires understanding the suitability and contraindications to therapy. Patient education will help to ensure the success of treatment. Finally, a team approach is necessary for managing these complex patients. The team members include the patient and family, physicians, a designated nurse, physician extenders such as physician assistants, and nurse practitioners, specialized pharmacies, pharmaceutical support systems, psychiatric support, and the use of support groups. Although the initial evaluation generally requires a specialist, the magnitude of this epidemic of liver disease suggests that, in the future, treatment management of these patients will have to be shared with a select group of knowledgable and committed primary care physicians and practitioners.

REFERENCES

1. Davis G, Lau J. Factors predictive of a beneficial response to therapy of hepatitis C. Hepatology 1997; 26(Suppl 1): 122S–127S.
2. McHutchison JG, Gordon SC, Schiff ER, et al. Interferon alfa-2b alone or in combinatin with ribavirin as initial treatment for chronic hepatitis C. International Hepatitis Interventional Therapy Group. N Engl J Med 1998; 339: 1485–1492.
3. Poynard T, Marcellin P, Lee SS, et al. Randomised trial of interferon alpha 2b lus ribavirin for 48 weeks or for 24 weeks versus interferon alpha2b plus placebo for 48 weeks for treatment of chronic infection with hepatitis C virus. International Hepatitis Interventinal Therapy Group. Lancet 1998; 352: 1426–1432.
4. Poynard T, McHutchison J, Goodman Z, et al. Is an "a la carte" combination interferon alfa-2b plus ribavirin regimen possible for the first line treatment in patients with chronic hepatitis C? Hepatology 2000; 31: 211–218.
5. Kawano T, Shigehira M, Uto H, et al. Retinal complications during interferon therapy for chronic hepatitis C. Am J Gastroenterol 1996; 91: 309–313.
6. Guyer DR, Tiederman J, Yannuzzi LA, et al. Interferon-associated retinopathy. Arch Ophthalmol 1993; 111: 350–356.
7. Chan HL, Ghany MG, Lok ASF. Hepatitis B. In: *Schiff's Diseases of the Liver* (Schiff ER, Sorrell MF, Maddrey WC, eds.), vol 1, 8th ed. Philadelphia: Lippincott-Raven, 1998, pp. 757–791.
8. Alter H. New kit on the block: evaluation of second-generation assay for detection of antibody to the hepatitis C virus. Hepatology 1992; 15: 350–353.
9. Younossi Z, McHutchison J. Serologic tests for HCV infection. Viral Hepatitis Rev 1996; 2: 161–173.
10. Toyoda H, Nakano S, Kumada T, et al. Comparison of serum hepatitis C virus RNA concentration by branched DNA probe assay with competitive reverse transcription polymerase chain reaction as a predictor of response to interferon-alpha therapy in chronic hepatitis C patients. J Med Virol 1996; 48: 354–359.
11. Simmons P. Variability of hepatitis C. Hepatology 1995; 21: 570–583.
12. Bukh J, Miller PH, Purcell RH. Genetic heterogeneity of hepatitis C virus, quasi-species and genotypes. Semin Liver Dis 1995; 15: 41–63.

13. Lee WM. Therapy of hepatitis C: interferon alfa-2a trials. Hepatology 1997; 26(Suppl 1); 89S–95S.
14. Hoofnagle JH, Peters M, Mullen KD, et al. Randomized, controlled trial of recombinant human alpha-interferon in patients with chronic hepatitis B. Gastroenterology 1988; 95: 1318–1325.
15. Perrillo RP, Schiff ER, Davis GL, et al. Randomized, controlled trial of interferon alfa-2b alone and after prednisone withdrawal for the treatment of chronic hepatitis B. The Hepatitis Interventional Therapy Group. N Eng J Med 1990; 323: 295–301.
16. Brook MG, Karayiannis P, Thomas HC. Which patients with chronic hepatitis B virus infection will respond to alpha-interferon therapy? A statistical analysis of predictive factors. Hepatology 1989; 10: 761–763.
17. National Institutes of Health Consensus Development Conference Panel Statement: Management of hepatitis C. Hepatology 1997; 26(Suppl 1): 2S–10S.
18. Hoofnagle JH. Hepatitis C: the clinical spectrum of disease. Hepatology 1997; 26 (Suppl 1): 15S–20S.
19. Di Bisceglie AM. Chronic hepatitis C viral infection in patients with normal serum alanine aminotransferases. Am J Med 1999; 107(Suppl): 53S–55S.
20. Chronic Hepatitis C: Current Disease Management, National Digestive Diseases Information Clearinghouse. Retrieved June 25, 1999 from World Wide Web: http://ww.niddk.nih.gov/health/digest/pubs/chrnhepc.htm.
21. Yano M, Kumada H, Kage M, et al. Long-term pathological evolution of chronic hepatitis C. Hepatology 1996; 23: 1334–1340.
22. Di Biceglie AM, Fong TL, Fried MW, et al. Randomized, controlled trial of recombinant alpha-interferon therapy for chronic hepatitis B. Am J Gastroenterol 1993; 88: 1887–1892.
23. Fried MW. Therapy of chronic viral hepatitis. Medi Clin North Am 1996; 80: 957–972.
24. Brumage LK, Wright TL. Treatment for recurrent viral hepatitis after liver transplantation. J Hepatol 1997; 26: 440–445.
25. Malik AH, Lee WM. Chronic hepatitis B virus infection: treatment strategies for the next millennium. Ann Intern Med 2000; 132: 723–731.
26. Dienstag JL, Schiff ER, Wright TL, et al. Lamivudine as initial treatment for chronic hepatitis B in the United States. New Engl J Med 1999; 341: 1256–1263.
27. Lai SL, Chien RN, Leung NW, et al. One-year trial of lamivudine for chronic hepatitis B. New Engl J Med 1998; 339: 61–68.
28. Poynard T, Bedossa P, Opolon P. Natural history of liver fibrosis progression in patients with chronic hepatitis C. The OBSVIRC, METAVIR, CLINIVIR, and DOSVIRC groups. Lancet 1997; 349: 825–832.
29. Okazaki T, Yoshihara H, Suzuki K, et al. Efficacy of interferon therapy in patients with chronic hepatitis C. Comparison between non-drinkers and drinkers. Scand J Gastroenterol 1994; 29: 1039–1043.
30. Ohnishi K, Matsuo S, Matsutani K, et al. Interferon therapy for chronic hepatitis C in habitual drinkers: comparison with chronic hepatitis C in infrequent drinkers. Am J Gastroenterol 1996; 91: 1374–1379.
31. Zdilar D, Franco-Bronson K, Buchler N, et al. Hepatitis C, interferon alfa, and depression. Hepatology 2000; 31: 1207–1211.
32. Maddrey WC. Safety of combintin interferon alpha-2b/ribavirin therapy in chronic hepatitis C-relapsed and treatment-naïve patients. Semin Liver Dis 1999; 19(Suppl): 67–75.
33. McHutchison JG, Poynard T. Combination therapy with interferon plus ribavirin for initial treatment of chronic hepatitis C. Sem Liver Dis 1999; 19(Suppl): 57–65.

34. Transplant Patient DataSource (2000, February 16). Richmond, VA: United Network for Organ Sharing. Retrieved August 15,2000 from the World Wide Web: http://207.239.150.13/tpd/.
35. Davis GL, Albright JE, et al. Projecting the future healthcare burden from hepatitis C in the United States (abstract). Hepatology 1998; 28: 390A.
36. Heathcote EJ, Shiffman ML, et al. Multinational evaluation of the efficacy and safety of once-weekly peginterferon alpha-2a(peg-inf) in patients with chronic hepatitis C (CHC) with compensated cirrhosis (abstract). Hepatology 1999, 30: 316A.
37. Shiffman ML, Hofmann CM, Contos MJ, et al. Randomized, controlled trail of maintenance interferon therapy for patients with chronic hepatitis C virus and persistent viremia. Gastroenterology 1999; 17: 1164–1172.
38. Fattovich G, Giustina G, Degos F, et al. Morbidity and mortality in compensated cirrhosis type C: a retrospective follow-up of 384 patients. Gastroenterology 1997; 112: 463–472.
39. Nelson DR, Lauwers GY, Lau JY, et al. Interleukin 10 treatment reduces fibrosis in patients with chronic hepatitis C: a pilot trial of interferon nonresponders. Gastroenterology 2000; Apr 118: 655–660.
40. Dieterich DT. Hepatitis C virus and human immunodeficiency virus: clinical issues in coinfection. Am J Med 1999; 107(Suppl); 79S–84S.

11 Supporting the Patient with Chronic Hepatitis During Treatment

*Nezam H. Afdhal, MD
and Tiffany Geahigan, PA-C*

CONTENTS

INTRODUCTION
PATIENT SELECTION
PRETREATMENT EVALUATION AND EDUCATION
SIDE EFFECTS MANAGEMENT
MONITORING OF THERAPY
MAINTENANCE THERAPY
REFERENCES

INTRODUCTION

Successfully managing the patient with chronic hepatitis C (CHC) can be a challenge to the physician. Not only does the patient with CHC impose a specific problem with therapy, but in addition the therapy itself is complex, and is associated with a multitude of side effects. This chapter examines strategies for the management of side effects in patients treated with both interferon (IFN) and IFN–ribavirin combination therapy. In the clinical trial scenario, approx 90% of patients can complete 6 mo of therapy with IFN and ribavirin, and 80% can complete a full 48 wk course of treatment *(1,2)*. This excellent level of compliance should be achievable in the office setting. Understanding and recognizing the side effects associated with IFN–ribavirin therapy will help the clinician in

From: *Clinical Gastroenterology: Diagnosis and Therapeutics*
Edited by: R. S. Koff and G. Y. Wu © Humana Press Inc., Totowa, NJ

educating the patient and family about the optimal strategies for successful therapy of CHC. Although this chapter focuses predominantly on IFN-based therapy, it also briefly discusses some of the newer treatments for hepatitis C virus (HCV), including pegylated IFNs.

PATIENT SELECTION

The initial selection of patients for therapy is an important determinant of the outcome of treatment. In a typical cohort of patients diagnosed with hepatitis C, approx one-third of patients are not candidates of therapy. Typically, in this third of patients are included those who are still actively using intravenous (iv) drugs, patients who are abusing alcohol, patients with concomitant serious medical illnesses, patients with advanced liver disease, and patients who decline therapy. In this latter group, both patient and physician bias can influence the choice of therapy. Patients may decline therapy because they believe it is not effective, or because they are worried about the side effects profile of treatment. Physicians are often influenced by their perception of the patient's individual commitment to a long course of treatment, and are frequently worried about the effect of therapy on the patient's quality of life. Recently, the authors evaluated 175 consecutive patients attending the liver clinics of an urban medical center, and discovered that 60% of patients received treatment for HCV *(3)*. In the remaining 40% of patients, depression and active alcohol abuse were the major determinants of whether treatment was recommended by the physician. Only eight patients, all with mild histological liver disease, declined therapy after discussion with the physician. Although these are important issues, the physician should select patients for treatment, based on the underlying severity of the chronic hepatitis and the absence of any absolute contraindications to therapy.

The major risk factors for CHC include blood transfusion prior to 1992 and use of iv drugs, even on one occasion *(4)*. In addition, approx 60% of new cases of CHC are related to use of iv drugs. Therefore, a major proportion of patients requiring treatment for CHC have had some experience with iv drug use *(5)*. More than one-third of these patients will have some underlying psychiatric problem, and this is one of the major issues that needs to be addressed at the onset of therapy by the clinician. In a recent Italian report *(6)*, 36.7% of patients suffered from some psychiatric disturbance. In the United States, various studies have reported a prevalence of depression and anxiety in HCV patients, from 11 to 57% *(7–9)*. When one examines all patients with CHC, it is clear that almost 50% of patients in certain situations are not candidates for antiviral therapy. The reasons why patients are excluded from therapy include active drug use, alcohol use, and underlying psychiatric illnesses. In fact, it has been estimated that, in certain situations, such as within the veterans population in the VA hospital system, and in the prison setting, only 20% of patients with HCV are suitable candidates for therapy *(10)*.

The authors do not routinely recommend therapy with IFN and ribavirin in patients who are actively drinking alcohol, or have used iv drugs within the preceding 6 mo. One of the key decisions is when to treat patients who have stopped drinking and are no longer using iv drugs. The authors' current recommendation is that there should be an alcohol- and drug-free period of no less than 6 mo prior to starting therapy. Some physicians do not like to treat patients who are on maintenance methadone therapy, but this would unnecessarily exclude many patients who require treatment. The authors will recommend treatment of patients on methadone, if they are attending a methadone clinic, and are currently on a stable dose of methadone. Their counselor at the methadone clinic will usually be contacted, and frequent spot testing for use of illicit drugs is recommended. In addition, it is wise to let the counselor know that these patients are starting therapy with IFN and ribavirin, because the fatigue associated with therapy may make compliance with the rules of the methadone clinic harder for the patient to accept.

The majority of patients treated for hepatitis C do not have severe underlying psychiatric problems, but frequently have a prior history of depression episodes. The physician must differentiate between situational depression, which is common in these patients, and ongoing severe depression illness. Many patients will have had psychiatric disturbances while using iv drugs, but, after rehabilitation, once their life-style situation has resolved, the psychiatric problems may no longer be as clinically relevant or so severe as to preclude treatment. Many of these patients will be seeing psychiatrists or drug counselors already, and discussion of the therapy plan with the psychiatrist or drug counselor is mandatory. Utilizing their help in getting the patient through therapy is critical to the success of any treatment schedule. The authors usually ask the psychiatrist to be available at short notice while the patient is on treatment with IFN and ribavirin. Most psychiatrists are now aware of the depression and irritability associated with IFN therapy, and are willing to give advice on the best pharmacological management of depression.

Patients with CHC already have underlying disturbances in their quality of life. Several studies, using quality-of-life questionnaires, such as the SF-36, have documented that patients with CHC have problems with psychosocial functioning, compared to a control population *(11–14)*. When these patients start therapy with IFN and ribavirin, a deterioration in quality of life should be expected in approx 70%. This deterioration is the major long-term side effects during therapy for chronic hepatitis, and provides multiple challenges for the treating physician. This chapter examines some of the specific side effects of therapy that lead to an overall reduction in the patients' quality of life, and discusses strategies to optimize management of these side effects and get patients through treatment.

PRETREATMENT EVALUATION AND EDUCATION

In the era of managed care, patient–physician contact tends to be brief, and, in many cases, complex decisions about treatment are made after only one or two visits to the physician. In the authors' practice, at the initial consultation, the patient is counseled about risk factors for the transmission of hepatitis C to family and friends. The second visit to the physician is usually for a percutaneous liver biopsy, and it is at the third visit that the major discussion about treatment takes place. Prior to that visit, the authors utilize available educational tools, such as patient information brochures and booklets, and videos about hepatitis C and its therapy, to give the patient some base-line understanding of the disease and its therapy. In addition, specific websites are recommended, such as those of the American Liver Foundation, that the patient can access for research into their disease. Unfortunately, since there is so much misinformation on the Web, recommending appropriate websites can prevent patients from receiving inaccurate or misleading information.

First, the authors like to establish the goals of therapy for each individual patient. The primary goal of therapy should be viral eradication that is sustained once treatment has stopped. Secondary goals of therapy include prevention of histological progression of disease and reduction of the risk of development of either liver failure or hepatocellular carcinoma. Education, so that the patient understands that the liver disease leads to significant morbidity and mortality, is of critical importance. The patient must understand that there is a significant benefit that can be obtained, even without viral eradication. This is particularly true for patients with advanced histological disease, who are at risk for the development of hepatocellular cancer.

Usually, on the visit to discuss therapy, the authors have all the information necessary to individualize the likelihood of treatment response for a given patient, particularly the viral genotype, viral load, and histological stage and grade of disease. Incorporating this information with the estimated duration of disease and the patient's sex enables prediction of both the estimated treatment response and duration of therapy. The authors like to discuss this prior to therapy with the patient, and to inform the patient about the time-points at which critical decisions, such as the continuation of therapy, will be made. Current practice is to inform the patient that, 3 mo into therapy, the viral load will be measured and that the authors looking for a minimum of a log-scale reduction in viral load or complete absence of virus. The authors recommend that only patients who achieve this degree of viral response continue on their initial course of therapy. Patients who fail to achieve this response are either discontinued, or their initial therapy is altered, either by increasing the dosage of IFN or, in some cases, by discontinuing ribavirin and continuing on IFN alone as a maintenance therapy for those with advanced histological disease. This may not be the current standard of care (see "Monitoring of Therapy", below), but is the authors' usual clinical practice: Patients must realize the rationale for therapy decisions prior to commencing treatment. Thus, from the onset of therapy, the patient understands both the short- and long-term goals of treatment, the clinical parameters upon which treatment decisions are based, and the proposed duration of therapy.

The next critical step in education is to reduce the anxiety the patient may feel about commencing an injection-based therapy, and to counsel on the management of side effects. The authors utilize both physician assistants and nurse practitioners to educate patients and families on self-injection techniques. The patient is usually requested to bring his significant other or family member to the initial session, where injection techniques are discussed. This also allows the opportunity to counsel the family member about side effects of therapy, and to advise them about the potential neuropsychiatric problems associated with IFN-based therapy. As discussed in, family members can be critical in both diagnosing and helping to manage these neuropsychiatric problems later, during therapy. The authors have found that the new self-injection pens or pre-filled syringes are associated with greater patient comfort and compliance. In particular, patients with a prior history of iv drug use do not like to use vial-based injection therapy, because it may remind them of their previous drug use. Utilization of videos and booklets can help the patient become familiar with self-injection, and, after the initial first few injections, most patients will lose their anxiety about self-injection. The authors recommend that injections of IFN be given 1–2 h before bedtime, and that the thigh region be the recommended site of injection. In very thin patients, who do not have much subcutaneous tissue, alternative sites of injection, including the abdominal area and the arms, may be utilized.

The nurse practitioner then discusses in detail, with the patient and family member, the major side effects of therapy with both IFN and ribavirin. The authors utilize a simple patient-education form, which lists these major side effects and suggested therapy to minimize them (Table 1). In particular, the patient is educated about the flu-like symptoms of IFN:

Table 1
Managing Side Effects of Rebetron Therapy

Side effects	Management
Flu-like symptoms	Take IFN injection shortly before bedtime
	Take acetaminophen one-half h–1 h prior to IFN injection.
	Drink plenty of water (10–16 full glasses/d).
Fatigue	Drink plenty of water.
	Get adequate amounts of sleep, which may be more than usual requirements.
	Perform light-to-moderate exercise regularly.
	Lessen work load, if possible.
Depression	Talk to friends, doctor, therapist.
	Join a local hepatitis support group.
	Consider use of antidepressant medication while on therapy.
Loss of appetite	Eat many small meals throughout the day.
	Attempt to eat more in the morning, when the appetite is likely to be the greatest.
Nausea/vomiting	If nausea occurs in the morning, eat dry crackers or toast. Consider antiemetics.
	Avoid stimuli, such as cooking odors or greasy food, which trigger nausea.
Dry, itchy skin	Change IFN injection sites frequently.
	Avoid taking long baths, which reduce skin moisture.
	Use moisturizing skin lotion.
Alopecia	Remember that the hair will grow back after therapy is finished.

fatigue and headache, depression and irritability, alopecia, nausea and vomiting, loss of appetite, insomnia, and the potential for disturbances in bone marrow and thyroid function. Ribavirin side effects, such as hemolysis and risk of teratogenicity, are discussed in detail. The patient is advised on the need for adequate contraception, and, if the patient is a female of childbearing potential, she is informed that monthly pregnancy tests will be performed while she is on therapy, and for 6 mo after stopping therapy. A detailed discussion of the authors' approach to these other side effects is found later in this chapter.

This is also an excellent time to discuss how to avoid potential hepatotoxic agents, such as alcohol. The authors recommend abstinence from alcohol, if possible, and, if not, then it is stressed that more than two alcohol drinks per week should not be taken, since not only will alcohol worsen the hepatic injury, but it may also diminish the response to IFN-based therapy. In addition, use of other medication is discussed, particularly the use of Tylenol and nonsteroidal anti-inflammatory drugs (NSAIDs). Tylenol is preferred as the drug of choice for the flu-like symptoms associated with IFN, and for the headaches, but many patients are worried about the use of Tylenol and need to be informed that up to 3 g/d has little liver toxicity. Patients are advised that, before they start any new therapy, they should inform their caregiver that they have chronic liver disease. Many patients are interested in the use of vitamin preparations and herbal remedies, which are discussed in Chapter 13. The authors do, however, recommend that patients should avoid iron-containing multivitamins and high doses of vitamin A. Antioxidant therapy, such as milk thistle (Silymarin) and vitamin E, are almost ubiquitously used by patients with CHC. The vitamin E is the preferred antioxidant, at a dose of 800 U/d. Many patients will not stop their herbal remedies, even when on treatment with IFN–ribavirin, but the authors do insist that they should bring all the tablets that they are taking to each follow-up visit, which occasionally allows identification of herbs that can worsen liver injury.

Finally, an opportunity is given to patients to express any anxiety they may have about therapy, and to ask further questions. This is a good time for the physician to address any life-style issues patients may have. The authors like to discuss how therapy may interfere with work habits of the patients. Patients who are in high-risk occupations for injury, such as construction workers, or patients who are involved in heavy physical labor, may not be able to continue with their usual employment. If there are issues with employment, a telephone call or a letter to the employer may help find a more suitable temporary position for the patient. The authors also discuss with the family member how best to cope with stress, irritability, and fatigue that the patient may experience in his home environment. The patient needs to feel a partnership with the physician in helping him through his therapy, and it is stressed that office staff and physician are available to help with further problems and questions, that the side effects profile of therapy is dynamic, and that the problems experienced with initiating therapy may not be those that cause a problem several months into therapy. Therefore, the authors stress that the patient must maintain the regular scheduled follow-up visits, initially 2 and 4 wk after starting therapy, then monthly until therapy is completed.

SIDE EFFECT MANAGEMENT

Side effect management is critical to getting the patient through therapy, and can be divided into general measures, as outlined above, then

Table 2
Adverse Events of IFN–Ribavarin in Patients Treated for 24 or 48 Wk

	% of Patients			
Adverse event	Intron A plus ribavirin	Intron A plus plus placebo	Dose-dependent Yes/No	Early/late
Application site disorders				
Injection site inflammation	13	14	–	Early/Late
Body as a whole: general disorders				
Headache	66	67	No	Early
Fatigue	70	72	No	Early
Rigors	42	39	No	Early
Fever	41	40	No	Early
Influenza-like symptoms	18	20	No	Early
Asthenia	9	9	No	Early
Chest pain	9	8	No	Early
Central and peripheral nervous system disorders				
Dizziness	23	19	No	Late
Neuropathy	<1	<1	No	Late
Gastrointestinal system disorders				
Nausea	46	35	Yes	Early
Anorexia	27	19	Yes	Early
Dyspepsia	16	9	Yes	Early
Vomiting	11	13	Yes	Early
Musculoskeletal system disorders				
Myalgia	64	63	No	Early
Arthralgia	33	36	No	Early
Musculoskeletal pain	28	32	No	Early
Psychiatric disorders				
Insomnia	39	30	Yes	Late
Irritability	32	27	Yes	Late
Depression	36	37	Yes	Late
Emotional lability	11	8	Yes	Late
Concentration impairment	14	14	Yes	Late
Nervousness	4	4	Yes	Late
Respiratory system disorders				
Dyspnea	19	10	Yes	Early
Sinusitis	10	14	No	Early
Skin and appendages disorders				
Alopecia	32	28	Yes	Late
Rash	28	9	No	Early/Late
Pruritus	21	9	No	Early/Late
Special senses, other disorders				
Taste perversion	8	4	No	–

specific problem management. The major side effects of IFN–ribavirin therapy are given in Table 2 *(15–20)*. This subheading discusses how the physician can manage these side effects of IFN–ribavirin therapy.

Flu-like Symptoms

Almost 80% of patients experience flu-like symptoms on commencing IFN therapy, but persistence of these symptoms beyond the twelfth week of therapy is seen in only 10% of patients. Onset of symptoms usually occurs 4–5 h after the IFN injection, and is dose-dependent. Symptoms can be minimized by taking the injection at night, taking Tylenol 30 min before the injection, and drinking plenty of fluids. If patients understand that the symptoms are worse at the beginning of therapy, and usually improve with time, the flu-like syndrome seldom needs any further therapy.

Headaches

Mild headaches, which are self-resolving, can be part of the initial flu-like syndrome, but 10% of patients may have severe, unrelenting headaches. The mechanism is unclear, but a migraine-like syndrome can also develop, which may require specific therapy, with agents such as mydrin or trazadone up to 150 mg po daily can help some patients with headache. Occasionally, control of headaches may require more analgesia than just Tylenol and NSAIDs, and codeine-based therapy, or even stronger analgesia, may be required.

Fatigue

One of the commonest symptoms of hepatitis C is fatigue, which is more common in patients with HCV, compared to a control population. In one controlled study *(21)*, fatigue was more common in patients with isolated hepatitis C than among those with isolated alcohol liver disease or hepatitis B (66 vs 30 and 29%, respectively). Fatigue has little correlation with either the degree of viremia or the alanine aminotransferase (ALT) level. However, in patients with advanced disease, such as cirrhosis, fatigue is even more common. IFN therapy is associated with fatigue in 23% of patients with HCV, and up to 90% of patients treated for melanoma. In the initial evaluation, it is important to determine what component of fatigue is related to IFN-induced depression or ribavirin-associated insomnia or anemia, since this type of fatigue will improve with treatment of the underlying cause. Fatigue is not dose-related, and can often worsen during the course of therapy, so that it strongly interferes with the patient's quality of life during the latter phase of treatment.

Treatment for fatigue includes conservation of energy by taking frequent rest periods, napping, if possible, and planning physical tasks and household tasks to be spread out over the course of the day. A gradual exercise-tolerance program, involving light exercise such as a daily walk, can be useful if initiated at the beginning of therapy, to condition patients to a higher level of activity and improve physical functioning, to better cope with fatigue. Adequate fluid balance is also critical in dealing with fatigue. IFN can affect the hypothalamic temperature center, resulting in an increase in core body temperature, which leads to low-grade fevers and fatigue. Adequate hydration with caffeine-free fluids can counterbalance this effect and lead to improvement in energy levels. A good rule of thumb is to divide the patient's weight by 2, which equals the daily recommended intake of fluids in fluid ounces (e.g., 160 lb woman = 80 fl oz/d).

Occasionally, fatigue is so severe that patients cannot perform routine daily functions. The authors often stop therapy at this level of fatigue, but recently have started to use Ritalin SL 20 mg/d for patients with severe fatigue and no contraindications to a trial of Ritalin. Although there are no controlled trials demonstrating benefit from Ritalin, anecdotal experience has shown this to be effective in a subset of patients.

Anorexia, Nausea and Vomiting

Anorexia is common in patients on IFN, with loss of appetite and associated early satiety. Patients are frequently told to expect a 5–10% weight loss while on treatment with IFN. In overweight patients with hepatic steatosis, this weight loss can actually be beneficial, but some patients, particularly those with cirrhosis and catabolic malnutrition, do poorly with this degree of weight loss. Frequent small meals and use of high-calorie nutritional supplements are occasionally necessary. If patients lose more than 10% body wt, or have any associated symptoms suggestive of more serious disease, then a clinically appropriate workup for occult malignancy may be necessary.

Nausea and vomiting are dose-dependent side effects of IFN therapy, and can be managed with dietary manipulation and use of antiemetics, such as Reglan or compazine, on a prn basis. In a small subset of patients, nausea and vomiting may be so severe that therapy must be stopped.

Respiratory Tract Symptoms

IFN has been associated with pulmonary infiltrates and a picture that clinically resembles fibrosing alveolitis. This type of clinical syndrome is rare and usually associated with high doses of iv IFN. More commonly, respiratory tract symptoms include a nonproductive cough and shortness of breath. Dyspnea is more common with Rebetron (19%), compared to IFN alone (9%). The etiology of these symptoms is unclear. Combination therapy with IFN and ribavirin has been shown to exacerbate the symptoms. Shortness of breath, within the first 3 mo of starting ribavirin therapy, is common, and is usually unrelated to the hemolytic anemia caused by ribavirin. A complete workup in these patients, including hemoglobin (Hb), chest X-ray, and pulmonary function tests, is usually unhelpful. There is frequently an associated cough, which occasionally will respond to therapy with histamine blockers. Sinusitis has also been reported with IFN therapy, and is no more common with the addition of ribavirin (10 vs 14%).

Eye Problems

IFN has been associated with multiple neurovisual complications. The most common ocular complication associated with IFN use has been the development of a mild-to-moderate ischemic retinopathy (22–27). On fundoscopy, this manifests as cotton-wool spots or hemorrhage, which is similar to diabetic retinopathy. The reported incidence of this retinopathy has varied greatly in different series (2–86%), but most cases are not associated with significant visual loss. Several cases of glaucoma have also been reported in association with IFN therapy, but a causative association remains unproven. Several case reports have also described a toxic effect of IFN on the optic nerve, in which patients presented with blurred vision similar to that seen with optic neuritis. Measurement of visually evoked response, in the subgroup of patients treated with chronic IFN therapy for hepatitis C, disclosed some patients with an increased latency in the visually evoked response (23). These patients had no visible pathology on ophthalmic examination. In none of the 11 patients with significant increases in visually evoked response were there associated visual symptoms. Therefore, the clinical significance of abnormal visually evoked response in patients with IFN should be interpreted with caution, and correlated to the presence of clinical symptoms. However, patients should be cautioned about the possibility of visual disturbance when they are treated with IFN therapy. In particular, patients with hypertension and diabetes should have fundoscopic examination performed at regular intervals, both prior to and during IFN therapy.

Dermatologic Complications

Multiple cutaneous lesions are associated with CHC (28). These include lichen planus, porphyria cutanea tarda, and vasculitic skin lesions, such as livedo reticularis, leukocytoclastic vasculitis, erythema nodosum, erythema multiforme, cryoglobulinemia, and polyarteritis nodosa.

IFN therapy has been associated with multiple autoimmune phenomena, and some of these may involve the skin. A list of the cutaneous lesions associated with IFN therapy is shown in Table 3.

Table 3
Dermatologic Manifestations of IFN

At injection site
  Erythema and induration
  Painful nodules with central vesiculation
  Ulceration/necrosis
  Contact allergy
Distant from injection site
  Psoriasis
  Lichen planus (skin, oral)
  Vitiligo
  Sarcoidosis
  Vasculitis
  Bullous pemphigus
  Raynauds

Adapted from ref *30*.

Injection-site inflammation can include simple erythema, induration, ulceration, necrosis, and even frank abscess formation. The newer pegylated IFNs have been associated with increased injection-site problems.

Patients with underlying psoriasis or lichen planus may have an exacerbation of their skin condition, when they are treated with IFN. In addition, IFN may cause the *de novo* development of both psoriasis and lichen planus. autoimmune alopecia may also be associated with IFN therapy: This is discussed in the next subheadings.

The commonest skin conditions associated with IFN–ribavirin therapy are nonspecific skin rashes, itchiness, or dry, thickened skin, which may resemble either drug eruptions or a nonspecific dermatitis. Skin rash is more common with combination therapy than with ribavirin alone (28 vs 8%). The rash can appear on any part of the body, and is frequently pruritic. In many cases, the rash is transient, and resolves over time, requiring no alteration of medication. In patients who have a major drug eruption, reduction in the dose of ribavirin, or even stopping ribavirin, may be necessary. In mild cases, a 0.05% steroid cream will improve the skin rash, and benadryl or other antihistamines can be used for the pruritis. Pruritus without skin rash is reported in 29% of patients taking Rebetron, compared to 9% on IFN. The dry skin can be treated by avoiding long baths or powerful soaps, and by using skin-moisturizing creams. Photo-allergic skin rash and sensitivity to UV light can be seen with ribavirin, which has been reported to act as a photosensitizer to UV-B light *(29)*.

Alopecia

IFN has been associated with an autoimmune alopecia areata *(30)*, but, more commonly, mild nonspecific hair loss occurs, which can be particularly disturbing to some patients, but will almost always resolve after cessation of IFN. Alopecia is no more common with rebetron combination therapy, and is seen to some degree in up to 32% of patients treated for 1 yr. The authors have seen one patient who lost all body hair, secondary to IFN, with normal return of hair after stopping IFN. Several hints for reducing the impact and degree of alopecia include placing a silk scarf on the pillow, or using satin pillowcases; low-pressure showers during hairwashing; trim longer, heavier hair, which will fall out more rapidly; avoid perms, gels, and mousses; and use wide-toothed combs or natural bristle brushes. The authors have not used agents such as minoxidil during IFN therapy, but this may be a reasonable approach in patients in whom hair loss is causing major emotional stress.

Thyroid Dysfunction

Thyroid dysfunction is a common occurrence in patients receiving IFN, with an incidence of 3–5% in patients treated for HCV *(31–33)*, but higher incidences associated with therapy of malignancy. Both the dosage and duration of therapy with IFN are associated with an increased incidence of thyroid problems *(34)*. Patients with antithyroglobulin or antithyroid peroxidase antibodies, prior to the start of IFN therapy, are at the highest risk of developing thyroid disease *(35,36)*. These antibodies are present in 16% of U.S. women and 1.5–3% of U.S. males, and are also the characteristic autoantibodies seen in Hashimoto's thyroiditis *(35)*. IFN causes an autoimmune destructive thyroiditis, which causes proteolysis and release of thyroid hormones, resulting in a clinically mild thyrotoxic state. As the gland is depleted of thyroid hormones, the persistent inflammation prevents further uptake of iodine and synthesis of thyroxine, resulting in hypothyroidism. Therefore, the commonest clinical manifestation of thyroid dysfunction is transient, mild hyperthyroidism, followed by hypothyroidism. The hypothyroidism can be transient, but resolution may take up to 18 mo after stopping IFN. Persistent hypothyroidism, requiring thyroid replacement therapy, will occur in one-half of patients.

A more aggressive syndrome of Graves' disease, with clinically active symptomatic hyperthyroidism, has been reported *(32,37)*, secondary to IFN therapy. Thyroid-stimulating immunoglobulins, directed at the thyroid-stimulating hormone (TSH) receptor, are diagnostic of this condition. Such patients will require therapy with antithyroid drugs, such as carbimazole or radioactive iodine therapy.

The authors recommend, for all patients receiving IFN, that a TSH is measured prior to therapy, every 6 mo on treatment, and up to 6 mo after treatment. Changes in TSH should be monitored by measuring thyroid function, but patients should be treated for hyperthyroidism only if they are clinically symptomatic. If hypothyroidism develops and fatigue is an issue, a low dose of thyroxine (50–75 mcg) can be used while therapy is continued. Once therapy is stopped, thyroid supplements can be discontinued, especially if autoantibodies are negative, but careful monitoring of TSH should be continued.

Glucose Metabolism

The association of hepatitis C with diabetes mellitus (DM) remains unclear, despite several cohort studies that suggest that HCV may be more common among patients with type II DM *(38,39)*. IFN therapy has been associated in isolated case reports *(35)* with the development of autoimmune DM, which may be mediated by the activation of interleukin-6 and IFN-γ in the pancreas, leading to β-islet cell destruction. More common, however, is the effect of IFN on glucose homeostasis in patients with established DM.

IFN can exacerbate DM and promote ketoacidosis in patients with type I DM, and convert patients with type II DM into requiring insulin for adequate glucose control. The authors recommend close monitoring of urine ketones and blood sugar in patients with DM, and informing patients of the disturbances that may occur in their glucose levels. In addition, patients with DM should have retinal examination annually, for IFN-induced exacerbation of retinopathy (*see* "Eye Problems").

Pregnancy

Counseling both male and female patients about the risks of pregnancy while on Rebetron therapy, or 6 mo after stopping treatment, is critically important for the caregiver, prior to starting treatment. IFN (5–10 mU) has been shown to cause abortion in pregnant rhesus monkeys, and there are no adequate and well-controlled studies in pregnant women. IFN is therefore not advisable in pregnancy. Ribavirin has produced significant embryonal or teratogenic effects in every animal species studied. Ribavirin is completely contraindicated in pregnancy, and any female that becomes pregnant on ribavirin should immediately notify her physician, and receive appropriate counseling about teratogenicity and the option for therapy abortion. Because the risk of transmission of defects, via the sperm in the male to the female is unknown, males should be advised not to impregnate their partners while on Rebetron. The authors advise all patients on Rebetron to practice at least two forms of contraception while on therapy, and for 6 mo after stopping ribavirin.

Hemolytic Anemia

The primary toxicity of ribavirin is hemolytic anemia, with a fall in Hb from 9.5 to 11 gm/dL seen in up to 32% of patients treated for 1 yr *(1,2, 20)*. Ribavirin is uniformly distributed through all cells in the body, and requires phosphorylation for excretion via the kidneys. The red cell is unable to phosphorylate ribavirin, and levels build within the erythrocyte, resulting in hemolysis. The hemolysis can be both sudden and severe. On average, Hb will fall by an average of 3 gm/dL in most patients treated with ribavirin. The fall in Hb occurs within the first 2–4 wk, and a nadir in Hb level is usually seen by wk 8. Most patients without underlying vascular or pulmonary disease will tolerate this level of reduction in Hb, but myocardial infarction and cardiac death has been reported in patients with underlying ischemic heart disease. All patients should be assessed for risk of cardiac disease prior to Rebetron therapy, and, if suspected, a stress test should be performed. The authors also recommend an EKG for all men over 40 and women over 50 yr of age, regardless of risk factors.

Several strategies have been developed to deal with hemolytic anemia. The most important is monitoring the Hb at wk 2 and 4, and monthly, while patients are on treatment. Because the hemolysis is dose-dependent, reduction of ribavirin dose is advisable when the Hb falls below 10 gm/dL. Patients on 1200 mg of ribavirin should reduce to 800 mg, and those on 1000 mg should reduce to 600 mg/d. The authors advise against attempting to increase the ribavirin dose after reduction, and there is evidence to suggest that the efficacy of ribavirin is still maintained with the reduced dose. If the Hb falls below 8.5 gm/dL, the authors recommend stopping ribavirin completely. In certain situations, such as in patients with HIV co-infection and cirrhosis, when continuation of therapy may be warranted, erythropoetin, 40,000 U/wk, can be used to maintain the Hb above 10 gm/dL, and should be started once the Hb falls below 10 gm/dL. The hemolytic effect of ribavirin can also be attenuated by the use of vitamin E, 800 U/d, which has been associated with an almost 50% reduction in hemolysis (Brass et al., unpublished observation). Biochemical abnormalities associated with the hemolytic anemia include unconjugated hyperbilirubinemia and elevations of uric acid.

Bone Marrow Toxicity

IFN has profound effects on the bone marrow that are dose-dependent, and include reduction of all cell-type precursors, resulting in a reduction of Hb, white cells, and platelets *(40)*. The bone marrow suppression is expected to be worse with the newer pegylated IFNs, since the marrow has less time to recover, because of the longer duration of IFN activity. The anemia associated with IFN is mild and much less significant than the hemolytic anemia caused by ribavirin. The average drop in Hb from 3 mU tiw of IFN is 10% of baseline, and is seen in 30% of patients treated with IFN. Fall in Hb below 10 gm/dL is seen in less than 1% of patients.

A reduction in the leukocyte count to between 2.0 and 2.9 ($\times 10^9$/L) is seen in 25–40% of patients, and to less than 1.0 in 1% of patients treated with IFN. More profound reduction in leukocytes has been reported in patients on PEG–IFN, or with higher daily dosing or induction therapy with standard IFNs. A reduction in neutrophil count of between 0.5 and 0.75, is seen in 9–14% of IFN-treated patients. Severe neutropenia below 0.5 is seen 11% of patients. Patients with cirrhosis and hypersplenism are at increased risk of neutropenia. The authors recommend that the IFN dose be halved at a total leukocyte count of 1.0, or a neutrophil count of 0.75, with complete cessation of therapy at a neutrophil count of 0.5.

Thrombocytopenia is the commonest hematologic complication of IFN therapy, and a reduction in platelet count below 100,000 is seen in up to 15% of patients at 3 mU tiw. Thrombocytopenia is common in advanced liver disease, because of a blunted response to thrombopoetin, and this response may be aggravated by IFN *(41,42)*. Severe thrombocytopenia, less than 50,000, is seen in less than 1% of patients, and is both dose-dependent and more common in patients with advanced fibrotic disease. The authors recommend halving the IFN dose at a platelet count of 50,000, and cessation of therapy at 30,000 platelets. We have not seen significant bleeding from thrombocytopenia, but have seen a patient with systemic lupus erythematosus, who had an autoimmune thrombocytopenia induced by IFN, with the development of antiplatelet antibodies and significant gastrointestinal bleeding. In patients who are on combination therapy, there appears to be a beneficial effect of ribavirin on the platelet count. The ribavirin-induced hemolysis is associated with a compensatory thrombocytosis, so that the fall in platelet count is frequently less than that seen with IFN monotherapy.

Neuropsychiatric Manifestations

A diverse constellation of neuropsychiatric symptoms are associated with the IFN component of therapy *(43)*. The major psychiatric disorders include insomnia (39%), irritability (32%), depression (37%), emotional lability (11%), concentration impairment (14%), nervousness (4%), dizziness (23%), and taste perversion (4%). These disorders are not dose-dependent, and can occur at any time during therapy, and even after therapy has been completed.

Insomnia is often related to ribavirin therapy, and the first step should be to advise patients to take their second ribavirin dose in the late afternoon, rather than at night. Insomnia can frequently exacerbate the fatigue that patients experience. If falling asleep is the major difficulty, then the newer sleeping pills, such as Ambien and Sonata, can be effective, with little hangover effect in the morning. Trazadone, starting at 50 mg and increasing to 150 mg, can also be effective. Valium and benzodiazepines should be avoided when possible, since they are metabolized by the liver, and can result in significant toxicity in patients with severe liver disease.

Irritability is one of the hardest side effects of IFN to deal with, and can be most disturbing to patients and their families. The authors strongly counsel patients and their families that irritability is common, and needs to be reported to the physician. Mild anxiolytic agents, such as Buspar, 5–10 mg bid or at night, can markedly improve the irritability associated with IFN. If the irritability progresses into severe mood swings and emotional lability, lithium can be used. If there is a component of depression with the irritability, Paxil, 20–40 mg/d, which is both an antidepressant and anxiolytic, can be useful.

Depression is the most important complication of therapy, and reported incidence varies from as low as 1% to as high as 44%, and the rate reported in the large Rebetron trial is 37%. A prior history of depression and a longer duration of therapy have been associated with the highest incidence of depression. Depression seldom is a major problem, if the clinician is aware of the signs and symptoms; the authors employ a simple questionnaire for the identification of occult depression (Center for Epidemiologic Studies Depressed Mood Scale, CES-D). Depression is usually mild, and can be managed with pharmaco-therapy *(44,45)*, allowing patients to complete therapy; but, occasionally, severe depression requiring hospitalization, suicidal ideation, or completed suicides have been reported. IFN may cause depression by alteration of neuroendocrine or neurotransmitter functions, or by modulating intracerebral cytokines. Serotonin depletion has been reported in the IFN dementia syndrome *(46)*. Selective serotonin transport inhibitors, which increase local concentration of serotonin, are the mainstay of anti-depression therapy. The therapy of depression induced by IFN has recently been reviewed *(43)*, and, although there are few published trials, certain recommendations about monitoring for depression and therapy for depression can be made.

The selective serotonin reuptake inhibitors (SSRIs) are the antidepressants of choice for treating IFN-induced depression. First, these agents appear to be well-tolerated and safe in patients with liver disease. Fluoxetine has a positive impact on the mental slowing associated with IFN, and venlafaxine and buprorion have stimulating effects that also help the mental slowing associated with IFN. Sertraline is easy to titrate, and very safe in liver disease, and citalopram has minimal drug–drug interactions. The clinician should become familiar with one or two the SSRIs, and use these, once depression is diagnosed. Tricyclic antidepressants, with their anticholinergic activity, are not recommended, particularly for patients with cirrhosis, since they may exacerbate cognitive dysfunction. Counseling and psychiatric consultation are advisable for all patients with more than mild depression.

MONITORING OF THERAPY

The patient with hepatitis C requires frequent visits while on IFN and ribavirin therapy, mainly for monitoring for side effects, and to aid in compliance with therapy. In the first 8 wk of therapy, monitoring for hemolysis, and helping the patient cope with the early side effects, is most important. After 12 wk, the major reason for monitoring is to ensure compliance, and to rule out neuropsychiatric problems. The authors recommend a visit at wk 2 and 4, then every 4 wk, while a patient is on therapy. In addition to a history and questioning about side effects, complete blood count (CBC), ALT, and pregnancy test are obtained at every visit, and every 12 wk, a TSH is performed.

Efficacy of therapy is usually determined by a polymerase chain reaction (PCR) test and ALT at either wk 12 or 24. If the goal of therapy is viral eradication, the authors suggest a quantitative PCR at wk 12. In patients on IFN monotherapy, failure to eradicate virus, with a positive PCR at 12 wk, indicates that the patient is highly unlikely (95%) to achieve a sustained virological response on that treatment regimen, and should probably discontinue therapy. PCR-negative patients should continue for a total of 48 wk of treatment. In patients on Rebetron, the standard of care is to perform a PCR at 24 wk, and to either continue therapy in those that are PCR-negative or stop therapy in those that are positive. Certain modifications to this approach have recently been proposed. In patients with genotype 2 and 3 disease, who also have low viral load (<2 million), no fibrosis on histological, female, and/or short duration of disease (<15 yr), 24 wk of therapy may be adequate.

A second modification is to obtain a quantitative PCR at 12 wk, and, if there is no change in viral load, to consider either discontinuation or modiification of therapy, by increasing IFN treatment to daily. These recommendations may all change with the advent of PEG–IFN plus ribavirin therapy.

Monitoring is also necessary once therapy has stopped, and the authors recommend a visit a wk 4, 12, and 24 posttreatment. Late-onset depression and suicides have been reported in patients who have completed treatment. The authors also continue to monitor pregnancy tests and TSH for 24 wk posttreatment. The critical time to determine the success of treatment is at wk 24 posttherapy. The absence of virus in serum, by a sensitive PCR test at this time-point, is referred to as a sustained response, and recently has been shown to correlate with long-term loss of virus *(47,48)*. These studies, with 5–10-yr follow-up, have confirmed that 95% of patients with a sustained response remain virologically, biochemically, and histologically free of liver disease *(47,48)*; Therefore, at this point, the authors talk to patients about cure of HCV. Once a patient has had a sustained response, the authors perform an annual ALT and PCR for 1–2 yr, to confirm the cure.

MAINTENANCE THERAPY

Even though 40% of patients will have a sustained response with IFN and ribavirin, that still leaves the majority of patients as nonresponders. A secondary goal of therapy is the prevention of progressive fibrosis, delaying decompensation of cirrhosis, and preventing hepatocellular carcinoma. There is a rationale to use pegylated-IFNs to achieve these goals, and clinical studies have commenced to examine these issues. However, many physicians, in practice, are already starting to use long-term IFN as maintenance therapy in selected nonresponders. Patients selected for maintenance therapy are usually nonresponders with severe histological liver injury, including advanced bridging fibrosis or compensated cirrhosis.

These patients may be taking IFN for up to 4 yr, and it is important to realize the end points that require monitoring. First, the dose of IFN should be well-tolerated, and is not necessarily equivalent to the dose required for attempted viral eradication (suggested dose for maintenance PEG–Intron, 0.5 mcg/kg/wk by sc injection). Therefore, looking for a virological response is not necessary. However, progressive liver fibrosis should be measured, either using serial liver biopsies or perhaps some of the newer serum markers of fibrosis.

REFERENCES

1. McHutchison JG, Gordon SC, Schiff ER, et al. Interferon alfa-2b alone or in combination with ribavirin as initial treatment for chronic hepatitis C. N Engl J Med 1998; 339: 1485–1492.

2. Poynard T, Marcellin P, Lee SS, et al. Randomised trial of interferon alfa-2b plus ribavirin for 48 weeks or for 24 weeks versus interferon alfa-2b plus placebo for 48 weeks for treatment of chronic infection with hepatitis C virus. Lancet 1998; 352: 1426–1432.
3. Afdhal NH, Keaveny AP, Nunes DP. Hepatitis C treatment of patients in an urban medical center. Hepatology 2000; 32: 565A
4. Alter MJ, Kruszon-Moran D, Nainan OV, et al. Prevalence of hepatitis C virus infection in the United States, 1988 through 1994. N Engl J Med 1999; 341: 556–562.
5. Fingerhood MI, Jasinski DR, Sullivan JT. Prevalence of hepatitis C in a chemically dependent population. Arch Intern Med 1993; 153: 2025–2030.
6. Taruschio G, Santarini F, Sica G, et al. Psychiatric disorders in hepatitis C virus related chronic liver disease (abstract). Gastroenterology 1996; 110: A1342.
7. Hunt CM, Dominitz JA, Bute BP, et al. Effect of interferon-α treatment of chronic hepatitis C on health-related quality of life. Dig Dis Sci 1997; 42: 2482–2486.
8. Lee DH, Jamal H, Regenstein FG, et al. Morbidity of chronic hepatitis C as seen in a tertiary care medical center. Dig Dis Sci 1997; 42: 186–191.
9. Singh N, Gayowski T, Wagener NM, et al. Quality of life, functional status, and depression in male liver transplant recipients with recurrent viral hepatitis C. Transplantation 1999; 67: 69–72.
10. Austin GE, Jensen B, Leete J, et al. Prevalence of hepatitis C virus seropositivity among hospitalized veterans. Am J Med Sci 2000; 319: 353–359.
11. Younossi ZM, Guyatt G. Quality-of-life assessments and chronic liver disease. Am J Gastroenterol 1998; 93: 1037–1041.
12. Foster GR, Goldin RD, Thomas HC. Chronic hepatitis C virus infection causes a significant reduction in quality of life in the absence of cirrhosis. Hepatology 1998; 27: 209–212.
13. Bonkovsky HL, Wooley JM, the Consensus Interferon Study Group. Reduction of health-related quality of life in chronic hepatitis C and improvement with interferon therapy. Hepatology 1999; 29: 264–270.
14. Koff RS. Impaired health-related quality of life in chronic hepatitis C: the how, but not the why. Hepatology 1999; 29: 277–279.
15. Dusheiko G. Side effects of alpha interferon in chronic hepatitis C. Hepatology 1997; 26(Suppl 1): 112S–121S.
16. Maddrey WC. Safety of combination interferon alpha-2b/ribavirin therapy in chronic hepatitis C-relapsed and treatment-naïve patients. Semin Liver Dis 1999; 19(Suppl 1): 67–75.
17. Kingsley D. Interferon alfa for chronic hepatitis C infection. Lancet 1999; 353–499.
18. Quesada JR, Talpaz M, Rios A, et al. Clinical toxicity of interferons in cancer patients: a review. J Clin Oncol 1986; 4: 234–243.
19. Okanoue T, Sakamoto S, Itoh Y, et al. Side effects of high-dose interferon therapy for chronic hepatitis C. J Hepatol 1996; 25: 283–291.
20. Rebetron Package Insert. Schering Plough, Kenillworth, NJ.
21. Barkhuizen A, Rosen HR, Wolf S, et al. Musculoskeletal pain and fatigue are associated with chronic hepatitis C. Am J Gastroenterol 1999; 94: 1355–1360.
22. Kawano T, Shigehira M, Uto H, et al. Retinal complications during interferon therapy for chronic hepatitis C. Am J Gastroenterol 1996; 91: 309–313.
23. Manesis EK, Moschos M, Brouzas D, et al. Neurovisual impairment: a frequent complication of alpha-interferon treatment in chronic viral hepatitis. Hepatology 1998; 27: 1421–1427.
24. Kuga K, Hasumura S, Nagamori S, et al. Intraocular hemorrhage developing during interferon therapy. Intern Med 1996; 35: 15–18.

25. Hayasaka S, Fujii M, Yamamoto Y, et al. Retinopathy and subconjunctival heamorrhage in patients with chronic viral hepatitis receiving interferon alfa. Br J Ophthalmol 1995; 79: 150–152.
26. Manesis EK, Petrou C, Brouzas D, et al. Optic tract neuropathy complicating low-dose interferon treatment. J Hepatol 1994; 21: 474–477.
27. Fortin E. Neurovisual complications of interferon-α therapy. Hepatology 1998; 27: 1441–1442.
28. Daoud MZ, Gibson LE, Daoud S, et al. Chronic hepatitis C and skin diseases. Mayo Clin Proc 1995; 70: 559–564.
29. Stryjek-Kaminska D, Olchsendorf F, Roder C, et al. Photoallergic skin reaction to ribavirin. Am J Gastroenterol 1999; 94: 1686–1688.
30. Kernland KH, Hunziker TH. Alopecia areata induced by interferon alpha? Dermatology 1999; 198: 418–419.
31. Lisker-Melman M, DiBisceglie AM, Usala SJ, et al. Development of thyroid disease during therapy of chronic viral hepatitis with interferon alfa. Gastroenterology 1992; 120: 2155–2160.
32. Watanabe U, Hashimoto E, Hisamitsu T, et al. Risk factor for development of thyroid disease during interferon-alpha therapy for chronic hepatitis C. Am J Gastroenterol 1994; 89: 399–403.
33. Preziati D, LaRosa L, Covini G, et al. Autoimmunity and thyroid function in patients with chronic active hepatitis treated with recombinant interferon alpha-2a. Eur J Endocrinol 1995; 132: 587–593.
34. Gisslinger H, Gilly B, Woloszczuk W, et al. Thyroid autoimmunity and hypothyroidism during long-term treatment with recombinant interferon-alpha. Clin Exp Immunol 1992; 90: 363–367.
35. Jones TH, Wadler S, Hupart KH. Endocrine-mediated mechanisms of fatigue during treatment with interferon-α. 1998; Semin Oncol 25(Suppl 1): 54–63.
36. Ronnblom LE, Alm GV, Oberg KE. Autoimmunity after alpha-interferon therapy of malignant carcinoid tumors. Ann Intern Med 1991; 115: 178–183.
37. Koizumi S, Mashio Y, Mizuto H, et al. Graves' hyperthyroidism following transient thyrotoxicosis during interferon therapy for chronic hepatitis type C. Intern Med 1995; 34: 58–60.
38. Caronia S, Taylor K, Luigi P, et al. Further evidence for an association between non-Insulin-dependent diabetes mellitus and chronic hepatitis C virus infection. Hepatology 1999; 30: 1059–1063.
39. Mason AL, Lau JY, Hoang N, et al. Association of diabetes mellitus and chronic hepatitis C virus infection. Hepatology 1999; 29: 328–333.
40. Toccaceli F, Rosati S, Scuderi M, et al. Leukocyte and platelet lowering by some interferon types during viral hepatitis treatment. Hepato-Gastroenterology 1998; 45: 1748–1751.
41. Peck-Radosavljevic M, Wichlas M, Pidlich J, et al. Blunted thrombopoietin response to interferon alfa-induced thrombocytopenia during treatment for hepatitis C. Hepatology 1998; 28: 1424–1429.
42. Martin TG, Shuman MA. Interferon-induced thrombocytopenia: is it time for thrombopoietin? Hepatology 1998; 28: 1430–1432.
43. Zdilar D, Franco-Bronson K, Buchler N, et al. Hepatitis C, interferon alfa and depression. Hepatology 2000; 31: 1207–1209.
44. Gleason O, Yates WR. Five cases of interferon-alpha-induced depression treated with antidepressant therapy. Psychosomatics 1999; 40: 510–512.
45. Levenson JL, Fallon HJ. Fluoxetine treatment of depression caused by interferon-α. Am J Gastroenterol 1993; 88: 760–761.

46. Brown RR, Ozaki Y, Datta SP, et al. Implications of interferon-induced trytophan catabolism in cancer, autoimmune diseases and AIDS. Adv Exp Med Biol 1991; 294: 425–435.
47. Marcellin P, Boyer N, Gervais A, et al. Long-term histologic improvement and loss of detectable intrahepatic HCV RNA in patients with chronic hepatitis C and sustained response to interferon-alpha therapy. Ann Intern Med 1997; 127: 875–881.
48. Lau DTY, Kleiner DE, Chany MG, et al. 10-year follow-up after interferon-alpha therapy for chronic hepatitis C. Hepatology 1998; 28: 1121–1127.

12 Complementary and Alternative Treatment of Liver Disease

Ken Flora, MD and Kent Benner, MD

CONTENTS

INTRODUCTION
TRADITIONS OF ALTERNATIVE MEDICINE
ALTERNATIVE THERAPY WITH HERBS
ADVERSE EFFECTS OF HERBAL THERAPY
CONCLUSION
REFERENCES

INTRODUCTION

In the broadest sense, complementary and alternative health treatments encompass health care provided outside the domain of conventional medicine. In the past decade, the proportion of Americans who report using alternative or complementary therapies has grown from 34 to 42%. During that interval, the projected number of total visits to alternative practitioners increased by 47%, from 427 million visits/yr in 1991 to 629 million visits/yr in 1997. It is estimated Americans paid, that year, $21.2 for alternative health services, most of which was out-of-pocket expenses ($12.2 billion), an amount comparable to out-of-pocket expenses paid for all U.S. physicians *(1,2)*. With the proliferation of nonconventional health care, patients, providers, and payers have increasingly adopted various forms of alternative therapy, thereby expanding the boundaries of "conventional" medicine. In response to these trends, Congress created the Office of Alternative Medicine (OAM) at the National Institutes of Health (NIH) in 1992, to perform research in complementary, alternative, and unconventional practices. NIH funding for research

From: *Clinical Gastroenterology: Diagnosis and Therapeutics*
Edited by: R. S. Koff and G. Y. Wu © Humana Press Inc., Totowa, NJ

in alternative medicine has steadily grown, from $2 million/yr in 1992 to a $68.7 million appropriation to the National Center for Complementary and Alternative Medicine (NICAM, formerly OAM) for fiscal year 2000, representing the largest annual increase among all NIH institutes (37% above 1999 spending).

Complementary and alternative medicine encompasses a broad spectrum of therapy, including acupuncture, homeopathy, herbal medicine, relaxation techniques, well-established therapy disciplines (chiropractic and osteopathy), and nonclinical self-care and life-style practices (e.g., massage, yoga, tai chi chuan, ayurvedic care, diet, exercise, and spiritual healing). In general, alternative therapy applies to those disciplines felt to be efficacious when used instead of, or as an alternative to, conventional or "allopathic" medicine. On the other hand, complementary therapy are those used along with other disciplines, including conventional medicine, in the treatment of disease. A rich history of alternative treatment systems in America, since the late 1700s, encompasses both indigenous traditions and those imported from Europe, Africa, and Asia, which offer distinctive approaches to therapy and physician–patient interactions. In the 1790s, Samuel Thompson formulated a program of botanical healing, emetics, and enemas, which was well received, by the early 1800s, as a less toxic, more natural alternative to prevailing practices by physicians of bleeding and purging. Homeopathy, a system formulated about the same time by Samuel Hahnemann, was based on a theory that remedies, which produce symptoms in healthy persons similar to those of illness, could be therapeutic, after being carried through a series of dilutions. The term "allopathic" (root "allo," meaning against) was coined by the homeopaths to denote conventional medicine, which uses medications against disease, rather than treatments based on the homeopathy "law of similars" (root "homo," meaning "same" or "with"). In the 1840s, hydrotherapy, imported from Austria, claimed to cure disease with a variety of therapy baths, combined with alterations of life-style. After the Civil War, mesmerism, a combination of magnetic healing and hypnosis, gained in popularity, and influenced Mary Baker Eddy, the founder of Christian Science. More recent arrivals on the alternative medicine scene include osteopathy, a technique of musculoskeletal manipulation originated by Andrew Taylor Still in the 1870s, and chiropractic, a method devised by Daniel David Palmer in the 1890s. In the last years of the nineteenth century, Benedict Lust developed an eclectic blend of manipulation procedures, hydrotherapy, herbal treatments, and other natural remedies that became the basis for naturopathy. More recently, eastern influences, since the 1970s, have resulted in the rediscovery of acupuncture in

Europe and the United States, and a growing interest in ayurveda, the ancient healing system of India *(3)*.

In a national survey of the use of unconventional medicine in the United States, which was instrumental in focusing attention on the widespread use of alternative therapy, 34% of 1539 adults questioned reported use of alternative treatments over the previous year. The most common therapy pursued were relaxation, chiropractic, and massage. However, most people who used alternative therapy visited conventional providers, and only one-third of persons were treated by alternative practitioners, most for chiropractic treatments or massage therapy *(2)*.

Several reasons have been cited for the public's apparent resurgent interest in alternative therapy, including dissatisfaction with limitations of conventional medicine, perception that the Western model of medicine tends to depersonalize patients and treats them as "mechanical processes," growing awareness of medical practices of other cultures, and increasing appreciation of the links of nutritional, emotional, and lifestyle factors to disease. Patients also increasingly express an expectation of wellness, demonstrate a growing interest in autonomy in health care decisions, and convey desire to reduce medications and their side effects. Recent support for alternative therapy by nationally known clinicians, and increased marketing by alternative practitioners and retailers, also probably play a role in the growing adoption of alternative treatments.

Several preliminary surveys, reported at a recent NIH-sponsored conference on complementary and alternative medicine in chronic liver disease, found that the use of alternative treatments, particularly use of herbal remedies, is common among patients visiting hepatology clinics around the United States. In a 1999 survey of 175 consecutive patients visiting the Hepatology Clinic at the Oregon Health Sciences University in Portland, OR, 42% reported using at least one of 24 different alternative treatments. Among hepatitis C virus (HCV)-infected patients, 56% (27/48) reported using alternative treatments, including milk thistle (48%), vitamins (8%), or thymus extract (4%). A minority of patients visited alternative practitioners that included herbalists (16%), naturopaths (15%), and chiropractors (4%): 36% of the patients reported that they believed that the alternative therapy that they were using was beneficial *(4)*.

The New Haven County Liver Study Group described the results of a population-based survey conducted in 1998–1999, among 79 consecutive patients with newly diagnosed chronic liver disease: 42% of the patients used 16 different remedies, including milk thistle (36%), ginseng (21%), and St. John's Wort (15%). The source of recommendations for alternative treatments included friends (58%), the lay press (15%), and naturopaths (15%); 54% of the patients in New Haven survey felt that alternative therapy was beneficial *(5)*.

A multicenter survey from six U.S. academic hepatology clinics, conducted over 3 mo in 1999, included 809 patients: 41% of patients reported use of herbal therapy. Alternative therapy use was favored by more highly educated and higher-income patients, and among women. Geographic variability was found in use of alternative treatments, highest in the Southern California sample (75%), and lower elsewhere (33–42%) *(6)*. Hepatology patients, particularly those with chronic hepatitis C infection, express several reasons for use of alternative treatment, including the limited success of conventional therapy in treating their illness, frustration with the uncertainty they perceive about the prognosis of HCV, concern about side effects of interferon (IFN)-based therapy, and a desire for a more "holistic" treatment approach, often in the context of recovery from substance abuse. The apparent motivation of many patients for using alternative treatments relates to perceived benefits of "natural" treatments and the appeal of alternative theories of wellness and disease, frustration with limitations of current conventional therapy, and interest in autonomy in their health care. Patients rarely cite demonstrated efficacy of alternative therapy for their liver diseases as an important factor in their decisions to use unconventional treatments.

Congress has mandated that the NIH, through the NICAM, facilitate evaluation of alternative medicine treatment modalities, investigate and evaluate the efficacy of alternative treatments, establish an information clearinghouse to exchange information with the public about alternative medicine, and support research training in alternative medicine practices *(7)*. Despite the suggestion that many types of alternative therapy may not be amenable to evaluation using the objective measurements and statistical interpretation of specific treatment interventions and outcomes, a recent NIH panel has recommended that application of precise research techniques are essential for defining the future role of alternative medicine *(8,9)*.

A rapidly growing literature on alternative therapy is developing, both in new alternative medicine journals and in the conventional medicine literature. However, several challenges face researchers who study the efficacy of alternative treatments. Because alternative treatments often target health maintenance, symptoms, rather than a specific disease process, or a general class of disorders, rather than a specific disease, the diseases under treatment are often poorly defined, based on criteria of conventional medicine. In addition, treatment interventions used in complementary and alternative medicine are often not discretely defined. Alternative therapy may consist of herbal compounds that contain contaminants or adulterants, involve variable doses of ingredients that are not well controlled, include multiple modalities used in combination, and can vary among persons with the same illness, depending on individual patient characteristics. Finally, assessment of the outcome of alternative therapy is often based on continued "wellness," improved sense of well being, decrease in symptoms, or improvement in biochemical parameters. Little data are currently available with respect to the effect of alternative treatments on objective measures that correlate with the virology or hepatic pathology of hepatitis C.

Clinicians must be aware of alternative therapy that patients are taking. This allows the provider to counsel concerning possible toxicity and drug interactions, to be aware of potential efficacy of alternative treatments, and to understand the concerns and motivations of patients with respect to their disease. A brief summary is provided below to familiarize clinicians with the major alternative therapy traditions or systems, including the theoretical basis of these practices, and the status of training and certification in each area. A discussion of several of the specific "herbal" treatments, more commonly used by patients with liver diseases, is followed by a review of toxicity of herbal agents, with emphasis on hepatotoxicity. More informed and detailed discussions are available in the references. This discussion is not meant to endorse the effectiveness of alternative treatments of liver disease.

TRADITIONS OF ALTERNATIVE MEDICINE

Traditional Chinese Medicine

A practitioner of traditional Chinese medicine views the patient's body as a reflection of the surrounding natural world. Many of the body's functions are described in terms of natural phenomena, such as rivers swelling, wind blowing, and so on. At the core of Chinese medicine is the concept that physical, emotional, genetic, and environmental influences exist in a balance, and that illness is a diversion from that balance. "Yin" and "yang" describe patterns of energy flowing through the body in a diametric relationship, similar to night and day and hot and cold. Yin is feminine and yang masculine, yin referring to the tissue of the organs, yang to their activities. The goal of Chinese medicine is to balance and strengthen the yin and the yang. All persons possess a unique life force, the "chi" (also spelled "qi"), which flows through the body in channels known as "meridians," which have been extensively mapped. Illness occurs when a blockage or imbalance develops in the flow of the chi, and acupuncture therapy and herbs can then be applied directly to the meridians. When sickness develops, the Chinese physicians attempts to determine

Table 1
Five Basic Elements and Their Relationship
to Organs, According to Chinese Medicine Philosophy

Element	Yin organs	Yang organs
Fire	Heart	Small intestine
Earth	Spleen	Stomach
Metal	Lungs	Large intestine
Water	Kidney	Bladder
Wood	Liver	Gall Bladder

the pattern of symptoms, and how they relate to the body as a whole. Extensive questioning is pursued regarding both physical and emotional aspects of the patient. This is supplemented by examination of the tone and strength of the voice, the complexion of the skin, the appearance of the tongue, smell of the body and secretions, and the pulses of the wrists and meridians, because all are effected by the flow of the chi.

The practice of Chinese medicine is primarily herbal, supplemented by acupuncture. However, acupuncture is often viewed as a medical discipline in itself. In acupuncture, the chi is broken down into five natural elements: fire, earth, metal, water, and wood. Ten of the organs have been characterized by which element most influences them (Table 1). The acupuncturist stimulates the meridians in an effort to realign the elements and the organs they represent. Chinese herbs are administered as teas, tablets, or extracts. Most of the traditional remedies consist of mixtures of herbal ingredients, and are individualized for each patient. Efficacy is ascribed to the actions of each component individually, and to the unique additive properties of the combined elements.

Practitioners of acupuncture are allowed to practice in all 50 states. Twenty-two states allow solo practice under a license or certificate; the majority of the remaining allow its practice only by MDs or DOs, or under the supervision of a licensed physician; 90% of the states that require certification recognize the examination conducted by the National Commission for Certification of Acupuncturists. This test includes both written and practical portions, including clean-needle techniques. Most schools of acupuncture require 3–4 yr of study.

Ayurveda

Ayurvedic medicine traces its roots back 5000 years. This knowledge was developed in ancient Hindu texts, the "Vedas." The four branches of the vedic sciences include self-knowledge, yoga, vedic astrology, and ayurveda, the science of healing with herbs, massage, and dietary manip-

Table 2
Ayurvedic Organization of Doshas

Vata	Pitta	Kapha
Thin and energetic	Medium, maintain steady weight	Heavy, obesity, strong
Cool, dry skin	Warm, ready, perspiring	Cool, thick, oily skin
Hyperactive, enthusiastic	Orderly, efficient	Slow, relaxed
Moody	Intense	High cholesterol
Imaginative	Short temper	Angers slowly, forgives easily
Nervous, anxiety	Passionate	
Constipation	Ulcers and GERD*	
	Hemorrhoids	
	Perfectionist	

*Gastroesophageal reflux disease (GERD).

ulations. One of the central concepts is the "prana," the vital force that all individuals have, akin to the Chinese chi. In ayurveda, the five major elements, earth, air, fire, water, and ether, are combined into three "doshas," vata (ether and air), pitta (fire and water), and kapha (earth and water). Each person is endowed with a unique balance of these, the pakriti, which governs physiological and psychological functions. Ayurvedic physicians attempt to identify abnormalities in the patient's pakritic pattern, and apply therapy to guide it back into balance. Patients' personalities and body characteristics are determined, according to which of the doshas is dominant (Table 2). Vata governs the circulation and the movement of materials through the body. It controls the movement of muscles and the functions of the hollow organs. Pitta governs digestion, body temperature, and other metabolic and enzymatic functions. Kapha provides the body's structural strength, and controls wound healing. Optimum health occurs when all of the functions, physical and spiritual, are in harmony. Ayurvedic medicine acknowledges that emotional state, environment, diet, seasons, and time of day are all important in affecting health, and classifies disease as psychological, physical, or spiritual. Ayurvedic diagnosis involves an evaluation of the tongue, pulses, eyes, and nails. Urine, blood, and fecal examinations are also undertaken.

There are four steps to ayurvedic therapy: detoxification, palliation, rejuvenation, and spiritual healing. Bowel purges, phlebotomy, enemas, and nasal douches are all utilized to purge impurities from each of the doshas. Diet, medications, herbs, and yoga are used to bring the now-cleansed doshas back into alignment. Once balanced, the body's functions are strengthened and rejuvenated with additional herbal and exercise treatments. Meditation, sound therapy, and gems, crystals, and metals are used to restore mental health.

Training in ayurvedic techniques can be undertaken both in the West and in India. In India, ayurveda is a five-and-one-half-yr degree, resulting in a Bachelor of Ayurvedic Medicine and Surgery. Western alternative schools tend to treat it as a subspecialty. In general, Western-educated practitioners have far less training than their Indian counterparts. It has been suggested that individuals have at least 3 yr of clinical experience, with supervised exposure to a minimum of 1000 patients, to be considered adequately trained. A number of institutions within the United States offer training in ayurvedic medicine, either alone or as part of a broader cur-riculum. However, at present, there are no standardized credentialing mechanisms, either of practitioners or the training programs. It has been pointed out that ayurvedic medicine tends to have little risk, given the minimal toxicity associated with ayurvedic agents.

Homeopathy

Homeopathy therapy can be traced to ancient Greece. Samuel Hahnemann developed the Law of Similars in Germany in the late 1700s, after observing that Peruvian bark used in the treatment of malaria also caused malaria-like symptoms when given to healthy subjects. He noted that other derivatives of plants, animals, and minerals also caused symptoms similar to many of the diseases for which they were administered. He believed that such treatments induced the body to respond better to disease, and this served as the basis of later work in vaccines. At the turn of the twentieth century, there were 22 homeopathic medicine schools in the United States.

Similar to Eastern practitioners, homeopaths believe that there is a vital source in all persons, which fights against illness and keeps one free of disease. Homeopathy practitioners seek to provoke or energize this force, to treat acute and chronic disease, and prophylax against future ailments. Homeopathy diagnosis involves attempting to identify the precise nature of the symptoms that the patient experiences, regardless of the underlying disease. Vast compendiums are consulted to identify which remedies most closely reproduce that symptom complex when administered. These remedies are then prepared through serial dilutions of individual agents in water or alcohol. The more dilute the remedy, the more potent its effects are believed to be. Most remedies are diluted beyond the point that any of the original substance can be detected within the solution. Homeopaths believe that there is a form of "molecular memory," and that the water molecules within the solution retain the electromagnetic signature of the therapy substance. These altered molecules are known as "clathrates." Most of the remedies are administered orally. The remedies may not be touched, and the patient is instructed not to eat, drink, or brush their teeth for 15–20 min after the remedy is taken. Because homeopathy remedies create the same symptoms as the diseases for which they are being prescribed, many patients worsen clinically before they get better. This is the "healing crisis," and it is considered to be a positive sign that the remedy is effective. Homeopathy therapy also involves the avoidance of "antidotes," substances that counteract the activities of the remedies. Antidotes include coffee, mint, and many prescription drugs.

The Council on Homeopathic Education is responsible for the accreditation of training programs in homeopathy medicine. At present, certified institutions are located in Oregon, Washington, Toronto, California, New England, and Virginia. In addition, courses in homeopathy are available, as part of the curriculum of most naturopathic training centers, and naturopaths are familiar with at least the basics of homeopathy techniques. There remains to be universally accepted standards for homeopathy practice; however, the American Board of Homeotherapeutics does conduct a competency examination that contains both written and practical components. The largest organization of homeopathy practitioners is the National Center for Homeopathy, headquartered in Alexandria, VA.

Naturopathy

Practitioners of naturopathic medicine generally believe in the six following principles: The body has considerable innate power to heal itself, and treatment should facilitate this ability; health and disease result from a complex interaction of physical, mental, emotional, genetic, social, and environmental forces; treating the cause of the illness is more important than treating the symptoms; prevention of disease is paramount; physicians must do no harm; and the role of the physician is to empower the patient through teaching. To accomplish all of these, most naturopaths utilize a combination of disciplines, including dietetics, acupuncture, homeopathy, and herbal therapy. Hydrotherapy, applying hot and cold moisture to the body, physical therapy, and massage are also commonly used. Most naturopathy is office-based, and relies heavily upon patient education and life-style modifications. Many conventional physicians are increasingly accepting of naturopathic beliefs, because of its common sense approach and its emphasis on preventive care. Naturopaths excel at dietary manipulation, and are responsible for the resurgence in natural childbirth.

At present, there are five institutes for the training of naturopathic physicians. They are located in Washington, Oregon, Arizona, Toronto, and New England. All of these are 4-yr programs that require an undergraduate degree prior to enrollment. Board certification is available to graduates, as is the Naturopathic Physician Licensing Examination. At the present time, fewer than 30% of states require credentialing as part of their licensing process. Most accredited practitioners are members of the American Association of Naturopathic Physicians.

ALTERNATIVE THERAPY WITH HERBS

In 1994, in response to over 4 million letters and faxes sent to congressional representatives, the U.S. Congress passed the Dietary Supplement Health and Education Act. This was a movement spearheaded by health food chains and the manufacturers of dietary supplements, to block Food and Drug Administration (FDA) proposals for setting standards for the manufacture and labeling of such products. This act places herbs within the category of "food supplements," and essentially allows producers to send products to market without the efficacy testing required of conventional therapeutic agents. The manufacturers are only required to provide reasonable assurance that their products are not associated with adverse effects. Under the law, no manufacturing standards for alternative agents are imposed, and, in effect, as long as a product does not claim to be a "cure" for a particular condition, it is allowed to remain within the food supplement category. Because of the lack of production standards, there is significant variability in the concentration of active ingredients within products produced by different manufacturers. An example of this is the variability in ginsenosides contained within 10 ginseng products manufactured in the United States and Korea, and analyzed by *Consumer Reports* magazine (Table 3). Among the 10 products labeled as containing between 100 and 648 mg ginseng per capsule, the concentration of ginsenosides range from 3 to 23.2 mg. In another example, analysis of the percentage of dehydroepiandrosterone (DHEA) found within 16 products, revealed that three contained no active ingredient, four contained less than 80% of the stated amount, and one contained 150% of the stated amount (Fig. 1). In addition to the variable content of active ingredients within the manufactured products, literature regarding the efficacy of these products provides no standard doses for treatment.

Milk Thistle (Silybum Marianum)

Milk thistle (*Silybum marianum*) has been utilized for medicine purposes for over 2000 yr. The ancient Greeks used it in the therapy of snake-

Table 3
Ginsenoside (Active Ingredient of Ginseng) Content of 10 Common Ginseng Products

Product	Ginseng/capsule (mg)	Ginsenosides/capsule (mg)
American ginseng	250	12.8
Ginsana	100	3.0
Herbal Choice Ginseng-7	100	6.5
KRG Korean Red ginseng	518	11.5
Natural Brand Korean	648	23.2
Naturally Korean	648	2.3
Nature's Resource	560	10.7
Rite Aid Imperial ginseng	250	0.4
Solgar Korean	520	10.6
Walgreen's Gin-zing	100	7.6

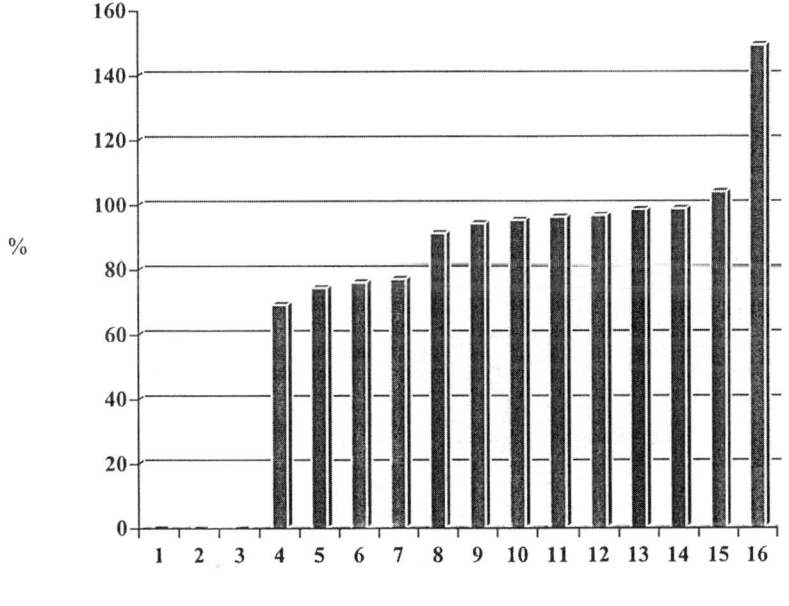

Fig. 1. DHEA: percentage of label claim. Adapted with permission from ref. *1*.

bites. Pliny the Elder (23–79 AD) touted silymarin's properties of "carrying off bile" in the treatment of jaundice. In the sixteenth century, silymarin was utilized for melancholy, and as an antidote to the effects of "black bile." Between the eighteenth century and the present, silymarin has been included in regimens as a "liver cleanser." Silymarin reportedly acts as an antioxidant, a stimulant of ribosomal RNA polymerase, iron chelation, reduction of tumor promoter activity, stabilization of mass cells, and protection against radiation-induced DNA injury.

Silymarin is extracted from the seeds or roots of the milk thistle plant, with absolute ethanol. Most preparations consist of the powdered product, which has been encapsulated, but it is also available as teas or alcohol-based extracts. The small number of subjects included in silymarin trials, and the variability in the etiologies and severity of liver diseases studied, flaw the majority of clinical trials of silymarin. Those trials, involving individuals consuming alcohol, were not controlled for alcohol abstinence, and heterogeneous dosing occurred in all of the studies. Statistically significant findings are unusual, and most authors appear to ignore the intrinsic ability of the liver to heal when an offending drug or substance, such as alcohol, is withdrawn. In an extensive review of the world's literature regarding silymarin, the San Antonio Evidence Based Practice Center found only 16 randomized double-blind placebo-controlled trials of silymarin, utilized for a variety of liver diseases. No placebo-controlled studies have been performed on patients with acute alcohol hepatitis; however, six addressed chronic alcohol liver disease. The issue of alcohol abstinence was inadequately addressed in all of these trials, and combined results suggest little difference in outcome between patients receiving silymarin and those treated with placebo. Only one study, which was not statistically significant, showed a trend toward improved survival with the herb *(10)*. Six silymarin studies *(10–15)* evaluated groups of patients affected by chronic liver diseases of mixed etiology. Findings were variable, and only two studies *(12,15)* revealed statistically significant improvements in serum alanine aminotransferase (ALT) levels in the groups treated with silymarin. One study *(16)* evaluated silymarin in 59 patients with acute viral hepatitis A or B, and found significant improvements in aspartate aminotransferase (AST) and bilirubin levels, and a trend toward improved ALT. Two studies *(17,18)* evaluated patients with chronic viral hepatitis, the first involving 20 patients with hepatitis B and/or hepatitis C. This study demonstrated significant improvement in AST, ALT, and serum glucose tolerance test levels with 7 d of therapy; however, the second study *(18)* showed only a trend in histologic improvement, with treatment and aminotransferase levels not evaluated. Neither of the studies evaluated the effect of silymarin on virologic measures of hepatitis B or hepatitis C (REF). Only one trial *(19)* utilized silymarin to treat drug-induced liver injury, including 60 patients on psychotropic drugs; there was significant improvement in malondialdehyde levels, but aminotransferases were unaffected. Overall, silymarin appears to be relatively free of adverse affects, the most common being gastrointestinal, with epigastric discomfort, nausea, and diarrhea.

Licorice (Glycyrrhizin)

Glycyrrhizin (licorice root extract) is extracted from the roots of the plant *Glycyrrhiza glabra*. Evidence of licorice root has been found in Egyptian tombs, and writings through the ages have described its use in suppressing cough, and soothing sore throats and upset stomachs. Because it is 50× sweeter than sucrose, its traditional use was as a sweetener of food and medications. A typical preparation contains between 5 and 25% percent of the product as glycyrrhizin. Reported healing properties include a reduction in inflammation via vasoconstriction, inhibition of inflammatory cell migration within tissues, and perhaps antiviral activities against a variety of viral agents, that may result from the induction of IFN-γ.

One trial *(20)*, which evaluated a glycyrrhizin-based compound against "other herbs," included 193 hepatitis C patients, followed prospectively for 2–16 yr for evidence of progression to cirrhosis or the development of hepatocellular carcinoma. Although glycyrrhizin appeared to slow the histological progression of the disease, both groups appeared to progress to carcinoma more frequently than in similar patients treated with IFN. Side effects attributed to glycyrrhizin included hypokalemia in 11% and hypertension (HT) in 3.6%. In a single randomized control study of iv glycyrrhizin vs placebo, among 58 IFN nonresponders or patients unlikely to respond (cirrhotic patients with genotype 1), the herb resulted in lower ALT, with no effect on HCV RNA levels *(21)*. The adverse effects of glycyrrhizin in humans are well-characterized. Glycyrrhizin inhibits 11-β-hydroxysteroid hydrogenase in the kidney, inhibiting the conversion of cortisol to cortisone. This results in a pseudohyperaldosteronism, leading to development of HT, hypokalemia, peripheral edema, headache, and metabolic alkalosis, especially if high doses of glycyrrhizin are administered. This has led to the recommendation that patients at risk for portal HT should avoid glycyrrhizin-based products, because of concerns of volume retention, and exacerbation of portal HT.

Thymosin (Thymic Gland Extract)

Thymosin extracts, derived from the thymic glands of humans and animals, stimulate T-cell maturation, natural killer cell activity, and appear to induce the production of IFNs. Two trials *(22,23)*, evaluating thymic

Table 4
Hepatotoxicity of Some Herbal Therapy

Constituent	Use	Adverse effect
Chaparral	Bronchitis, pain	Centrilobular necrosis
Pyrrolizidine alkaloids (comfrey, senecio, heliotropium)	Liver disorders, wounds	Veno-occlusive disease
Valerian, Skullcap	Sedative	Acute hepatitis
Germander	Antiseptic	Centrilobular necrosis, chronic hepatitis
Pennyroyal oil	Abortifacient	Centrilobular necrosis
Jin Bu Huan	Sleep, pain relief	Acute hepatitis, cholestatic hepatitis
Ma Huang (ephedra)	Weight reduction	Acute hepatitis, chronic hepatitis
Sassafras	Herbal tea	Potential hepatic carcinogen

Adapted with permission from ref. 40.

extracts for the treatment of chronic hepatitis B found that aminotransferase levels improved more quickly, and that the virus was cleared more often, among those on therapy, compared to placebo; a third trial (24) showed no improvement in efficacy, compared to IFN therapy. When used alone in the treatment of hepatitis C, thymosin appears to be ineffective (25–27). However, in one trial (28), patients treated with thymosin α 1, in combination with IFN, cleared HCV RNA more often, compared to patients receiving IFN alone or patients treated with placebo (37 vs 16 vs 3%, respectively). However, sustained virologic response rates were not shown to be different in this trial (28).

ADVERSE EFFECTS OF HERBAL THERAPY

Although protected from FDA regulation, many of the substances utilized in alternative therapy regimens have physiologic activities, and the Western medicine literature is becoming increasingly prolific regarding the adverse effects of these agents (Table 4). Adverse events can be either directly related to the alternative agent(s) used, or indirectly attributed to use of alternative therapy when they delay or replace more effective forms of conventional treatment.

The adverse events directly related to herbal therapy are generally of four types (29). First, predictable reactions to alternative treatments, which are generally dose-dependent and occur shortly after initiation of the therapy. Indeed, homeopathy therapy is based on this type of reaction, because agents are specifically chosen for the predictable side effects that they cause in an individual patient. Second, idiosyncratic adverse reactions are not predicted, and may occur at any point during a course of therapy. Allergic reactions are generally of this type. The third type of adverse event results from effects of the agent, which develop during long-term courses of therapy, such as hypokalemia and HT associated with prolonged-administration glycyrrhizin therapy *(30,31)*. Fourth, unexpected and delayed side effects, such as teratogenicity or carcinogenicity, may occur. For example, extracts of sassafras root have been shown to increase the likelihood of hepatocellular carcinoma in laboratory animals *(32)*.

Herbal remedies may be toxic for other reasons. For example, toxic substances, i.e., heavy metals, or substitutes such as nonsteroidal anti-inflammatory medications, may contaminate herbal products and cause adverse events. An additional area of concern is the interactions between herbal remedies and medications. Chinese herbal drugs have been found to increase the activity of coumarin; other plants high in vitamin K reduce the drug's effectiveness *(33)*. A recent letter to the editor *(34)* stated that eight patients taking St. John's Wort developed breakthrough bleeding, despite being on oral contraceptives. Because of its efficacy in treatment of mild depression, St. John's Wort has been suggested as a possible addition to IFN regimens, because IFN treatment is associated with the development of depression. This has raised concerns that St. John's Wort therapy may result in unwanted pregnancy. This is of concern to hepatologists, because patients on IFN therapy are mandated to utilize adequate contraception, which may be hindered by this herbal agent. Therefore, it is suggested that caution be utilized if St. John's Wort is administered to prophylaxis against IFN-induced adverse events.

The incidence of the adverse effects associated with alternative therapy is not insignificant *(35)*. A list of reported adverse effects on the liver from herbal treatments are noted in Table 4. A retrospective study *(36)*, including 2695 patients admitted to a Taiwanese medicine ward, found that 4% of the admissions were because of drug-related problems, and that herbal adverse effects ranked among the top three among the drug categories. A survey of 1701 patients hospitalized in Hong Kong *(37)* found that 0.2% of all admissions resulted from adverse effects of Chinese herbal regimens. A British poison control unit discovered that, between the years of 1983 and 1991, they had received over 1000 inquiries related to herbal regimens *(38)*. Abbott et al. *(39)* queried 400 users of complementary medicine and discovered that 8% of those who utilized alternative agents had experienced side effects of some degree. Given that so many patients are hesitant to discuss their alternative regimens with their primary physicians, the adverse effects of these agents are probably significantly underreported.

CONCLUSION

Patients with liver disease are increasingly embracing alternative and complementary methods, as part, or all, of their therapy. Complementary and alternative medicine currently accounts for a significant portion of the dollars spent on their health care. The variety of disciplines, techniques, and agents is broad, and although most do not present significant risk to patients, care must be taken to avoid unforeseen effects or interactions. This is especially important, because there is little FDA regulation of the administration and manufacture of complementary and alternative medicine agents and the educational and professional backgrounds of the practitioners. There is a historic basis for the use of much of complementary and alternative medicine therapy, but most of it has not been rigorously tested. However, in this era of multidisciplinary approaches to chronic disease, complementary and alternative medicine plays a role, and it is probable that at least some of the techniques and agents utilized will be found to be of some benefit in some patients.

REFERENCES

1. Eisenberg DM, Ettner SL. Trends in alternative medicine use in the United States, 1990-1997. JAMA 1998; 280: 1569–1575.
2. Eisenberg DM, Kessler RC, Foster C, et al. Unconventional medicine in the United States. Prevalence, costs, and patterns of use (see comments). N Engl J Med 1993; 328: 246–252.
3. Whorton JC. History of complementary and alternative medicine. In: *Essentials of Complementary and Alternative Medicine* (Jonas WB, Jeffry S., eds.), Philadelphia: Lippincott Williams & Wilkins, 1999, pp. 16–30.
4. Berk BS, Chaya C, Benner KG, Flora KD. Comparison of herbal therapy for liver disease (abstract). Hepatology 1999; 30: 478A.
5. Navarro V, Heye C, Kunze K, et al. The New Haven County liver study: the use of herbal remedies in patients with recently diagnosed chronic liver disease. Complementary and alternative medicine in chronic liver disease (abstract). NIH 1999; 8: 100.
6. Strader D, Bacon B, Hoofnagle J, et al. Use of CAM by patients in liver disease clinics. Complementary and alternative medicine in chronic liver disease (abstract). NIH 1999; 8: 47.
7. Jonas WB. Researching alternative medicine. Nat Med 1997; 3: 824–827.
8. Levin JS, Glass TA, Kushi LH, et al. Quantitative methods in research on complementary and alternative medicine. A methodological manifesto. NIH Office of Alternative Medicine. Med Care 1997; 35: 1079–1094.
9. Vickers A, Cassileth B, Ernst E, et al. How should we research unconventional therapies? A panel report from the Conference on Complementary and Alternative Medicine Research Methodology, National Institutes of Health. Int J Technol Assess Health Care 1997; 13: 111–121.
10. Benda L, Dittrich H, Ferenzi P, et al. [The influence of therapy with silymarin on the survival rate of patients with liver cirrhosis (author's transl)]. Wien Klin Wochenschr 1980; 92: 678–683.
11. Fintelmann V. Zur therapie der fettleber mit silymarin. Therapiewoche 1970; 20: 23.

12. Fintelmann V, Albert A. Double blind trial of silymarin sodium in toxic liver damage. Therapiewoche 1980; 30: 5589–5584.
13. Tanasescu C, Petrea S, Baldescu R, et al. Use of the Romanian product Silimarina in the treatment of chronic liver diseases. Med Intern 1988; 26: 311–322.
14. Ferenci P, Dragosics B, Dittrich H, et al. Randomized controlled trial of silymarin treatment in patients with cirrhosis of the liver. J Hepatol 1989; 9: 105–113.
15. Marcelli R, Bizzoni P, Conte D, et al. Randomized controlled study of the efficacy and tolerability of a short course of IdB1016 in the treatment of chronic persistent hepatitis. Eur Bull Drug Res 1992; 1: 131–135.
16. Magliulo E, Gagliardi B, Fiori GP. [Results of a double blind study on the effect of silymarin in the treatment of acute viral hepatitis, carried out at two medical centres (author's transl)]. Med Klin 1978; 73: 1060–1065.
17. Buzzelli G, Moscarella S, Giusti A, et al. Pilot study on the liver protective effect of silybin- phosphatidylcholine complex (IdB1016) in chronic active hepatitis. Int J Clin Pharmacol Ther Toxicol 1993; 31: 456–460.
18. Kiesewetter E, Leodolter I, Thaler H. [Results of two double-blind studies on the effect of silymarine in chronic hepatitis (author's transl)]. Leber Magen Darm 1977; 7: 318–323.
19. Palasciano G, Portincasa P, Palmier V, et al. Effect of silymarin on plasma levels of malon-dialdehyde in patients receiving long-term treatment with psychotropic drugs. Curr Ther Res Clin Exp 1994; 55: 537–545.
20. Arase Y, Ikeda K, Murashima N, et al. The long term efficacy of glycyrrhizin in chronic hepatitis C patients. Cancer 1997; 79: 1494–1500.
21. van Rossum TG, Vulto AG, Hop WC, et al. Intravenous glycyrrhizin for the treatment of chronic hepatitis C: a double-blind, randomized, placebo-controlled phase I/II trial. J Gastroenterol Hepatol 1999; 14: 1093–1099.
22. Mutchnick MG, Appelman HD, Chung HT, et al. Thymosin treatment of chronic hepatitis B: a placebo-controlled pilot trial [see comments]. Hepatology 1991; 14: 409–415.
23. Mutchnick MG, Lindsay KL, Schiff ER, et al. Treatment of chronic hepatitis B: a multicenter, randomized, placebo-controlled, double-blind study (abstract). Gastroenterology 1995; 108: A1127.
24. Andreone P, Cursaro C, Gramenzi A, et al. Randomized controlled trial of thymosin-alpha1 versus interferon alfa treatment in patients with hepatitis B e antigen antibody- and hepatitis B virus DNA-positive chronic hepatitis B. Hepatology 1996; 24: 774–777.
25. Andreone P, Cursaro C, Gramenzi A, et al. Double-blind, placebo-controlled, pilot trial of thymosin alpha 1 for the treatment of chronic hepatitis C. Liver 1996; 16: 207–210.
26. Rezakovic I, Zanaglia C, Botelli R, et al. Pilot study of thymosin alpha-1 therapy in chronic active hepatitis C (abstract). Hepatology 1993; 18: 252A.
27. Raymond R, Fallon M, Abrams G. Oral thymic extract for chronic hepatitis C in patients previously treated with interferon. Ann Intern Med 1998; 129: 797–800.
28. Sherman KE, Sjogren M, Creager RL, et al. Combination therapy with thymosin alpha-1 and interferon for the treatment of chronic hepatitis C infection: a randomized, placebo-controlled double-blind trial. Hepatology 1998; 27: 1128–1135.
29. De Smet PA. Health risks of herbal remedies. Drug Safety 1995; 13: 81–93.
30. Soma R, Ikeda M, Morise T, et al. Effect of glycyrrhizin on cortisol metabolism in humans. Endocr Regul 1994; 28: 31–34.
31. Bernardi M, D'Intino PE, Trevisani F, et al. Effects of prolonged ingestion of graded doses of licorice by healthy volunteers. Life Sci 1994; 55: 863–872.

32. Segelman A, Segelman F, Karliner J, Sophia R. Sassafras and herb tea. potential health hazards. JAMA 1976; 236: 447.
33. Brinker F. Modifying the effects of prothrombopenic anticoagulants. In: *Herb Contraindications and Drug Interactions.* Sandy, OR: Eclectic Medical, 1998, pp. 166–169.
34. Ingram K, Dragosavac G, Benner K, Flora K. Risks of drug interactions with St. John's Wort. Am J Gastroenterol 2000; 95: 3323,3324.
35. Ernst E. Harmless Herbs? A review of the recent literature. Am J Med 1998; 104: 170–178.
36. Lin SH, Lin MS. Survey on drug related hospitalisation(sic) in a community teaching hospital. Int J Clin Pharmacol Ther Toxicol 1993; 31: 66–69.
37. Chan T, Chan A, Critchley J. Hospital admissions due to adverse reactions to Chinese herbal medicines. J Trop Med Hyg 1992; 95: 296–298.
38. Perharic L, Shaw D, Colbridge L, et al. Toxicological problems resulting from exposure to traditional remedies and food supplements. Drug Safety 1994; 11: 284–294.
39. Abbot N, White A, Ernst E. Complementary medicine. Nature 1996; 381: 361.
40. Consumer Reports. November 1996.

13 Drugs and Chronic Viral Hepatitis

*Ajay Batra, MD,
Richard W. Lambrecht, PHD,
and Herbert L. Bonkovsky, MD*

CONTENTS

INTRODUCTION AND OVERVIEW
BRIEF OVERVIEW OF HEPATIC DRUG METABOLISM
MAJOR TYPES OF INJURY RESULTING FROM DRUGS
   AND TOXINS
ROLE OF ALCOHOL
EFFECTS OF CHRONIC VIRAL HEPATITIS ON DRUG
   METABOLISM OR HEPATOTOXICITY
SUMMARY AND RECOMMENDATIONS
ACKNOWLEDGMENTS
REFERENCES

INTRODUCTION AND OVERVIEW

This is a medicinal age. Indeed, it appears that it has always been so, because human kind, even in antiquity and prehistoric times, appears to have been fascinated with exogenous chemicals and xenobiotics that affect the mind and body. However, advances in therapeutics have been truly remarkable within the past one or two generations. Increasingly, new drugs are being developed, based on biochemical and structural knowledge of specific targets, such as site-directed inhibitors of enzymes in host human beings, or in infectious agents. Other drugs are targeted at specific receptors such as the histamine type-1 and -2 receptors, the several types of serotonin receptors, and so on.

From: *Clinical Gastroenterology: Diagnosis and Therapeutics*
Edited by: R. S. Koff and G. Y. Wu © Humana Press Inc., Totowa, NJ

Another reason for the widespread and increasing use of medicines is to be found in the heavy advertising now carried out by pharmaceutical companies. Such advertising is present in virtually all medical journals that enjoy wide readership by clinicians who may prescribe such medicines. In addition, in the past few years, there has been steadily increasing advertising directly to patients and their families and acquaintances, which now takes the form of advertisements for prescription drugs shown during prime-time popular television, and in newspapers and magazines.

Another reason for the increased use of drugs, both licit and illicit, is to be found in the affluence of modern American and other Western societies. Most people now have disposable income that they can use for the purchase of drugs, or herbal remedies, if they so choose. Indeed, such expenditures are one of the main reasons why total expenditure on health and beauty products in the United States takes up such a remarkably large percentage of gross domestic product (~15–20%).

Accompanying the increased awareness of orthodox drugs, there has been an increasing fascination with so-called "natural" or "herbal" remedies. This is part of the contemporary zeitgeist of seeking succor or benefit in alternative or complementary approaches to personal health care and treatment of disease. Patients with liver disease seem at least as interested in such alternative approaches and herbal remedies as are patients with other chronic diseases. Because current treatments for chronic hepatitis B and C (CHC) fall far short of the ideal, it is not surprising that so many patients with chronic viral hepatitis are taking herbal remedies, or have taken them in the past. For example, many (perhaps most) of the patients seen at our center with CHC have taken milk thistle, despite lack of evidence of its benefit in the treatment for chronic viral hepatitis. Further discussion of herbal remedies can be found in Chapter 12.

The other side of the coin is to stress caution in the use of drugs and chemicals in patients with liver diseases, including those with chronic viral hepatitis. Such caution is appropriate, because of the central role played by the liver in the metabolism of most drugs and chemicals, and because drug-induced hepatotoxicity remains a major risk. Such risk is by no means limited to prescription drugs, but also exists for numerous herbal remedies.

Although there is no evidence that allergic or idiosyncratic drug reactions are more likely to occur in patients with chronic viral hepatitis or other forms of chronic liver disease, such reactions, if they occur, may be more severe, and even fatal, in patients with advanced underlying liver disease. There probably is an increased but low risk of toxicity developing from certain potential hepatotoxins, such as acetaminophen or isoniazid. As is described in more detail below, acetaminophen is an example of a drug or chemical that normally is detoxified by conjugation to glutathione (GSH). Levels of GSH have been found to be decreased in livers of patients with CHC, even when the disease was not particularly advanced. It appears that CHC increases oxidative stress in hepatocytes, and it is this stress that causes partial depletion of stores of GSH.

This chapter first provides an overview of hepatic drug metabolism and the major forms of toxicity or injury caused by drugs and xenobiotics; it then considers the role of alcohol, the effects of chronic viral hepatitis, and the effects of therapy for viral hepatitis on drug metabolism. The authors conclude with summary recommendations.

BRIEF OVERVIEW OF HEPATIC DRUG METABOLISM

The liver is the primary site for the metabolism of a variety of endogenous and exogenous compounds. Typically, these compounds have mol wt of 300 or greater; they are lipophilic (more soluble in butanol than in water); and they are often tightly bound to plasma proteins (e.g., bilirubin and many therapeutic agents). The liver is able to remove these compounds from the circulation, because of the presence of receptors on the surface of hepatocytes, which allow the import of these compounds into the cells. Once inside the hepatocytes, a variety of biotransformation reactions occur, with the net effect of increasing the water solubility of the modified products. These modified products are then secreted into the bile and eliminated in the feces, or they are secreted back into the plasma, and eliminated by the kidney into the urine.

The hepatic biotransformation reactions can be divided into phase I reactions (the oxidation of the compound, often by hydroxylation) and phase II reactions (the conjugation of the oxidized product, especially at the newly formed hydroxylation site, to further enhance the water solubility of the modified compound).

Phase I reactions are carried out by the mixed-function oxidase system, whose enzymes are mostly located in the smooth endoplasmic reticulum. Cytochromes P-450 (a superfamily of hemoproteins, each with individual, but overlapping, substrate specificities) are the terminal components of an electron transport chain, and they are the enzymes that actually hydroxylate the substrates. These hydroxylations require reduced nicotinamide adenine dinucleotide phosphate (NADPH) (a source of electrons) and molecular oxygen. One oxygen atom is incorporated into the substrate, and the other is reduced to water, according to the formula:

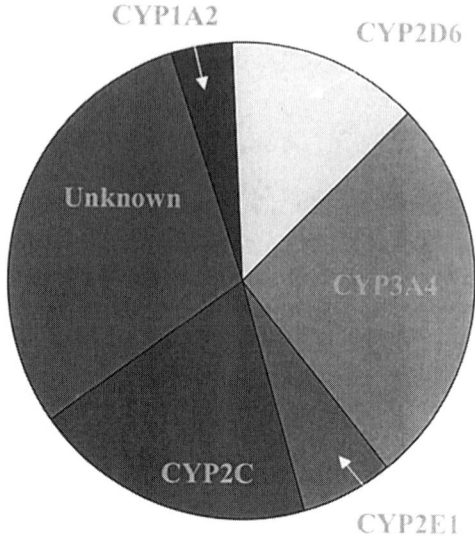

Fig. 1. Major forms of cytochromes P450 involved in human drug metabolism.

$$RH + O_2 + NADPH + H^+ \rightarrow ROH + H_2O + NADP^+$$

NADPH-cytochrome reductase is primarily responsible for supplying electrons to cytochrome P-450, but NADH and cytochrome b5 sometimes play supporting roles in supplying these electrons. Cytochromes P-450 participate in repeated cycles of reduction/oxidation as the substrates undergo hydroxylation reactions. A summary of the major human cytochromes P-450 that are involved in drug metabolism is shown in Fig. 1.

After the drug has been hydroxylated by cytochrome P-450, the phase II reactions come into play, and are summarized in Table 1.

MAJOR TYPES OF INJURY RESULTING FROM DRUGS AND TOXINS

Mechanisms of Drug-induced Hepatic Injury

OVERVIEW: TWO TYPES OF DRUG-INDUCED LIVER DISEASE

Although not all hepatic drug reactions fit neatly, it is useful, heuristically, to consider such reactions to be of two types: those that are predictable or dose-dependent, and those that are idiosyncratic or dose-independent *(1)*. These can be further characterized as toxic vs allergic-type injuries, respectively (*see* Table 2). In the presence of liver disease, the transformation of various drugs, from pharmacologically active to inactive compounds, may be impaired *(2)*.

Table 1
Summary of Phase II Drug Metabolism

Phase II reaction	Enzyme responsible	Conjugating moiety
Glucuronidation	Glucuronyl transferase	Uridine diphosphoglucuronic acid
Sulfation	Sulfotransferases	3'-phosphoadenosine-5'-phosphosulfate (PAPS)
GSH conjugation	GSH transferases	Reduces GSH
Epoxide hydration	Epoxide hydrolase	Water

Table 2
Key Features Differentiating Toxic from Allergic or Idiosyncratic-type Drug-induced Injury

Feature	Dose-dependent, toxic reaction	Allergic, idiosyncratic type reaction
Effects dose-related	Yes	No
Incidence	Occurs in virtually 100% of subjects, if enough chemical is administered	Rare and unpredictable
Effects can be produced in experimental animals with regularity.	Yes, predictably	No
Associated with fever, chills, eosinophilia, skin rash, or other signs of allergy	Not usually	Frequently
Effects reversible, if exposure stopped	Yes, although irreversible non-inflammatory damage may persist (e.g., cirrhosis or cancer)	Usually; but, rarely, inflammation persists and appears to be self-perpetuating.
Pathology of "pure" case	Parenchymal necrosis, fatty change, zonal degeneration, little inflammatory reaction	Lesions indistinguishable from viral hepatitis; some agents give rise usually to hepatocellular reactions; others to cholestatic. Fat is rare; granulomas, eosinophils common.
Examples of inciting compounds	Halogenated hydrocarbons, e.g., CCl_4, $CHCl_3$; aromatic hydrocarbons, e.g., bromobenzene; yellow phosphorus; senecio; toxins from amanita mushrooms; vinyl chloride; 17-alkyl androgens; acetaminophen; furosemide; halothane, in the presence of hypoxia	α-methyldopa; benzodiazepines; fluothane, isoniazid; hypoglycemic agents; oxyphenasitin; phenothiazines; thiazolidine diones (any drug or herbal remedy may be suspect in an individual case)

DOSE-DEPENDENT, TOXIC-TYPE HEPATOTOXICITY

The number of drugs that fall into the predictable category is small, partly because the usual doses of drugs result in plasma and tissue concentrations of the drugs or their metabolites, which are well below toxicity levels for most patients. However, attempts at keeping drug levels "safe" can fail for several reasons, including advanced age, genetically altered metabolism, interactions with other drugs, or underlying liver disease (e.g., chronic viral hepatitis). These conditions may interfere with normal drug clearance, resulting over a period of time in toxic concentrations. Such alterations are called "pharmacokinetic" changes *(1)*.

It should be noted that dosage and duration of therapy are not the only factors involved in drug toxicity that may be caused by the so-called "predictable" toxins. Other individual metabolic aberrations, which are poorly understood and unknown in most individual cases, probably account for many of the infrequent clinical manifestations of toxicity due to these agents *(1)*.

The presence of underlying liver diseases, such as chronic viral hepatitis, may predispose patients to greater dose-dependent toxicity, unless drug dosage is adjusted downward. This is especially true if the margin of safety between therapeutic and toxic concentrations is relatively small. The concept that antecedent liver disease puts patients at increased risk for drug-induced toxicity applies, of course, only to those drugs that depend on the liver for metabolism and elimination. It also assumes that the parent drugs, or one of their early metabolites, are toxic, and that the liver is damaged enough to impair drug elimination *(1)*. For example, a diseased liver may have decreased GSH stores or decreased GSH-generating capacity, making an individual more susceptible to the toxic effects of drugs such as acetaminophen. In other situations, prior liver damage may lessen the risk of drug-induced hepatotoxicity, because it may reduce the formation of toxic metabolites.

Chronic liver disease, including chronic viral hepatitis, can result in low serum albumin concentrations. Many drugs are highly bound to albumin, and, with a lower serum albumin, there is decreased drug binding and greater availability of free, unbound drugs to target tissues. This may result in greater drug effect and toxicity, and may be another effect of underlying chronic liver disease to increase the risk of drug toxicity *(1,3,4)*. Altered pharmacodynamics may also play a role in drug toxicity in patients with chronic liver disease. This toxicity may be exerted at the receptor level. The precise mechanism(s) of the adverse effects resulting from this are unclear, and warrant further study *(1,5)*.

Dose-independent
(Idiosyncratic or Allergic-type) Drug Toxicity

The majority of hepatic injury resulting from drugs is not dose-dependent. Rather, it seems to occur in individuals with a genetic susceptibility for generating an unusual metabolite, and/or who develop an immune response to the parent drug or a metabolite (usually the latter). This so-called idiosyncratic drug toxicity presents a challenge, because such reactions generally have not been observed in early phases (1–3) of drug testing, nor can individuals at risk be identified beforehand. The problem is usually only detected in phase 4 large-population, postmarketing surveys. Because, in most cases, the toxic effect is probably mediated by a drug metabolite, rather than by the parent drug, liver impairment does not promote toxicity. Indeed, it may even decrease the risk of occurrence. However, the liver may be more susceptible to damage secondary to decreased defenses resulting from underlying disease *(1,2)*. Currently, there are few examples of idiosyncratic drug reactions that are known to be enhanced by the presence of underlying liver disease *(1,6,7)*.

ROLE OF ALCOHOL

Alcohol is one of the most commonly used drugs in the United States. It is also one of the most abused substances in this country, with an estimated 15.3 million people suffering from alcoholism *(8)*. Alcohol alone, and in conjunction with other drugs, can play a major role in worsening liver disease in patients with chronic viral hepatitis, and, unfortunately, those with such hepatitis are more likely to abuse alcohol than the general population.

Alcohol contributes to progression of liver disease in viral hepatitis patients in several ways. The liver is the primary site of ethanol (EtOH) metabolism. Within the liver, EtOH is oxidized by three enzyme systems: the alcohol dehydrogenases, the microsomal ethanol-oxidizing system (MEOS, analogous to mixed-function oxidase system described above), and catalase. When hepatic levels of EtOH exceed 50 mg/dL, the MEOS contributes appreciably to EtOH oxidation. A critical component of the MEOS system is cytochrome P-450 2E1 (CYP2E1). This enzyme not only catalyzes EtOH oxidation, but also the metabolism of drugs such as acetaminophen and nitrosamines. With chronic alcohol consumption, there is upregulation of CYP2E1 *(8)*.

EtOH causes liver injury through several proposed mechanisms. One of these processes is an increase in oxidant stress. EtOH oxidation leads to formation of several free-radical species in hepatocytes, including the hydroxyethyl radical, the superoxide anion, and the hydroxyl radical.

These free radicals inflict oxidative damage on a wide range of intracellular compounds. They initiate a chain reaction of peroxidation of unsaturated lipids. In animal models of EtOH-induced liver injury, hepatic lipid peroxidation is associated with acute liver injury and fibrosis. In these models, lipid peroxidation is enhanced by adding polyunsaturated fat to the diet. These fats themselves are inducers of CYP2E1, and have the added effect of altering hepatic membrane lipid composition in favor of peroxidation *(8)*.

DNA is also sensitive to oxidant stress, and mitochondrial DNA is more susceptible to oxidative damage than nuclear DNA. Oxidants can cause both deletions and mutations in mitochondrial DNA, which can result in dysfunction of these critical organelles. Whether EtOH induces sufficient free-radical production to cause liver injury remains unclear, but the effects of radicals may be amplified if EtOH also reduces antioxidant defenses. Chronic EtOH consumption can also lead to the depletion of several hepatic antioxidants, including vitamins A and E, and GSH. Vitamin A depletion causes lysosomal damage, and vitamin E deficiency can enhance hepatic lipid peroxidation. GSH depletion induced by alcohol occurs selectively in hepatic mitochondria, and impairs their function *(8)*.

EtOH and Increased Acetaminophen Toxicity

Acetaminophen in low doses (≤ 2.5 g/d) is not absolutely contraindicated in patients with underlying liver disease. However, in conjunction with chronic alcohol consumption, enhanced metabolism of usually safe doses of acetaminophen to a toxic derivative may occur *(1,9)*. The mechanisms by which this occurs are shown in Fig. 2.

Acetaminophen is well-absorbed from the gastrointestinal tract, and is uniformly distributed throughout most body fluids. Conjugation occurs in the liver, mostly with glucuronic acid, and, to a smaller extent, with phosphoadenosine phospho-sulfate (PAPS) (Table 1; Fig. 2). 80% is excreted in the urine after hepatic conjugation. Hepatotoxicity caused by overdose results from the formation of a highly reactive intermediary metabolite of acetaminophen, N-acetyl-p-benzoquinoneimine, produced by the action of cytochromes P450, especially CYP 2E1 and CYP 1A1/2. As described above, chronic heavy EtOH induces CYP2E1, thus increasing formation of acetaminophen's toxic metabolite. Heavy EtOH use also depletes GSH. Then, too, persons who drink heavily often eat poorly, and this may cause further depletion of GSH. Thus, the combination of large amounts of EtOH and acetaminophen, as well as chronic EtOH consumption and acetaminophen, should be avoided in all patients, particularly those with chronic liver disease, such as chronic viral hepatitis.

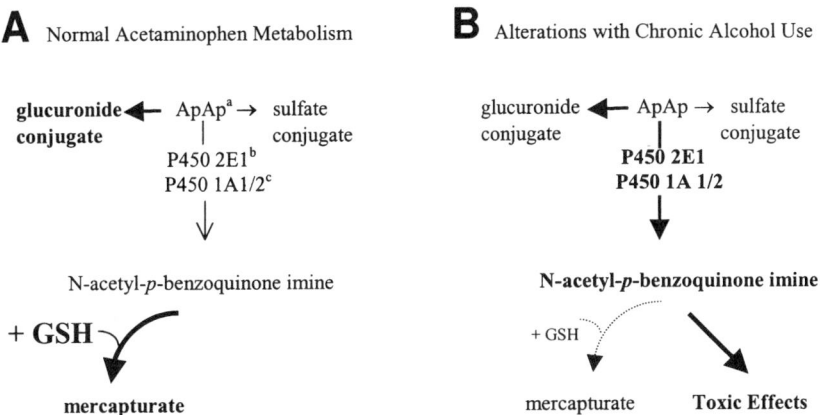

Fig. 2. Effects of chronic alcohol use on acetaminophen (Ap Ap) metabolism and toxicity.

EtOH and Increased Methotrexate Toxicity

Methotrexate (MTX) may induce liver damage. The pathogenesis of hepatotoxicity with MTX is poorly understood. Some patients may develop fibrosis or cirrhosis, following long-term treatment with MTX. However, several studies, with serial liver biopsies during continued treatment, have shown that MTX-induced liver cirrhosis is not of an aggressive nature. Alcohol has been cited as a major contributing factor to development of cirrhosis in patients treated chronically with MTX *(10,11)*. There is a strong association with previous or concurrent heavy EtOH intake and host susceptibility to injury by MTX *(12)*. Pre-existing hepatic injury, as may be seen with chronic viral hepatitis, may also contribute to injury with MTX *(12)*. Whenever chronic MTX use is contemplated, discontinuation of alcohol use should be recommended.

In addition, careful patient screening and selection are advisable. Patients should be screened, at baseline, for potential risk factors for liver disease, including chronic viral hepatitis. The American College of Rheumatology recommends routine periodic measurement of serum aspartate aminotransferase (AST), alanine aminotransferase (ALT), alkaline phosphatase, albumin, total bilirubin, hepatitis B and hepatitis C serologies, complete blood count, and serum creatinine in all patients receiving MTX. A pretreatment liver biopsy is recommended for patients with prior excessive alcohol consumption, persistently abnormal baseline serum AST or ALT values, and/or chronic hepatitis B and/or CHC infections. Serum AST, ALT, and albumin levels should be monitored at 4- to 8-wk intervals during MTX therapy. The American College of Rheumatology recommends liver biopsy, if 5/9 AST determinations within a 12-

mo interval are abnormal, or there is a decrease in serum albumin below the normal range. Based on the findings at liver biopsy, there are criteria to help decide whether MTX should be continued or discontinued. In patients with persistent liver test abnormalities, or who refuse biopsy, current recommendations are to discontinue MTX *(12)*.

EtOH and Increased Damage Caused by Iron Overload

Excessive iron (Fe) in the body is toxic to many cells. High Fe levels *per se* (as in hemochromatosis) can cause cirrhosis, liver failure, and hepatocellular carcinoma *(13,14)*. There is also growing evidence that only mildly increased, or even normal, amounts of Fe can cause or enhance hepatic injury in the presence of alcohol. Evidence is now accumulating that Fe can also potentiate hepatotoxicity caused by other etiologies, such as chronic viral hepatitis *(13)*. In addition, Fe overload may facilitate or exacerbate microbial infections, and suppress the ability of the host's immune system to overcome such infections. Abnormalities in serum parameters of Fe status (ferritin, transferrin saturation) are common in patients with chronic viral hepatitis, probably because of the release of Fe from injured hepatocytes. The increased, metabolically active Fe, in turn, may increase the severity of chronic viral hepatitis and the degree of hepatocyte damage *(13)*. Some of the proposed mechanisms to account for this include nonspecific effects, such as increased oxidative stress, enhanced lipid peroxidation, depletion of hepatoprotective factors, and exacerbation of immune-mediated tissue inflammation *(15)*. Other possible mechanisms include enhancement of rates of viral replication and increased rates of viral mutation. Fe may also impair host cellular immunity through several means, including impairment of antigen-presenting cells, impairment of T-lymphocyte proliferation and maturation, as well as other possibilities *(15)*.

In patients with chronic viral hepatitis, somewhat higher levels of hepatic Fe have been associated with a decreased likelihood of response to therapy with interferon-α2b (IFN-α2b). Recent evidence indicates that Fe-depletion therapy, prior to IFN therapy, increases the likelihood of a favorable response to IFN *(13,16,17)*.

EtOH may play a role in enhancing the deleterious effects of Fe. A synergism between Fe and alcohol has been shown clearly in experimental studies. For example, the livers of EtOH-fed rats were more susceptible to Fe-catalyzed lipid peroxidation and hepatic fibrogenesis. In these EtOH-fed animals, accentuated liver injury and fibrogenesis were associated with relatively small increases in liver Fe concentrations, which were near the upper limit of normal for human subjects. Thus, it is tempting to speculate that the threshold concentration of hepatic Fe for developing liver damage is lower in patients with alcohol liver disease than in those without *(18)*. This may also have significance for patients with chronic viral hepatitis. In the study on rats mentioned above, worsening of liver damage by alcohol and Fe occurred in animals receiving a diet high in saturated fat *(18)*. Such animals probably have increased oxidative stress related to fatty livers, which is potentiated by Fe overload. They resemble humans with fatty livers, in whom there are increased risks of developing cirrhosis, especially with the addition of alcohol and Fe overload.

Alcohol and Chronic Viral Hepatitis

The most common form of nonalcohol-induced liver disease seen in patients with alcoholism is CHC *(7)*. In patients with CHC, chronic alcoholism has been shown to cause more severe and rapidly progressive liver disease. This can lead more frequently to cirrhosis of the liver and hepatocellular carcinoma. Alcohol intake in excess of 10 g/d has been associated with increased serum hepatitis C viral RNA and aminotransferase levels *(7)*. The mechanisms of these increases are poorly understood, but, as mentioned, Fe may enhance viral replication and/or reduce immune-dependent viral killing. The histological picture in hepatitis C patients with chronic alcohol abuse is usually indistinguishable from that in CHC patients who do not use EtOH. In alcoholic patients, compared with nonalcoholic patients, IFN therapy has been shown to be less effective, even after a period of abstinence. Alcohol intake should be restricted to 10 g/d or less in patients with CHC. If cirrhosis is present, or IFN therapy is planned, abstinence should be encouraged *(7)*.

Several studies *(6,19)* have shown that heavy alcohol intake, particularly more than 60 g/d, may enhance the viral inflammatory changes in the liver of patients with persistent hepatitis B antigenemia.

EFFECTS OF CHRONIC VIRAL HEPATITIS ON DRUG METABOLISM OR HEPATOTOXICITY

Dose-dependent Hepatotoxicity

Chronic Viral Hepatitis Is not Unique Among Liver Diseases

As already described, in patients with advanced chronic liver disease, there clearly are increased risks of hepatotoxicity or other toxicity effects caused by drugs and other xenobiotics. Some clinically important examples are listed in Table 3. More extensive lists may be found in refs. *9* and *20*.

Few studies of drug metabolism or population-based surveys of hepatotoxicity have been carried out in patients with chronic viral hepatitis. There is no recognized unique aspect of chronic viral hepatitis known to be a predisposing cause of increased drug- or toxin-dependent hepatotoxicity.

Table 3
Selected Dose-dependent, Drug-induced Toxicity in Chronic Liver Disease

Agent	Risk factors	Comments
Acetaminophen	Induction of CYP1A1, 2E (chronic alcohol) Co-existing cardio or respiratory disease (decreased pO_2 in liver) Nutritional state (decreased GSH in liver)	Risks are greatest in chronic alcohol abusers.
Aminoglycosides	High drug levels; chronic use Hypotension	Severe renal effects likely in advanced liver disease (early hepatorenal syndrome)
Aspirin	High drug level Presence of rheumatoid disease Use of other drugs that inhibit 3A4 Hypoalbuminemia Hyperbilirubinemia (decreased albumin binding)	Severe renal effects likely in advanced liver disease (early hepatorenal syndrome)
Benzodiazepines	Decreased CYP activities Increased central nervous system sensitivities Possible endogenous or "natural" drug-like compounds	Oxazepam metabolism less affected, because phase 2 only
Cyclosporine	High drug level CYP3A4 phenotype Use of other drugs that inhibit CYP3A4	Konazole-type antifungals and macrolide antibiotics are potent inhibitors of CYP3A4
Methotrexate	Total dose Alcohol use Concomitant fatty liver (alcoholism, diabetes mellitus, NASH, obesity)	Risks higher in psoriatics than rheumatoids
NSAIDs	High drug levels Hypoalbuminemia Hyperbilirubinemia (decreased albumin binding)	Severe renal effects likely in advanced liver disease (early hepatorenal syndrome)

CYP, Cytochrome P-450; GSH, reduced glutathione; NASH, nonalcoholic steatohepatitis; NSAIDs, nonsteroidal anti-inflammatory drugs.

Thus, for the present, one should assume that patients with chronic viral hepatitis will respond to drugs and toxins like other patients with chronic liver disease of similar severity, regardless of cause.

INTERPLAY OF FACTORS INFLUENCES DOSE-DEPENDENT HEPATOTOXICITY

When one considers that 3–4 million Americans have CHC infections, and that the use of many over-the-counter and prescription drugs and natural products continues to grow steadily, it is remarkable that dose-dependent hepatotoxicity is reported so rarely. The reasons for this are not entirely clear. Perhaps many instances are unrecognized, with episodic rises in serum liver enzymes being wrongly ascribed to fluctuations in the activity of the underlying chronic hepatitis, or to alcohol use. Doubtless, an important reason is that, for most drugs, the doses commonly used are relatively low, and the therapeutic indices are high. As discussed above, in many instances in which toxicity is mediated by a toxic metabolite, the presence of liver disease may decrease the rate or extent of formation of the metabolite, and actually exert a protective effect. Then, too, most authorities advise all patients with chronic liver disease not to drink alcohol (or to drink only occasionally, and not more than one drink per day). This decreases the induction of CYP2E and minimizes alcohol-dependent toxicity.

On the whole, a complex, variable, and poorly defined interplay of factors, including the inciting drug or chemical, the host, and the environment, leads to the final outcome of toxicity or lack of toxicity in patients (Fig. 3).

Idiosyncratic (Unpredictable) Hepatotoxicity

As already described, the great majority of liver injury caused by drugs and chemicals falls into this category. Indeed, virtually every systemically absorbed drug has been implicated in producing hepatic injury. As a result, package inserts of most drugs contain warnings recommending avoidance of the drugs in patients with chronic liver disease.

Although this is the safest course of action, it should not be applied only to patients with underlying liver disease. Drugs should be avoided by everyone, unless their use is clearly indicated. In fact, there is no credible evidence that underlying chronic liver disease increases the risk of development of an idiosyncratic drug reaction. However, there can be little doubt that, if such an untoward hepatic reaction occurs, the effects on the patient are likely to be worse if the patient has underlying advanced liver disease. The addition of an idiosyncratic drug reaction may be the straw that breaks the camel's back.

INTERPLAY OF FACTORS INFLUENCES ALLERGIC OR IDIOSYNCRATIC HEPATOTOXICITY

As for dose-dependent hepatotoxicity, in all likelihood, a complex interplay of host and environmental factors influences the development and evolution of allergic or idiosyncratic hepatitis (Fig. 4).

A priori, there is simply no way to anticipate which patients will develop such toxicity, nor is any test or group of tests likely to provide such

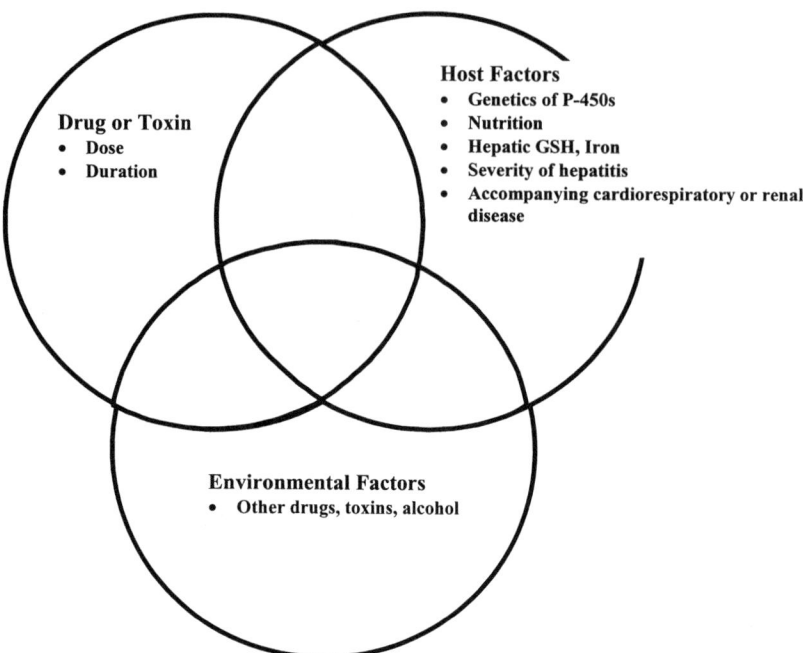

Fig. 3. Interplay of factors that influence dose-dependent hepatotoxicity in patients with viral hepatitis.

prospective information in the foreseeable future. It does seem likely that patients with strong family or personal histories of allergic diatheses are at increased risk for developing allergies to drugs. However, because the actual development of such allergies is infrequent, specific drugs are not contraindicated for such patients, unless they have convincing histories of prior allergy to the same or related drugs.

Effects of Current Therapy of Chronic Viral Hepatitis on Drug Metabolism

INTERFERONS

IFN-α and other type-1 IFNs have been shown to affect phase I drug metabolism, potentially increasing the risk of adverse drug interactions. Not unexpectedly, these effects depend on the particular isoenzyme of cytochrome P-450 that is under consideration. Horsmans et al. *(21)* investigated the effect of IFN-α on the cytochrome P-450-mediated metabolism of ^{14}C-aminopyrine, in patients with CHC. They found a

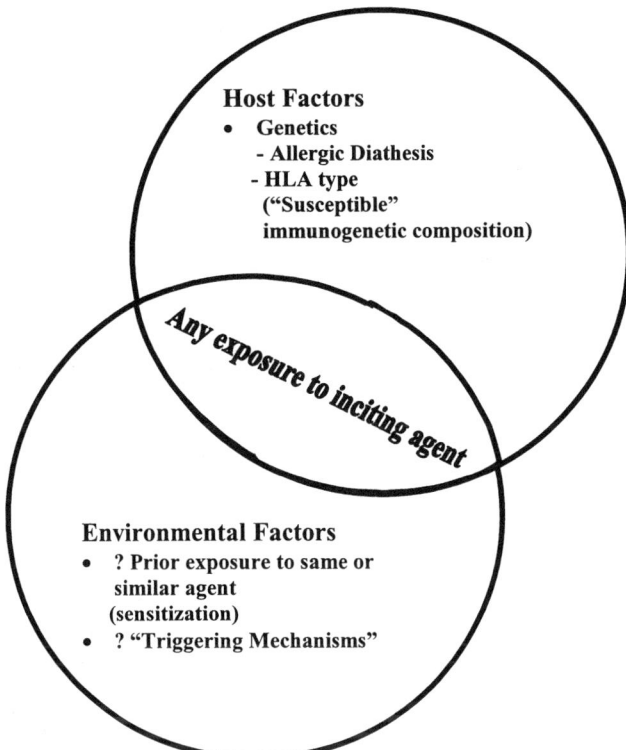

Fig. 4. Interplay of factors that influence allergic or idiosyncratic responses to drugs or toxins in patients with viral hepatitis.

significant transient inhibition of this cytochrome P-450 activity, and they recommended that this finding be taken into account when prescribing concurrent therapy with drugs that are metabolized by this pathway. However, since the *N*-demethylation of aminopyrine is efficiently catalyzed by a number of human cytochromes P-450, including CYP2C19, 2C8, 2D6, 2C18, and 1A2 *(22)*, the task of predicting the effect of IFN on metabolism of concurrently administered drugs is complicated.

In a recent study, Pageaux et al. *(23)* studied the effects of IFN-α on in vivo caffeine metabolism (as a measure of CYP1A2 activity) and in vivo cortisol metabolism (as a measure of CYP3A activity) in patients with CHC. They found no significant changes in either of these activities, and concluded that drugs that are metabolized by these isoenzymes can be used together with IFN-α, without a significant risk of adverse drug interactions.

The mechanisms by which type-1 interferons affect the regulation of cytochromes P-450 are often unclear, and they may vary with the specific isoenzyme of cytochrome P-450. Delaporte and Renton *(24)* report that rats treated with polyinosinic acid-polycytidylic acid (an inducer of both IFN-α and IFN-β) had decreased transcription rates for CYP1A1 and CYP1A2, and increased rates of degradation of hepatic CYP1A1 and CYP1A2 mRNAs. These results support the involvement of both transcriptional and posttranscriptional mechanisms in the loss of these cytochromes P-450 mediated by IFN.

The possible role of nitric oxide in the downregulation of cytochrome P-450 has been examined. Carlson and Billings *(25)* found that the downregulation of cytochrome P-450 by two cytokines (tumor necrosis factor-α and interleukin-1 β) in vitro was directly associated with nitric oxide production. By contrast, Hodgson and Renton *(26)* found no evidence in mice that the downregulation of cytochrome P-450 by IFN or its inducers involves nitric oxide as a required intermediary. A role for xanthine oxidase in the loss of cytochrome P-450 mediated by IFN in the livers of hamsters has also been proposed *(27)*.

There have been a number of reported examples of IFN–drug interactions. Treatment with IFN-α was reported to potentiate the anticoagulant effects of warfarin (coumadin) in a woman with CHC *(28)*. Also, influenza vaccination, which is known to increase endogenous production of IFNs, was reported to increase the anticoagulant effect of warfarin *(29)*. IFN-α slows the clearance of some highly metabolized drugs, such as theophylline *(30)*; for example, the clearance of theophylline was reduced by 33% in cancer patients treated with IFN-α *(31)*.

In addition to causing adverse drug reactions secondary to modulations of phase I metabolism, IFNs sometimes cause autoimmune diseases. Bell et al. *(32)* found that low-titer autoantibodies were a risk factor for the development of autoimmune disease during treatment with IFN-α for CHC infections. They also report that patients with no detectable autoantibodies have a low risk for developing autoimmune complications during treatment with IFN-α *(33,34)*. Although IFN frequently induces the formation of autoantibodies, the presence of these autoantibodies, either before or after IFN treatments, should not be considered a contraindication to interferon therapy *(33,34)*.

Ribavirin

Ribavirin induces hemolysis *(35)*, which can lead to subsequent increases in hepatic Fe stores *(36)*, particularly in hepatocytes *(37)*. The combination of treatment with ribavirin plus other drugs that increase hemolysis, or with a partial deficiency of glucose-6-phosphate dehydrogenase, significantly increases the development of symptomatic anemia. The clinically significant adverse events associated with ribavirin treatment include anemia and depression *(38,39)*. In the authors' clinical experience of treating several hundred patients with IFN plus ribavirin for CHC, the most important side effects of ribavirin have been anemia, which has been particularly severe among men treated with high doses (1200 mg/d), depression and development of a pruritic, scaling skin rash (Bonkovsky, unpublished observation). These have required dose reduction or cessation of ribavirin therapy in ~20% of treated patients *(39)*.

DRUGS OF SPECIAL IMPORTANCE IN PATIENTS WITH CHRONIC VIRAL HEPATITIS

Drugs Used in Therapy of Tuberculosis. Antimycobacterial drugs (INH, rifampin, pyrazinamide) are well-known for their propensity to cause elevations of serum aminotransferases and idiosyncratic liver injury, particularly in older women. A recent study from Hong Kong *(40)*, in patients given antituberculous drugs, reported that the incidence of worsening serum aminotransferases was significantly greater in patients treated with these drugs who also had chronic hepatitis B (15/43, 35%) than in those without (26/276, 9%).

Highly Active Antiretroviral Therapies (HAART). Many of the nucleoside analogs, protease inhibitors, and other newer drugs used for therapy of human immune deficiency virus (HIV) infection, cause hepatotoxicity *(41)*. Large numbers of patients are co-infected with HIV and with HBV, HCV, and/or hepatitis D virus. Although a reasonable hypothesis is that such co-infected patients might experience greater hepatotoxicity than those infected only with HIV, this hypothesis has not yet been tested rigorously, either with retrospective case-control or prospective, broad-based observational studies. Even if it were shown to be true, given the serious nature of uncontrolled HIV infection, it would still be medically necessary to treat such patients with HAART, with frequent, careful follow-up of liver chemicals and symptoms.

SUMMARY AND RECOMMENDATIONS

Adjustments in Drug Doses in Chronic Viral Hepatitis or Other Chronic Liver Disease

The need for adjustments in drug doses depends on the drug and the severity of liver disease. In general, adjustments are not needed for the minority of drugs that are not metabolized by the liver, unless there is concomitant renal insufficiency. Functional renal insufficiency is, of course, common in severe, advanced liver disease.

Table 4
Summary Recommendations for Drug Use and Dose Adjustments in Chronic Viral Hepatitis or other Chronic Liver Diseases

Whenever possible:
 Use drugs that do not require hepatic metabolism.
 Use drugs that do not require phase 1 hepatic metabolism.
 Use drugs that do not have high hepatic extraction (little or no "first-pass" metabolism).
When drugs that require hepatic metabolism are needed;
 adjust doses based on Childs-Turcotte-Pugh scores;
 5–6 (Class A): No adjustment.
 7–9 (Class B): Decrease dose by 25–33%.
 10–15 (Class C): Decrease dose by 50%.
Observe patients with advanced liver disease closely and frequently, whenever new drugs are started.
Primum nil nocere: First, do no harm.
 The best drugs are often those that are withheld.

Most drugs do undergo hepatic biotransformation. As already described, hepatic phase 2 (conjugation) reactions are maintained more nearly normally than are phase 1 (CYP-dependent hydroxylation) reactions in patients with chronic liver disease. Therefore, whenever possible, drugs that do not require phase 1 metabolism are to be preferred (e.g., oxazepam in pref-erence to diazepam, or most other benzodiazepines).

The other major factors that affect hepatic drug metabolism are binding to serum proteins (especially albumin), hepatic blood flow, and accessibility of drugs in the liver to functional hepatocytes. Drugs that are are highly extracted are generally affected most markedly by advanced chronic liver disease, because of marked decreases in first-pass metabolism due to portosystemic shunts, intrahepatic shunts, and capillarization of the space of Disse, all of which diminish the exposure of the drug to functional hepatocytes and their receptors and drug transporters.

In view of such complexities, and in absence of a simple, widely available, well-validated approach for estimating hepatic function, it is currently possible only to offer general guidelines for adjustments of drug doses in chronic viral hepatitis or other chronic liver diseases (Table 4). The need for care, and circumspection in prescribing, increases markedly as the severity of liver disease increases. Although patients with decompensated, end-stage cirrhosis have many symptoms, and often feel miserable, it is unwise to prescribe sedatives or strong analgesics, because of the risk of precipitating or worsening encephalopathy. Close observation and follow-up are mandatory for all such patients, but especially whenever new drugs are prescribed. Fortunately, most patients with chronic viral hepatitis are well-compensated (Childs-Turcotte-Pugh score 5–6), and drugs can be used in them with greater freedom.

ACKNOWLEDGMENTS

The authors thank Jan Smith, Cathy DeCaire, and Mary Taubert for help with typing the manuscript and preparing figures. Supported by grants and contracts from National Institutes of Health (R01-DK38825 and N01-DK-9-2326, to H. L. B. and DK56665-01 to R. W. L.). The opinions expressed in this chapter are those of the authors, and do not necessarily reflect the official views of the University of Massachusetts Medical School, the U.S. Public Health Service, or the National Institutes of Health.

REFERENCES

1. Schenker S, Ralston R, Hoyumpa AM. Antecedent liver disease and drug toxicity. J Hepatol 1999; 31: 1098–1105.
2. Hoyumpa AM, Schenker S. Influence of liver disease on the disposition and elimination of drugs. In: *Diseases of the Liver* (Schiff L, Schiff ER, eds.), 7th ed. Philadelphia: JB Lippincott, 1993, pp. 784–824.
3. Greenblatt DJ, Koch-Weser J. Clinical toxicity of chlordiazepoxide and diazepam in relation to serum albumin concentration: a report from the Boston Collaborative Drug Surveillance Program. Eur J Clin Pharmacol 1974; 7: 259–262.
4. Roberts MS, Rumble RH, Wanwimolruk DT, et al. Pharmacokinetics of aspirin and dalicylate in elderly subjects and in patients with alcoholic liver disease. Eur J Clin Pharmacol 1983; 25: 253–261.
5. Branch RA. Is there increased cerebral sensitivity to benzodiazepines in chronic liver disease? Hepatology 1987; 7: 772–776.
6. Murata T, Hideki T, Watanabe S, et al. Enhancement of chronic viral hepatic changes by alcohol intake in patients with persistent HBs-antigenemia. Am J Clin Pathol 1990; 94: 270–273.
7. Schiff ER. Hepatitis C and alcohol. Hepatology 1997; 26(Suppl 1): 39S–42S.
8. Maher J. Alcoholic liver disease. In: *Gastrointestinal and Liver Disease* (Sleisenger MH, Fordtran JS, eds.), 6th ed. Philadelphia: Saunders, 1998, pp. 1199–1202.
9. Westphal JF, Brogard JM. Drug administration in chronic liver disease. Drug Safety 1997; 17: 47–73.
10. Zachariae H, Sogaard H. Methotrexate-induced liver cirrhosis. Dermatologica 1987; 175: 178–182.
11. West SG. Methotrexate hepatotoxicity. Rheum Dis Clin NA 1997; 23: 883–914.
12. Lewis JH, Schiff E. Methotrexate-induced chronic liver injury: guidelines for detection and prevention. Am J Gastroenterol 1988; 88: 1337–1345.
13. Bonkovsky HL, Banner BF, Lambrecht RW, et al. Iron in liver diseases other than hemochromatosis. Sem in Liver Dis 1996; 16: 65–82.
14. Barton JC, Edwards CQ, eds. Part V of Hemochromatosis: Genetics, Pathophysiology, Diagnosis, and Treatment. Cambridge UK: Cambridge University Press, 2000, pp. 229–328.

15. Bonkovsky HL, Banner BF, Rothman AL. Iron and chronic viral hepatitis. Hepatology 1997; 25: 759–768.
16. Fong TL, Han SH, Tsai NC, et al. Pilot randomized, controlled trial of the effect of iron depletion on long-term response to alpha-interferon in patients with chronic hepatitis C. J Hepatol 1998; 28: 369–374.
17. Fontana RJ, Israel J, LeClair P, et al. Iron reduction prior to and during interferon therapy of chronic hepatitis C: results of a multi-center, randomized, controlled trial. Hepatology 2000; 31: 730–736.
18. Tsukamoto H, Horne W, Seiichiro K, et al. Experimental liver cirrhosis induced by alcohol and iron. J Clin Invest 1995; 96: 620–630.
19. Kondili LA, Tosti ME, Szklo M, et al. Relationships of chronic hepatitis and cirrhosis to alcohol intake, hepatitis B and C, and delta virus infection: a case-control study in Albania. Epidemiol Infect 1998; 121: 391–395.
20. Farrell, GC. Drug Induced Liver Disease. Melbourne: Churchill Livingstone, 1994.
21. Horsmans Y, Brenard R, Geubel AP. Short report: interferon-alpha decreases 14C-aminopyrine breath test values in patients with chronic hepatitis C. Aliment Pharmacol Ther 1994; 8: 353–355.
22. Niwa T, Sato R, Yabusaki Y, et al. Contribution of human hepatic cytochrome P450s and steroidogenic CYP17 to the N-demethylation of aminopyrine. Xenobiotica 1999; 29: 187–193.
23. Pageaux GP, le Bricquir Y, Berthou F, et al. Effects of interferon-alpha on cytochrome P-450 isoforms 1A2 and 3A activities in patients with chronic hepatitis C. Eur J Gastroenterol Hepatol 1998; 10: 491–495.
24. Delaporte E, Renton KW. Cytochrome P4501A1 and cytochrome P4501A2 are downregulated at both transcriptional and post-transcriptional levels by conditions resulting in interferon-alpha/beta induction. Life Sci 1997; 60: 787–796.
25. Carlson TJ, Billings RE. Role of nitric oxide in the cytokine-mediated regulation of cytochrome P-450. Mol Pharmacol 1996; 49: 796–801.
26. Hodgson PD, Renton KW. Role of nitric oxide generation in interferon-evoked cytochrome P450 downregulation. Int J Immunopharmacol 1995; 17: 995–1000.
27. Moochhala SM, Renton KW. Role for xanthine oxidase in the loss of cytochrome P-450 evoked by interferon. Can J Physiol Pharmacol 1991; 69: 944–950.
28. Adachi Y, Yokoyama Y, Nanno T, et al. Potentiation of warfarin by interferon. Br Med J 2000; 311: 292.
29. Kramer P, Tsuru M, Cook CE, et al. Effect of influenza vaccine on warfarin anticoagulation. Clin Pharmacol Ther 1984; 35: 416–418.
30. Dorr RT. Interferon-alpha in malignant and viral diseases. A review. Drugs 1993; 45: 177–211.
31. Israel BC, Blouin RA, McIntyre W, et al. Effects of interferon-alpha monotherapy on hepatic drug metabolism in cancer patients. Br J Clin Pharmacol 1993; 36: 229–235.
32. Bell TM, Bansal AS, Shorthouse C, et al. Low-titre auto-antibodies predict autoimmune disease during interferon-alpha treatment of chronic hepatitis C. J Gastroenterol Hepatol 1999; 14: 419–422.
33. Clifford BD, Donahue D, Smith L, et al. High prevalence of serological markers of autoimmunity in patients with chronic hepatitis C. Hepatology 1995; 21: 613–619.
34. Heller J, Musiolik J, Homrighausen A, et al. Occurrence and significance of autoantibodies in the course of interferon therapy of chronic hepatitis C. Dtsch Med Wochenschr 1996; 121: 1179–1183.
35. Di Bisceglie AM, Shindo M, Fong TL, et al. Pilot study of ribavirin therapy for chronic hepatitis C. Hepatology 1992; 16: 649–654.

36. Di Bisceglie AM, Bacon BR, Kleiner DE, et al. Increase in hepatic iron stores following prolonged therapy with ribavirin in patients with chronic hepatitis C. J Hepatol 1994; 21: 1109–1112.
37. Fiel MI, Schiano TD, Guido M, et al. Increased hepatic iron deposition resulting from treatment of chronic hepatitis C with ribavirin. Am J Clin Pathol 2000; 113: 35–39.S
38. Maddrey WC. Safety of combination interferon-alfa-2b/ribavirin therapy in chronic hepatitis C-relapsed and treatment-naive patients. Semin Liver Dis 1999; 19: 67–75.
39. Bonkovsky HL, Stefancyk D, Tortorelli K, et al. Comparative effects of different doses of ribavirin (600 vs. 1000–1200 mg per day) plus interferon alpha-2b for therapy of chronic hepatitis C: results of a controlled, randomized trial, submitted, 2000.
40. Wong W-M, Wu P-C, Yuen M-F, et al. Antituberculosis drug-related liver dysfunction in chronic hepatitis B infection. Hepatology 2000; 31: 201–206.
41. Hanna GJ, Hirsch MS. Antiretroviral therapy of human immunodeficiency virus infection. In: *Principles and Practice of Infectious Diseases* (Mandell GL, Bennett JE, Dolin R, eds.), 5th ed. Philadelphia: Churchill Livingstone, 2000, pp. 1479–1499.

14 Chronic Viral Hepatitis and Liver Transplantation

Aijaz Ahmed, MD and Emmet B. Keeffe, MD

CONTENTS

INTRODUCTION
INDICATIONS FOR LIVER TRANSPLANTATION
CHRONIC VIRAL CO-INFECTION
CHRONIC HEPATITIS B VIRUS INFECTION
CHRONIC HEPATITIS C VIRUS INFECTION
CONCLUSION
REFERENCES

INTRODUCTION

End-stage liver disease, secondary to chronic hepatitis C virus (HCV) infection, is the most common indication for liver transplantation worldwide. Historically, the first liver transplantations, for decompensated cirrhosis caused by chronic viral hepatitis, were performed in the 1970s, in patients with chronic hepatitis B virus (HBV) infection. According to data from the United Network of Organ Sharing (UNOS), of the more than 4000 liver transplantations performed annually in the United States from 1994 to 1998, 23% were for chronic hepatitis C (CHC), 16% for alcoholic cirrhosis, 7% for both alcoholic cirrhosis and hepatitis C, 4% for chronic hepatitis B, and 4% for acute liver failure, including hepatitis A or hepatitis B *(1)*. Liver transplantation for chronic viral hepatitis has evolved rapidly over the past two decades, with reduced re-infection rates and improved outcomes for patients with end-stage chronic hepatitis B,

From: *Clinical Gastroenterology: Diagnosis and Therapeutics*
Edited by: R. S. Koff and G. Y. Wu © Humana Press Inc., Totowa, NJ

and the rise of CHC as the most common indication for liver transplantation. The optimal management of the patient with moderate or severe recurrent hepatitis C after liver transplantation is the focus of intense study, but continues to remain uncertain.

In the United States, the expected overall 1-yr survival rate after liver transplantation for chronic viral hepatitis is 85–90%, and the majority of patients who survive have excellent quality of life, and are able to resume full-time activities at work or at home *(1,2)*. These improved results are a reflection of multiple medical and surgical factors, including more effective prophylaxis against re-infection, in the case of liver transplantation for chronic hepatitis B. With the use of newer immunosuppressive drug regimens, rejection is now seldom a cause of early or late graft failure. The major problem in patients with chronic viral hepatitis, who undergo liver transplantation, is the management of recurrent viral infection with allograft dysfunction.

INDICATIONS FOR LIVER TRANSPLANTATION

The selection and listing of patients with UNOS for liver transplantation has become more standardized over the past several years. The primary criterion for placement of a patient on the liver transplantation waiting list is an estimated 1-yr survival from chronic liver disease of less than 90%, which is the expected outcome with liver transplantation at most centers *(3)*. This criterion is based on a Child-Turcotte-Pugh (CTP) score of ≥7 for patients with cirrhosis, i.e., CTP class B or C. Cirrhotic patients who have experienced gastrointestinal bleeding caused by varices, or a single episode of spontaneous bacterial peritonitis, have reduced survival, and are also considered to meet minimal criteria for transplant listing, irrespective of their CTP score.

CHRONIC VIRAL CO-INFECTION

Patients with HBV and hepatitis D virus (HDV) co-infection demonstrate more rapid progression to cirrhosis, compared to patients with isolated HBV infection *(4)*. However, after liver transplantation, the outcome is favorable in patients who are co-infected prior to liver transplantation, in part because HDV downregulates HBV replication. Patients who are co-infected with HBV and HDV usually develop HDV infection of the liver allograft early posttransplant, without markers of HBV infection *(4)*. The course of isolated HDV infection after liver transplantation is indolent, and usually results in spontaneous resolution, except when HBV recurs.

Between 10 and 20% of patients with chronic hepatitis B have detectable anti-HCV *(4,5)*. Alternatively, 2–10% of patients with anti-HCV demonstrate markers of HBV infection. Co-infection with HBV and HCV results in more severe liver disease, compared to patients with isolated HBV or HCV infection. Posttransplant, HCV suppresses HBV, and thereby improves the clinical outcome of patients co-infected with HBV and HCV, compared to patients with isolated HBV infection. Retrospective observation of liver transplantation recipients, with HBV, HCV, and HDV co-infection, demonstrates suppression of HCV replication and a mild necroinflammatory response on biopsy *(5)*. Hepatitis G virus (HGV) is a RNA virus that is parenterally transmitted, and can be frequently found in patients with chronic HCV infection. Infection with HGV is often persistent, but the association of HGV with liver disease is controversial. The HGV persists in patients with HCV and HGV co-infection after liver transplantation, but appears to have no influence on the posttransplant course of recurrent hepatitis C *(6)*.

This chapter focuses on a practical discussion of current knowledge of liver transplantation (indications, management, and outcomes) in the care of patients with chronic hepatitis B and CHC.

CHRONIC HEPATITIS B VIRUS INFECTION

Chronic hepatitis B is a major global public health problem. There are an estimated 350 million chronic HBV virus carriers worldwide. The prevalence rate of chronic hepatitis B is as high as 15–20% in some countries in Asia. Chronic HBV infection may cause advanced liver disease. Once decompensated end-stage liver disease develops, prognosis is poor, with 5-yr survival rates decreasing, from 84% in patients with compensated cirrhosis, to 14% in patients with decompensated disease *(7)*. Moreover, patients with compensated chronic hepatitis B associated with active viral replication are more likely to have progressive disease and a poorer prognosis than patients with inactive replication. Ultimately, many patients with advanced HBV infection become potential candidates for liver transplantation.

Chronic HBV infection is the most common cause of hepatocellular carcinoma worldwide. The principal treatment for cure is resection, in suitable candidates with acceptable hepatic function (CTP class A) and a technically accessible lesion, or liver transplantation. Unfortunately, less than one-third of patients are candidates for either resection or liver transplantation at the time of clinical presentation *(8)*. Hepatocellular carcinoma causes few or no symptoms; therefore, screening with abdominal ultrasound and α-fetoprotein, every 6 mo in cirrhotic patients, is crucial for early diagnosis, with the potential option for cure.

Liver Transplantation for HBV

The long-term outcome after liver transplantation for chronic HBV infection with cirrhosis is excellent, but this has not always been the case; in fact, in the early 1990s, patients with chronic hepatitis B were generally regarded as poor candidates for liver transplantation. The initial experience with liver transplantation for hepatitis B was associated with a disappointing 50% survival after 3 yrs of follow-up *(9)*. The reason for this relatively poor survival was that HBV re-infection with detectable hepatitis B surface antigen (HBsAg) occurred in 80% of patients, usually within the first year. In many instances, recurrent HBV infection had an aggressive course, with rapid progression to cirrhosis and death. Histologically, a pattern of fibrosing cholestatic hepatitis was recognized as an unusual, but rapidly progressive, and usually fatal, form of liver disease associated with HBV re-infection that occurred in some recipients after liver transplantation *(10,11)*. High levels of immunosuppression appear to play a role in facilitating the development of this syndrome, as may infection with the pre-core HBV variant associated with active viral replication and production of anti-HBe, but not hepatitis B e antigen (HBeAg) *(12)*. Based on this earlier experience, it was apparent that effective HBV antiviral prophylactic therapy was needed to prevent recurrent HBV infection and lead to a successful outcome of liver transplantation.

Hepatitis B Immune Globulin Prophylaxis for HBV Re-Infection

A major breakthrough was reported in 1993, when the European Concerted Action on Viral Hepatitis Study showed that patients who received prophylactic hepatitis B immunoglobulin (HBIg) perioperatively, and long-term, after liver transplantation, had a lower incidence of recurrent HBV and improved survival rate *(13)*. This study showed that patients with evidence of active viral replication before liver transplantation, i.e., detectable serum HBeAg and/or HBV DNA, were at an increased risk for recurrent HBV infection (Table 1). On the other hand, patients without active viral replication, transplanted for fulminant hepatitis rather than cirrhosis, or co-infected with HDV, had a lower incidence of HBV recurrence. Several studies from the United States later confirmed that the administration of high-dose intravenous HBIg, after liver transplantation, reduces the incidence of recurrence to 20–30% or less *(14–17)*. The finding that some patients without recurrence of HBsAg, the routine test used to diagnose HBV infection, have detectable HBV DNA in the liver or blood by polymerase chain reaction (PCR) indicates low-grade

Table 1
Factors Associated with HBV
Re-Infection after Liver Transplantation

Lower re-infection
  Absence of HBeAg
  Absence of HBV DNA
  Fulminant HBV
  HDV co-infection
  ? Lower levels of immunosuppression
Higher re-infection
  ? Pre-core stop codon mutant
  ? Asian vs Caucasian race

persistent HBV infection even when HBsAg is not detectable and thus the need to use HBIg long-term, which is the current standard of care *(15)*. Most centers administer HBIg intravenously post-transplant, once monthly long-term, although individualized and less-frequent dosing may be achievable. At most centers, HBIg, at a dose of 10,000 IU, is given intravenously, starting intraoperatively, for 6 consecutive d, then monthly. After the first year, the dosing interval is adjusted to 4–8 wk, to maintain a trough hepatitis B surface antibody level of >500 mIU/mL.

In the mid-1990s, there was a common belief that Asians with chronic hepatitis B and cirrhosis have a poorer outcome after liver transplantation, compared with non-Asians. This was largely based on a report from the University of California at Los Angeles of an analysis of 16 Asians and 29 non-Asians transplanted between 1984 and 1993, most of whom did not receive long-term HBIg prophylaxis *(18)*. That study showed that Asians had a higher postoperative mortality rate of 31 vs 3.4%, a higher incidence of HBV recurrence (72 vs 32%), and a higher risk of dying from recurrent HBV (87 vs 22%). In contrast, in the authors' study *(19)* of 15 Asians and 20 non-Asians transplanted between 1988 and 1994, many without long-term prophylactic HBIg, Asian patients were found to have had a similar HBV recurrence rate (64 vs 50%) and a lower late mortality from recurrent HBV, compared with non-Asians (14 vs 40%). On the other hand, late referral and more advanced chronic liver disease, at the time of liver transplantation, appeared to be the major reason why Asian patients had a higher perioperative mortality rate. More recent data from the authors' institution *(16)* confirmed that the outcome of liver transplantation in Asians is similar to non-Asians. In 27 consecutive patients transplanted between 1994 and 1997, and treated with long-term, high-dose HBIg, results were excellent. The 3-yr actuarial patient survival rate was 100% in both Asians and non-Asians, with 26 patients remaining seronegative for HBsAg after liver transplantation. Thus, in order to obtain the best transplant outcomes, it is important that patients be referred early for evaluation and listing for liver transplantation and receive HBIg posttransplant.

Lower-than-usual doses of immunosuppressive drugs may also be an important factor in achieving a low HBV re-infection rate posttransplant *(20)*. If high doses of immunosuppressive drugs are used, altered host responsiveness may allow HBV re-infection, despite of administration of HBIg. Lowering serum HBV DNA levels before liver transplantation may also minimize the risk of recurrence in the subgroup of patients with pretransplant evidence of active viral replication, i.e., detectable HBeAg and high HBV DNA levels (Table 1). In recent years, lamivudine, an oral nucleoside analog and potent inhibitor of HBV replication, has been used to treat patients who are HBV DNA-positive and are awaiting liver transplantation *(21)*. After liver transplantation, it remains uncertain if lamivudine should be discontinued in these patients, if they received long-term HBIg treatment or continued long-term, as further prophylaxis against HBV re-infection.

With the use of long-term HBIg prophylaxis after liver transplantation, patients with a low viral load before liver trans-plantation (serum HBV DNA-negative) have a low risk (probably less than 5%) for HBV recurrence *(14)*. Although patients with a high viral load before liver transplantation (serum HBV-DNA- or HBeAg-positive) have an increased risk of developing recurrent HBV, based on the analysis of Samuel et al. *(13)*, later reports showed that the incidence of HBV re-infection could be less than 20% *(14,16)*. McGory et al. *(14)* reported a recurrence rate of 17% with HBIg treatment alone, and, at this center, the recurrence rate was only 7% in HBV-DNA-positive patients treated with lamivudine before liver transplantation and long-term HBIg after liver transplantation *(16)*. Pretransplant infection with the pre-core HBV mutant was originally thought to be associated with a high HBV re-infection rate, but a more recent study shows no difference in posttransplant HBV recurrence rate or survival, with the administration of long-term HBIg prophylaxis *(22)*.

LAM Prophylaxis for HBV Re-Infection

HBIg prophylaxis is expensive, poorly tolerated in some patients, periodically unavailable, and associated with HBV recurrence rates of ~20% *(13,23)*. Lamivudine has been investigated as a prophylactic therapy option for HBV re-infection. In various open-label studies of patients with advanced chronic hepatitis B undergoing liver transplantation *(24–26)*, lamivudine was administered before and after liver transplantation. Efficacy was assessed by improvement in serological markers of HBV. In the largest of these studies, 47 of the enrolled patients underwent liver transplantation *(26)*. Of the 34 patients with available data at 1 yr after liver transplantation, 24 (71%) were HBsAg-negative and 10 (29%) patients were HBsAg-positive, seven of whom were also HBV DNA-positive. Analysis carried out for 5/7 HBV-DNA-positive patients showed that three had detectable tyrosine-methionine-asparate-aspartate amino acid motif of HBV polymerase (YMDD) variant HBV.

The results of this study indicated that, although recurrent HBsAg occurred in close to 30% of patients, most were clinically stable at 1 yr after liver transplantation. Similar findings were observed in other studies *(24,25)*. In all studies, lamivudine therapy was generally well-tolerated. Thus, although lamivudine monotherapy has moderate efficacy for prophylaxis against HBV recurrence following liver transplantation, viral breakthrough with the development of YMDD-variant HBV does occur.

Combination Prophylactic Therapy: LAM and HBIg

The combination of lamivudine with HBIg may be synergistic following liver transplantation. Because lamivudine is a potent inhibitor of viral replication, it is less likely that the viral-binding capacity of HBIg would be overwhelmed. Additionally, HBIg may provide humoral immunity, and therefore limit viral spread, thus indirectly inhibiting viral replication and reducing the likelihood of YMDD variants emerging.

A number of studies *(25–31)* have investigated the combination of lamivudine and HBIg given long-term as prophylaxis against recurrent HBV infection in patients undergoing liver transplantation. All of these studies demonstrated that the combined prophylactic regimen of HBIg and lamivudine was highly effective in preventing recurrent HBV infection in the allograft. Following liver transplantation, the majority of patients remained seronegative for HBsAg and/or HBV DNA (median follow-up, 5–35 mo). Furthermore, only one patient had evidence of escape mutants with the combined regimen *(28)*. These data suggest that HBIg and lamivudine prophylaxis is synergistic in prevention of recurrent HBV infection after liver transplantation.

The optimal regimen for lamivudine and HBIg use remains the subject of ongoing investigation. To minimize the disadvantages associated with HBIg therapy, particularly high cost, the efficacy of the combination of short-term HBIg and long-term lamivudine therapy has been investigated *(32)*. Of 52 patients studied, 29 patients received HBIg monotherapy as long-term prophylaxis, and 23 patients received lamivudine with short-term HBIg given for 6 mo after liver transplantation. At 2-yr follow-up, there was no evidence of HBV recurrence in patients who received combination prophylaxis; 22% of patients who received HBIg monotherapy developed recurrent infection, a difference that was not statistically significant. Thus, the combination of lamivudine with short-term HBIg was at least as effective in preventing HBV recurrence as HBIg monotherapy. Pharmacoeconomic analyses *(33)* support the contention that combined short-term HBIg and lamivudine prophylaxis is cost-effective.

Treatment of Recurrent HBV Infection Posttransplant with LAM

Despite prophylaxis with HBIg, lamivudine, or a combination of these treatments, 10–30% of patients will develop recurrent HBV infection after liver transplantation, and a small percent of patients transplanted for other diseases develop *de novo* HBV infection *(13,23)*. Based on historical data, recurrent HBV infection may be accelerated, leading to liver failure.

Interferon (IFN) has limited efficacy for recurrent HBV infection, and may be poorly tolerated *(34)*. Attention thus focused on the use of the nucleoside analogs, including ganciclovir, famciclovir, and lamivudine. Ganciclovir was the first of these agents to be used, but efficacy was limited by its relatively modest antiviral activity, and intravenous administration was required *(35)*. Famciclovir also has some antiviral activity against HBV, but histological improvement has not been well-documented *(36)*.

Preliminary studies indicated that the use of lamivudine, a more potent nucleoside analog against HBV, was a promising therapy approach in this setting *(37–39)*. In one of these studies *(38)*, early initiation of lamivudine treatment, following the detection of HBsAg posttransplant, induced sustained inhibition of viral replication. Patients rapidly became HBV-DNA-negative, with subsequent normalization of serum alanine aminotransferase (ALT) levels within 24 wk in all patients. Loss of serum HBsAg occurred in 7/12 patients (64%).

These initial promising results were subsequently confirmed in a large, multicenter study *(40)*. 52 transplant recipients received lamivudine, 100 mg/d, for 1 yr, following a diagnosis of recurrent HBV infection. At follow-up, 60% of patients had lost detectable serum HBV DNA, 31% of the initially positive patients had lost HBeAg, and 71% had normalized serum ALT. Treatment was also associated with a significant improvement in liver histology, including portal, periportal, and lobular necrosis. Although YMDD variants were detected in 27% of patients, there was no consistent evidence that the presence of such variants was associated with the progression of hepatic disease. Overall, these data indicate that lamivudine is an effective oral therapy for the treatment of recurrent HBV infection after liver transplantation.

Finally, the role of retransplantation for recurrent HBV infection has been evaluated. In the past, the management of patients with severe recurrent hepatitis B with retransplantation was poor *(41)*. A more recent study *(42)* showed that retransplantation, using high-dose, long-term HBIg treatment, can also result in good long-term success.

CHRONIC HCV INFECTION

CHC with end-stage liver disease is the leading indication for liver transplantation in the United States *(1,43)*. The World Health Organization estimates that 120 million people worldwide are infected with HCV, and that 20% of these will develop cirrhosis. Most cases of hepatocellular carcinoma not associated with HBV are caused by HCV. In the United States, 1.8% of the population, or 4 million Americans, have been infected with HCV, and about 8000 die each year from this infection. Approximately 25% of all liver transplantations in the United States are performed for end-stage liver disease secondary to HCV infection, and this percentage will increase, based on the large number of patients with CHC on the waiting list. Liver transplantation is the best treatment for decompensated cirrhosis caused by HCV infection, but HCV re-infection poses important clinical problems that may appear either early or late after liver transplantation *(44,45)*.

Liver Transplantation for HCV

Like hepatitis B, the natural history of HCV infection in liver transplantation recipients is often accelerated, and the spectrum of recurrent disease ranges from asymptomatic mild hepatitis to severe chronic hepatitis and cirrhosis. Re-infection with HCV after liver transplantation is virtually universal, occurring in more than 95% of cases *(44–46)*. Acute lobular hepatitis is seen in up to 75% of the patients, at a median of 4 mo after liver transplantation. Fortunately, approx 85% of patients with recurrent HCV generally do well, with only mild manifestations of re-infection, but an unpredictable 15% of patients have a more severe course, with rapidly recurrent disease and progression to cirrhosis.

The most sensitive method of detecting HCV infection after liver transplantation is measurement of HCV RNA. A common problem facing transplant physicians and pathologists is the differentiation of recurrent HCV infection from acute allograft rejection. Since the majority of patients with recurrent HCV infection have mild aminotransferase elevations, similar to those seen in acute rejection, patterns of liver enzyme tests can rarely be used to separate one diagnosis from the other. In addition to the similarities between the serum enzyme patterns of injury, many of the liver biopsy features of recurrent HCV infection resemble those seen in acute allograft rejection *(46)*.

Most studies that have analyzed the survival of patients with recurrent HCV infection after liver transplantation have failed to show significant differences, compared to those transplanted for other causes of cirrhosis *(44)*. However, the usual average follow-up in published studies has been only 5 yr or less, and it is possible that longer follow-up, with the persistence of posttransplant hepatitis, will result in reduced survival.

Risk Factors for Recurrent HCV in Transplant Recipients

The underlying cause for recurrence of HCV infection with progressive liver disease is probably multifactorial and largely undefined *(47–67)*. However, certain characteristics associated with the virus, the recipient, and the type of immunosuppressive therapy have been identified as possibly influencing the course of posttransplant HCV infection, and warrant further investigation (Table 2). HCV genotype 1b has been associated with progression of liver injury after liver transplantation, in some *(44,47,48)*, but not all, trials *(49)*. Some European studies have suggested that HCV genotype 1b is associated with more severe recurrent HCV, but this association has not been confirmed by more recent studies in the United States *(49)*. Additional risk factors for recurrent HCV include age and absence of pretransplant co-infection with HBV *(47)*. Pretransplant serum HCV RNA level is associated with more rapid disease progression and lower survival *(50,53)*. The results of trials that studied early serum HCV RNA level after transplant, and disease severity, show higher HCV viral load to be associated with more severe disease *(54,55)*. Fibrosing cholestatic hepatitis is the severest form of HCV recurrence after transplant, and is associated with high viral loads. Reducing the level or dosage of immunosuppression more rapidly than usual after liver transplantation is crucial to limit HCV replication posttransplant *(56,57)*. There is growing evidence that relates a higher likelihood of HCV recurrence with intense posttransplant immunosuppression. Methylprednisone boluses, cumulative steroid doses, neuromonab-CD3 (OKT3), and mycophenolate use are all risk factors for severe recurrence of HCV and rapid progression *(55,58)*.

Table 2
Factors Associated with More Severe
Recurrence of HCV after Liver Transplantation

Factor	Ref.
Viral	
Genotype 1b	(44,47–52)
High (> 1×10^6 Eq/mL) pretransplant HCV RNA levels	(50,53)
High serum or liver, early posttransplant HCV RNA viral load	(54,55)
CMV viral co-infection	(59,61,66)
Absence of pretransplant co-infection with HBV	(47)
Allograft recipient	
HLA matching	(62)
Age	(47)
Nonwhites	(50,53)
Early posttransplant histologic injury	(54,63,65)
Immunosuppression	
High level of immunosuppression	(53,58,63,67)
Episodes of rejection	(58,63,67)
Mycophenolate use	(53)
OKT3 use	(58,63,64,67)
Methylprednisone boluses	(58,63,67)
High cumulative steroid dose	(55)

Treatment of Recurrent HCV

Unfortunately, in contrast to the success in preventing HBV re-infection after liver transplantation, there is as yet no effective antiviral treatment to prevent HCV re-infection. Recurrent HCV may be accelerated in immunosupressed liver transplantation recipients, progressing to cirrhosis in 8–16% of patients within 5 yr, in some reports *(44)*. The rapid rate of progression to liver failure has been observed in a subset of HCV-infected transplant recipients who develop a cholestatic pattern of liver injury *(42,56,57)*. Cholestatic hepatitis is an infrequent cause of jaundice in HCV-infected liver transplantation patients, and should be a diagnosis of exclusion *(68)*. Cholestatic hepatitis C ranges in severity, and does not always signal impending graft failure. The natural history of cholestatic hepatitis C differs dramatically from that of cholestatic hepatitis B, which has been shown to lead to death or need for retransplantation within several weeks *(9)*.

There are numerous emerging antiviral treatment strategies that have been suggested for recurrence of HCV after liver transplantation (Table 3). Most of the literature on preemptive antiviral therapy consists of anecdotal case reports and uncontrolled, nonrandomized trials with a small

Table 3
Treatment Options
for Recurrence of HCV after Transplant

Preemptive antiviral therapy
Pretransplant treatment
Early posttransplant treatment
Treatment of recurrent HCV
Selection of immunosuppressive agents
Retransplantation

number of patients. Therefore, it is recommended that patients be enrolled in clinical trials, and not be treated based on limited experience. IFN is poorly tolerated in patients who have decompensated end-stage liver disease, and often in patients in the early posttransplant period, and IFN can also precipitate further worsening of liver disease in this setting.

Treatment of HCV recurrence with IFN has resulted in a biochemical response, with normalization of serum ALT levels in only 10–30% of patients *(69–71)*. Similar to nontransplant patients, patients with low titers of HCV RNA appear to respond more favorably than those with more severe disease and higher viral titer *(44)*. Sustained biochemical (normal serum ALT levels) and virological (undetectable HCV RNA) responses are uncommon, probably because of the presence of continued replication of the virus or to the level of immunosuppression. Infection also causes an upregulation in the expression of human lymphocyte antigen (HLA) antigens in the liver graft and predisposition to rejection. An increased incidence of rejection has been reported to occur in up to 35% of recipients treated with IFN after liver transplantation *(71)*.

Recently, the use of IFN with ribavirin, an oral antiviral agent that increases the effectiveness of IFN, was shown to achieve better control of HCV infection after liver transplantation *(72,73)*. In 21 patients with recurrent HCV treated with combination IFN-α (3 MU, 3× wk) and ribavirin (1200 mg/d) for 6 mo, followed by ribavirin alone for another 6 mo, 48% cleared serum HCV RNA *(73)*. Serum ALT levels returned to normal in almost all patients with IFN therapy alone, no patient developed rejection. Ribavirin was stopped in three patients, because of the development of hemolytic anemia. Patients who failed to show a biochemical response are rebiopsied, then placed on combination IFN and ribavirin therapy.

The initial reported outcome of retransplantation for recurrent HCV, particularly within the first year after the initial transplant, was poor, with less than 50% surviving more than 1 yr *(74,75)*. A recent study suggested that, if patients with graft failure secondary to recurrent HCV infection posttransplant are retransplanted prior to development of infection and renal failure, the outcome is more favorable *(76)*.

CONCLUSION

Advances in immunosuppressive therapy, recognition of prognostic markers, operative techniques, and perioperative management have resulted in long-term patient survival, approaching 90% following liver transplantation for chronic viral hepatitis *(77,78)*. HBV infection was previously thought to be a contraindication for liver transplantation, because of the high recurrence rate. However, with the administration of prophylactic long-term HBIg, with or without lamivudine, and avoiding high levels of immunosuppression, the recurrence rate is less than 20%. Both long-term patient survival and quality of life are generally excellent after liver transplantation for patients with both chronic hepatitis B and CHC *(79)*. The recurrence rate of HBV is probably not different in Asians, compared with non-Asians, but Asian patients tend to be sicker at presentation for liver transplantation, because of late referral. Long-term treatment with new antiviral agents, such as lamivudine in combination with, or instead of, HBIg, are being studied to reduce the cost associated with maintenance HBIg therapy.

The large number of referrals for liver transplantation reflects the impact of chronic HCV infection as cause of end-stage liver disease. Unlike hepatitis B, there is still no effective treatment in preventing recurrent hepatitis C after liver transplantation. The spectrum of allograft injury, related to universal HCV infection recurrence, ranges from no evidence of histologic injury to mild inflammation to severe disease with allograft failure, in a small portion of patients. Various factors may explain these differing outcomes, including degree of pretransplant viremia, HLA compatibility, presence of more pathogenic HCV genotypes, integrity of cellular immune response, and type of immunosuppression. Fortunately, patient survival does not seem to be affected short-term, although the long-term outcome of liver transplantation for CHC is uncertain *(80,81)*. Combination therapy with IFN and ribavirin, appears to be a promising treatment strategy for posttransplant-recurrent HCV. Pegylated IFN may improve these results. Histopathologically documented recurrent HCV hepatitis in liver transplantation recipients is associated with impairment in quality of life, inferior physical condition, and higher incidence of depression, compared with patients who did not have HCV, and in those without HCV recurrence *(82,83)*.

Chronic viral hepatitis, predominantly chronic hepatitis C virus infection, will continue to be the most common indication for liver transplantation in the future. Patients should be referred to liver transplantation centers at the first sign of decompensated, for transplant evaluation and listing, particularly with the longer waiting time on the liver transplantation list and the shortage of donors.

REFERENCES

1. Seaberg EC, Belle SH, Beringer KC, et al. Liver transplantation in the United States from 1987-1998: updated results from the Pitt-UNOS liver transplant registry. In: *Clinical Transplants* (Cecka JM, Terasaki PI, eds.), 14th ed. Los Angeles: UCLA Tissue Typing Laboratory, 1998, pp. 17–37.
2. Bravata DM, Olkin I, Barnato AE, et al. Health-related quality of life after transplantation: a meta-analysis. Liver Transpl Surg 1999; 5: 318–331.
3. Lucey MR, Brown KA, Everson GT, et al. Minimal criteria for placement of adults on the liver transplant waiting list: a report of a national conference organized by the American Association for the Study of Liver Diseases. Liver Transpl Surg 1997; 3: 628–637.
4. Colantoni A, Hassanein T, Idilman R, et al. Liver transplantation for chronic viral disease. Hepatogastroenterology 1998; 45: 1357–1363.
5. Taniguchi M, Shakil AO, Vargas HE, et al. Clinical and virologic outcomes of hepatitis B and C viral coinfection after liver transplantation: effect of viral hepatitis D. Liver Transpl 2000; 61: 92–96.
6. Bizollon T, Guichard S, Ahmed SN, et al. Impact of hepatitis G virus co-infection on the course of hepatitis C virus infection before and after liver transplantation. J Hepatol 1998; 29: 893–900.
7. de Jongh FE, Janssen HLA, De Man RA, et al. Survival and prognostic indicators in hepatitis B surface antigen-positive cirrhosis of the liver. Gastroenterology 1992; 103: 1630–1635.
8. Esquivel CO, Keeffe EB, Garcia G, et al. Resection versus transplantation for hepatocellular carcinoma. J Gastroenterol Hepatol 1999; 14(Suppl): S37–S41.
9. Todo S, Demetris AJ, Van Thiel D, et al. Orthotopic liver transplantation for patients with hepatitis B virus-related liver disease. Hepatology 1991; 13: 619–626.
10. Davies SE, Portmann BC, O'Grady JG, et al. Hepatic histological findings after transplantation for chronic hepatitis B virus infection, including a unique pattern of fibrosing cholestatic hepatitis. Hepatology 1991; 13: 150–157.
11. Benner KG, Lee RG, Keeffe EB, et al. Fibrosing cytolytic liver failure secondary to recurrent hepatitis B after liver transplantation. Gastroenterology 1992; 103: 1307–1312.
12. Fang JWS, Tung FYT, Davis GL, et al. Fibrosing cholestatic hepatitis in a transplant recipient with hepatitis B virus precore mutant. Gastroenterology 1993; 105: 901–904.
13. Samuel D, Muller R, Alexander G, et al. Liver transplantation in European patients with the hepatitis B surface antigen. N Engl J Med 1993; 329: 1842–1847.
14. McGory RW, Ishitani MB, Oliveira WM, et al. Improved outcome of orthotopic liver transplantation for chronic hepatitis B cirrhosis with aggressive passive immunization. Transplantation 1996; 61: 1358–1364.
15. Terrault NA, Zhou S, Combs C, et al. Prophylaxis in liver transplant recipients using a fixed dosing schedule of hepatitis B immunoglobulin. Hepatology 1996; 24: 1327–1333.

16. So SKS, Esquivel CO, Imperial JC, et al. Does Asian race affect hepatitis B virus recurrence or survival following liver transplantation for hepatitis B cirrhosis? J Gastroenterol Hepatology 1999; 14(Suppl): S48–S52.
17. Nymann T, Shokouh-Amiri MH, Vera SR, et al. Prevention of hepatitis B recurrence with indefinite hepatitis B immune globulin (HBIG) prophylaxis after liver transplantation. Clin Transplant 1996; 10: 663–667.
18. Jurim O, Martin P, Shaked A, et al. Liver transplantation for chronic hepatitis B in Asians. Transplantation 1994; 57: 1393–1411.
19. Ho BM, So SK, Esquivel CO, et al. Liver transplantation in Asian patients with chronic hepatitis B. Hepatology 1997; 25: 223–225.
20. Gish RG, Keeffe EB, Lim J, et al. Survival after liver transplantation for chronic hepatitis B using reduced immunosuppression. J Hepatol 1995; 22: 257–262.
21. Keeffe EB. End-stage liver disease and liver transplantation: role of lamivudine therapy in patients with chronic hepatitis B. J Med Virol 2000; 61: 403–408.
22. Naumann U, Protzer-Knolle U, Berg T, et al. Pretransplant infection with precore mutants of hepatitis B virus does not influence the outcome of orthotopic liver transplantation in patients on high dose anti-hepatitis B virus surface antigen immunoprophylaxis. Hepatology 1997; 26: 478–484.
23. Terrault NA. Hepatitis B virus and liver transplantation. Clin Liver Dis 1999; 3: 389–415.
24. Grellier L, Mutimer D, Ahmed M, et al. Lamivudine prophylaxis against reinfection in liver transplantation for hepatitis B cirrhosis. Lancet 1996; 348: 1212–1215.
25. Markowitz JS, Martin P, Conrad AJ, et al. Prophylaxis against hepatitis B recurrence following liver transplantation using combination lamivudine and heptitis B immune globulin. Hepatology 1998; 28: 585–589.
26. Perrillo RP, Schiff ER, Dienstag JL, et al. Lamivudine for prevention of recurrent hepatitis B after liver transplantation: final results of a U.S./Canadian multicenter trial (abstract). Hepatology 1999; 30: 222A.
27. Han S-H, Martin P, Markowitz J, et al. Long-term combination HBIG and lamivudine is highly effective in preventing recurrent hepatitis B in orthotopic liver transplant (OLT) recipients (abstract). Hepatology 1998; 28: 222A.
28. Marzano A, Debernardi-Venon W, Actis GC, et al. Efficacy of lamivudine treatment associated with low-dose immunoprophylaxis on HBV recurrence after liver transplantation (abstract). J Hepatol 1999; 30: 80.
29. Roche B, Samuel D, Roque AM, et al. Intravenous anti HBsIg combined with oral lamivudine for prophylaxis against HBV recurrence after liver transplantation (abstract). J Hepatol 1999; 30: 80.
30. McCaughan GW, Spencer J, Koorey D, et al. Lamivudine therapy in patients undergoing liver transplantation for hepatitis B virus precore mutant-associated infection: high resistance rates in treatment of recurrence but universal prevention if used as prophylaxis with very low dose hepatitis B immune globulin. Liver Transpl Surg 1999; 5: 512–519.
31. Yoshida EM, Erb SR, Partovi N, et al. Liver transplantation for chronic hepatitis B infection with the use of combination lamivudine and low-dose hepatitis B immune globulin. Liver Transpl Surg 1999; 5: 520–525.
32. Terrault NA, Wright TL, Roberts JP, Ascher NL. Combined short-term hepatitis B immunoglobulin (HBIG) and long-term lamivudine (LAM) versus HBIG monotherapy as hepatitis B virus (HBV) prophylaxis in liver transplant recipients (abstract). Hepatology 1998; 28: 389A.
33. Pasha TM, Douglas DD, Krom RA, Wiesner RH. Cost-effectiveness of lamivudine and hepatitis B immunoglobulin after liver transplantation for hepatitis B (abstract). Hepatology 1998; 28: 348A.

34. Perrillo RP. Interferon in the management of chronic hepatitis B. Dig Dis Sci 1993; 38: 577–593.
35. Gish RG, Lau JYN, Brooks L, et al. Ganciclovir treatment of hepatitis B virus infection in liver transplant recipients. Hepatology 1996; 23: 1–7.
36. Krüger M, Tillmann HL, Trautwein C, et al. Famciclovir treatment of hepatitis B virus recurrence after liver transplantation: a pilot study. Liver Transpl Surg 1996; 2: 253–262.
37. Ben-Ari Z, Shmueli D, Shapira Z, et al. Beneficial effect of lamivudine in recurrent hepatitis B after liver transplantation. Transplantation 1997; 63: 393–396.
38. Andreone P, Caraceni P, Grazi GL, et al. Lamivudine treatment for acute hepatitis B after liver transplantation. J Hepatol 1998; 29: 985–989.
39. Nery JR, Weppler D, Rodriguez M, et al. Efficacy of lamivudine in controlling hepatitis B virus recurrence after liver transplantation. Transplantation 1998; 65: 1615–1621.
40. Perrillo R, Rakela J, Dienstag J, et al. Multicenter study of lamivudine therapy for hepatitis B after liver transplantation. Hepatology 1999; 29: 1581–1586.
41. Crippin J, Foster B, Carlen S, et al. Retransplantation in hepatitis B: a multicenter experience. Transplantation 1994; 57: 823–826.
42. Ishitani M, McGory R, Dickson R, et al. Retransplantation of patients with severe posttransplant hepatitis B in the first allograft. Transplantation 1997; 64: 410–414.
43. Bzowej NH, Wright TL. Viral hepatitis and liver transplantation. J Gastroenterol Hepatol 1999; 14(Suppl): S53–S60.
44. Gane EJ, Portmann BC, Naoumov NV, et al. Long-term outcome of hepatitis C infection after liver transplantation. N Engl J Med 1996; 334: 815–820.
45. Ferrell LD, Wright TL, Roberts J, et al. Hepatitis C viral infection in liver transplant recipients. Hepatology 1992; 16: 865–876.
46. Dickson RC, Caldwell SH, Ishitani MB, et al. Clinical and histologic patterns of early graft failure due to recurrent hepatitis C in four patients after liver transplantation. Transplantation 1996; 61: 701–705.
47. Feray C, Caccamo L, Alexander GJ, et al. European colloborative study on factors influencing outcome after liver transplantation for hepatitis C. European Concerted Action on Viral Hepatitis (EUROHEP) Group. Gastroenterology 1999; 117: 619–625.
48. Pageaux GP, Ducos J, Mondain AM, et al. Hepatitis C virus genotypes and quantitation of serum hepatitis C virus RNA in liver transplant recipients: relationship with severity of histological recurrence and implications in the pathogenesis of HCV infection. Liver Transpl Surg 1997; 3: 501–505.
49. Zhou S, Terrault NA, Ferrell L, et al. Severity of liver disease in liver transplantation recipients with hepatitis c virus infection: relationship to genotype and level of viremia. Hepatology 1996; 24: 1041–1046.
50. Charlton M, Seaberg E, Wiesner R, et al. Predictors of patient and graft survival following liver transplantation for hepatitis C. Hepatology 1998; 28: 823–830.
51. Feray C, Gigou M, Samuel D, et al. Influence of genotypes of hepatitis C on the severity of recurrent liver disease after liver transplantation. Gastroenterology 1995; 108: 1088–1096.
52. Gayowski T, Singh N, Marino IR, et al. Hepatitis C virus genotypes in liver transplant recipients: impact on posttransplant recurrence, infections, and response to interferon-alpha and outcome. Transplantation 1997; 64: 422–426.
53. Berenguer M, Ferrell L, Watson J, et al. Fibrosis progression in recurrent hepatitis C Virus (HCV) dsiease: differences between the U.S. and Europe (abstract). Hepatology 1998; 28: 220A.

54. DiMartino V, Saurini F, Samuel D, et al. Long-term longitudinal study of intrahepatic hepatitis C virus replication after liver transplantation. Hepatology 1997; 26: 1343–1350.
55. Schluger LK, Sheiner PA, Thung SN, et al. Severe recurrent cholestatic hepatitis C following orthotopic liver transplantation. Hepatology 1996; 23: 971–976.
56. Gretch DR, Bacchi C, Corey L, et al. Persistent hepatitis C virus infection after liver transplantation: clinical and virological features. Hepatology 1995; 22: 1–9.
57. Pessoa MG, Bzowej N, Berenguer M, et al. Evolution of hepatitis C virus quasispecies in patients with severe cholestatic hepatitis after liver transplantation. Hepatology 1999; 30: 1513–1520.
58. Berenguer M, Prieto M, Cordoba J, et al. Early development of chronic active hepatitis in recurrent hepatitis C virus infection after liver transplantation: association with treatment of rejection. J Hepatol 1998; 28: 756–763.
59. Berenguer M, Terrault NA, Piatak M, et al. Hepatitis G virus infection in patients with hepatitis C virus infection undergoing liver transplantation. Gastroenterology 1996; 111: 1569–1575.
60. Casavilla A, Rakela J, Kapur S, et al. Clinical outcome of patients infected with hepatitis C virus infection on survival after primary liver transplantation under tacrolimus. Liver Transpl Surg 1998; 4: 448–454.
61. Huang EJ, Wright TL, Lake JR, et al. Hepatitis B and C coinfections and persistent hepatitis B infections: clinical outcome and liver pathology after transplantation. Hepatology 1996; 23: 396–404.
62. Manez R, Mateo R, Tabasco J, et al. Influence of HLA donor-recipient compatibility on the recurrence of HBV and HCV hepatitis after liver transplantation. Transplantation 1995; 59: 640–642.
63. Prieto M, Berenguer M, Rayon JM, et al. High incidence of allograft cirrhosis in hepatitis C virus genotype 1b infection following liver transplantation: relationship with rejection episodes. Hepatology 1999; 29: 250–256.
64. Rosen HR, Shackleton CR, Higa L, et al. Use of OKT3 is associated with early and severe recurrence of hepatitis C after liver transplantation. Am J Gastroenterol 1997; 92: 1453–1457.
65. Rosen HR, Gretch DR, Oehlke M, et al. Timing and severity of initial hepatitis C recurrence as predictors of long-term liver allograft injury. Transplantation 1998; 65: 1178–1182.
66. Rosen HR, Chou S, Corless CL, et al. Cytomegalovirus viremia. risk factor for allograft cirrhosis after liver transplantation for hepatitis C. Transplantation 1997; 64: 721–726.
67. Sheiner PA, Schwartz ME, Mor E, et al. Severe or multiple rejection episodes are associated with early recurrence of hepatitis C after orthotopic liver transplantation. Hepatology 1995; 21: 30–34.
68. Cotler SJ, Taylor SL, Gretch DR, et al. Hyperbilirubinemia and cholestatic liver injury in hepatitis C-infected liver transplant recipients. Am J Gastroenterol 2000; 95: 753–759.
69. Wright HI, Gavaler JS, Van Thiel DH, et al. Preliminary experience with α-2b-interferon therapy of viral hepatitis in liver allograft recipients. Transplantation 1992; 53: 121–124.
70. Wright TL, Combs C, Kim M, et al. Interferon-α therapy for hepatitis C virus infection after liver transplantation. Hepatology 1994; 20: 773–779.
71. Féray C, Samuel D, Gigou M, et al. Open trial of interferon alfa recombinant for C after liver transplantation hepatitis: antiviral effects and risk of rejection. Hepatology 1995; 22: 1084–1089.

72. Mazzaferro V, Regalia E, Pulvirenti A, et al. Effect of interferon and ribavirin prophylaxis after liver transplantation in HCV-RNA positive patients. Hepatology 1995; 22: 287A.
73. Bizollon T, Palazzo U, Ducerf C, et al. Pilot study of the combination of interferon alfa and ribavirin as therapy of recurrent hepatitis C after liver transplantation. Hepatology 1997; 26: 500–504.
74. Casavilla FA, Lee R, Lim J, et al. Outcome of liver retransplantation (ReOLTx) for recurrent hepatitis C infection. Hepatology 1995; 22: 153A.
75. Féray C, Habsanne A, Samuel D, et al. Poor prognosis of patients retransplanted for recurrent liver disease due to hepatitis C virus. Hepatology 1995; 22: 135A.
76. Sheiner PA, Schluger LK, Emre S, et al. Retransplantation for recurrent hepatitis C. Liver Transpl Surg 1997; 3: 130–136.
77. Dodson SF, Issa S, Bonham A. Liver transplantation for chronic viral hepatitis. Surg Clin North Am 1999; 79: 131–145.
78. Mutimer D. Long term outcome of liver transplantation for viral hepatitis: is there a need to re-evaluate patient selection? Gut 1999; 45: 475–476.
79. Dickson RC, Wright RM, Bacchetta MD, et al. Quality of life of hepatitis B and C patients after liver transplantation. Clin Transplant 1997; 11: 282–285.
80. Boker KH, Dalley G, Bahr MJ, et al. Long-term outcome of hepatitis C virus infection after liver transplantation. Hepatology 1997; 25: 203–210.
81. Weinstein JS, Poterucha J, Zein N, et al. Epidemiology and natural history of hepatitis C infections in liver transplant recipients. J Hepatol 1995; 22(Suppl 1): 154–159.
82. Paterson DL, Gayowski T, Wannstedt CF, et al. Quality of life in long-term survivors after liver transplantation: impact of recurrent viral hepatitis C virus hepatitis. Clin Transplant 2000; 14: 48–54.
83. Singh N, Gayowski T, Wagener MM, et al. Quality of life, functional status, and depression in male liver transplant recipients with recurrent viral hepatitis C. Transplantation 1999; 67: 69–72.

15 Viral Hepatitis and Pregnancy

Rene Davila, MD *and Caroline A. Riely,* MD

CONTENTS

INTRODUCTION
ACUTE VIRAL INFECTIONS
CHRONIC VIRAL INFECTIONS
DIFFERENTIAL DIAGNOSIS OF LIVER DISEASE IN PREGNANCY
CONCLUSION
REFERENCES

INTRODUCION

Because viral hepatitis is the most prevalent liver disease worldwide, it occurs frequently in pregnancy. This can be as acute viral hepatitis during a previously normal gestation, or as pregnancy occurring in a woman with chronic hepatitis. In either situation, special concerns for both mother and child must be considered. In addition, the liver diseases unique to pregnancy can present in the guise of viral hepatitis, providing problems in differential diagnosis.

The aim of this chapter is to describe the risk of perinatal transmission of viral hepatitis, the effects of pregnancy on the course of liver disease, the effects of viral hepatitis on the course of pregnancy, and the management of viral hepatitis in pregnancy. Liver disease in pregnancy may be caused by acute or chronic viral infections, drug-induced hepatotoxicity, or diseases unique to pregnancy, such as cholestasis of pregnancy, hemolysis, elevated liver enzymes, and low platelet count (HELLP) syndrome, and acute fatty liver of pregnancy (AFLP). The differential diagnosis of fulminant liver failure in pregnancy includes hepatitis E virus (HEV) infection, herpes simplex virus infection, AFLP, drug-induced

From: *Clinical Gastroenterology: Diagnosis and Therapeutics*
Edited by: R. S. Koff and G. Y. Wu © Humana Press Inc., Totowa, NJ

hepatotoxicity, and Budd-Chiari syndrome. The clinician must recognize the clinical, biochemical, and serological differences that will allow for a correct diagnosis and treatment.

ACUTE VIRAL INFECTIONS

Pregnant women may experience acute viral infections that result in varying degrees of liver injury. In addition to the hepatitis A, B, C, D, and E viruses, herpes simplex virus, cytomegalovirus and Epstein-Barr virus are also known to affect the liver during pregnancy.

Hepatitis A

The hepatitis A virus (HAV) is an RNA picornavirus that is enterically transmitted. Affected adults usually develop mild-to-moderate generalized symptoms, such as malaise, anorexia, and nausea. Peak aminotransferase (AT) (alanine AT, aspartate AT) levels range from 500 to 5000 U/L. Patients experience complete clinical and biochemical recovery within 3–6 mo. Perinatal transmission of HAV, although rare, has been associated with blood or fecal contact during delivery *(1)*.

Pregnancy does not appear to affect the natural course of the infection. Similarly, hepatitis A is not thought to affect the course of pregnancy, although the authors reported *(2)* two patients who experienced third trimester premature delivery during the course of severe hepatitis A. The treatment of HAV infection in affected children is supportive. Prevention of infection transmission is achieved by immunization of women in endemic areas with inactivated HAV vaccine or by postexposure use of immunoglobulin.

Hepatitis E

The HEV is an RNA virus that is enterically transmitted. It is widely distributed in the developing world, but rare in the United States. The clinical presentation of acute HEV hepatitis during pregnancy is that of liver failure, with high AT levels and increased prothrombin time. Acute HEV infection during the third trimester of pregnancy may result in up to 20% mortality caused by fulminant liver failure *(3)*. It is believed that the fulminant course of HEV during pregnancy may result from some pregnancy-induced abnormality, perhaps some partial immunodeficiency, that alters the usually benign course of the infection in nonpregnant individuals. HEV infection has also been associated with reported cases of intrauterine deaths, but it is not clear whether this is related to maternal factors or direct fetal effects. Maternal–fetal transmission of HEV, resulting in neonatal symptomatic hepatitis, has been reported *(4)*. There are no therapeutic agents currently available to prevent vertical transmission of the virus.

Herpes Simplex Virus

Herpes simplex virus hepatitis is common and subclinical during primary infection, but only becomes clinically evident when the patient is immunosuppressed or pregnant. Partial immunosuppression induced by pregnancy is believed to be the underlying condition that renders pregnant women susceptible to herpes simplex virus hepatitis. Affected pregnant women present with high AT levels and prolongation of the prothrombin time. Subtle vesicular lesions of the oropharynx and genital areas are suggestive of the correct diagnosis (in contrast to typical cold sores or genital sores of recurrent or secondary infection). Herpes simplex virus infection during the third trimester of pregnancy may result in fulminant hepatitis accompanied by encephalopathy. The encephalopathy may be exacerbated by the development of encephalitis. Serologic tests may be useful, but are usually not readily available. Liver histology is diagnostic, revealing typical inclusion bodies. Acyclovir is usually an effective treatment of the infection, and it appears to prevent transmission of the virus to the fetus *(5)*.

CHRONIC VIRAL INFECTIONS

Worldwide, the majority of cases of chronic hepatitis are caused by to viral infections with the hepatitis B, C, and D viruses. These chronic viral infections in turn account for the majority of cases of chronic liver disease that require liver transplantation. The presence of chronic viral hepatitis in pregnancy must be recognized early, to set in motion mechanisms to prevent transmission of disease related to prenatal, peripartum, and postpartum events.

Hepatitis B

The hepatitis B virus (HBV) is a DNA virus belonging to the hepadnavirus family. The viral nucleocapsid (core) is comprised of double-stranded circular DNA and the hepatitis B core antigen. The hepatitis B e antigen (HBeAg) is a derivative of hepatitis B core antigen. The surface antigen (HBsAg) comprises the outer shell of the virus. HBV affects humans and chimpanzees.

In the United States, approx 20,000 infants are born to HBsAg-positive mothers each year. HBV-infected individuals exhibit high viral concentrations in blood, and lower levels in tears, saliva, synovial fluid, vaginal fluid, semen, stool, and breast milk. Cases of intrauterine transmission of HBV have been reported, but this does not seem to be a significant source. Perinatal transmission of HBV occurs as a result of exposure to maternal blood. Exposure of infant traumatized surfaces or intact mucous membranes to maternal fluids, as well as to placental tears, appear to be the routes of perinatal transmission of HBV.

ACUTE HBV INFECTION

Acute HBV infection during pregnancy does not appear to adversely affect the clinical course of the gestation. The risk of infectivity to the neonate, however, appears to be related to the time of acute HBV infection. Acute maternal infection during the third trimester of pregnancy markedly increases the risk of HBV vertical transmission. All neonates born to infected mothers, regardless of the time of infection, ought to receive the transmission-preventive treatment discussed later.

CHRONIC HBV INFECTION

Chronic HBV infection has little effect on the pregnancy. Female HBV carriers usually have less liver inflammation than male carriers, and are less likely to develop liver cirrhosis. Consequently, most young female HBV carriers have a lower risk to develop hepatic failure, or any other decompensation of liver disease, during pregnancy or delivery. Pregnancy has no adverse effects on the course of HBV infection, and does not result in meaningful changes in AT levels.

Interferon is not used in pregnancy to treat chronic hepatitis B virus infection. Lamivudine (LAM), a nucleoside analog useful in the treatment of hepatitis B, has been used in pregnancy for the treatment of HIV infection. Concentrations of LAM in maternal serum, amniotic fluid, and neonatal serum are similar, probably because of free transplacental diffusion of the drug. LAM has also been found in breast milk *(6)*. Adverse pregnancy outcomes, such as frequent prematurity or biliary malformations caused by use of LAM have been reported *(7)*. Based on those reports, the use of LAM for treatment of HBV infection in pregnancy cannot be recommended, until further data are obtained.

VIRAL TRANSMISSION

Vertical transmission of HBV is responsible for the majority of cases of the chronic-carrier state worldwide, particularly in endemic areas, such as Southeast Asia and Africa *(8)*. Consequently, it is essential that all infected mothers are identified prior to or at the time of delivery, in order to take appropriate measures to prevent transmission to the neonate.

Many countries recommend testing pregnant women for HBsAg. Approximately one-half of those who are found to be positive, on routine testing, do not fit into any high-risk groups, and could potentially be missed, if more universal testing is not implemented.

The HBsAg carrier rate in pregnant women varies widely, from 0.15% in white U.S. women, to 8.9% in Asian women born outside the United States (9). The AT levels may be normal or only slightly elevated in many HBsAg-positive individuals. For epidemiologic purposes, persons with detectable HBsAg should be considered infectious. Mothers who are HBsAg-positive should not be discouraged from breastfeeding, as long as the infant has received prophylactic treatment.

Individuals who are HBeAg-positive usually have higher viremia levels, and have higher rates of vertical HBV transmission (10). Mothers who are hepatitis B e antibody-positive may also transmit HBV to their neonates, but at a much lower rate (11). If untreated, approx 90% of infants born to HBeAg-pos-itive mothers, compared to 10% of infants born to HBeAg-negative mothers, will become infected with HBV.

The majority of HBV-infected infants are asymptomatic, and become HBsAg-positive several weeks to months postpartum. When HBsAg is detectable in the neonate at birth, transplacental infection is suspected (10). Prophylactic treatment is not effective in this group of infants, and chronic infection is likely to develop. It is possible, that in infants, some degree of immune tolerance to the viral antigens results in a significantly decreased response to the prophylactic treatment (12).

Prophylactic Treatment

Multiple studies have been conducted using different doses and regimens of HBV vaccine in combination with hepatitis B immunoglobulin. The combination prophylactic treatment is approx 95% effective in preventing HBV infection in the neonate exposed at birth. Premature neonates exhibit rates of response comparable to that in full-term infants. Prophylactic treatment started at birth provides prolonged protection.

Studies of prophylactic treatment, with the HBV vaccine alone, have provided promising results. In one study (13), the vaccine was 85% successful in preventing infection. Another study (14) revealed good results with a combined intramuscular–intradermal vaccination regimen. In another study (15), infants were vaccinated within 1 wk of birth, regardless of maternal HBsAg status. The prevalence of HBsAg was 4–5× greater in nonimmunized infants than in vaccinated ones after 1 yr. The above findings suggest that, in poor countries, it may be more cost-efficient to vaccinate all neonates, rather than to test the mothers for the presence of HBV.

The majority of the world's countries test pregnant women for HBsAg. Infants born to HBsAg-positive mothers receive hepatitis B immunoglobulins at birth. They should also be immunized with the HBV vaccine at d 1, mo 1, and mo 6 after birth *(16)*. Side effects of the vaccine are uncommon, and include irritability, mild fever, and local irritation at the injection site.

The goal of immunization is to develop a protective hepatitis B surface antibody level above 100 IU/L. The rate of decline of antibody titer is well-known, with a titer of 100 IU/L falling to less than 10 IU/L in approx 5 yr. There are no universal recommendations regarding routine follow-up of antibody levels in infants or women of childbearing age.

In 1991, the Centers for Disease Control and Prevention of the U.S. Public Health Service recommended the vaccination of all infants against HBV infection. Two yr later, two-thirds of U.S. infants were being immunized with the HBV vaccine, along with the other regularly scheduled childhood vaccinations. By then, one-half of all U.S. hospitals were offering HBV vaccines at birth.

The World Health Organization recommended the universal HBV vaccination of all infants to all countries, starting in 1992. In 1994, a goal of reducing the incidence of newly infected children by 80% by the year 2001 was established. Many nations adopted the routine HBV immunization of children; other nations elected to vaccinate only infants born to HBsAg-positive mothers. The tidal wave of new data revealing the efficacy of universal immunization should convince the latter nations to change their immunization policies and follow WHO recommendations.

Adverse effects following HBV vaccination of children have been reported in recent years. Allergic reactions, such as urticaria, ocular inflammation, and asthma, appear to be the most commonly reported HBV-vaccine-induced effects. There have also been reports of delayed neurologic development in children who received the vaccine, although a causal relationship has not been proven. These adverse effects have been attributed to the presence of the preservative, thimerasol, a mercury derivative, in the vaccine preparation *(17)*. Newer HBV vaccines are free of thimerasol or any other mercury derivative.

HEPATITIS C

The hepatitis C virus (HCV), an RNA virus in the flavivirus family, is the etiologic agent in the majority of cases of what was previously referred to as non-A, non-B hepatitis. It is also the virus responsible for the majority of cases of posttransfusion hepatitis in the United States, and the predominant bloodborne virus in injection drug users who share equipment. In excess of 170 million people worldwide have chronic HCV infection. Children can be infected by vertical spread from infected mothers, and evidence for sexual transmission has been documented. Sporadic infection without an identifiable risk factor is also responsible for some infections. Since the introduction of donor screening in 1990, transfusion-associated HCV infection has declined dramatically.

ACUTE INFECTION

Data on acute HCV infection in pregnancy are scarce. Recent polymerase chain reaction (PCR) and HCV antibody data have been available for both mother and infant. Some reports have identified PCR and antibody-positive infants born to mothers who had acute HCV in the last trimester. Other reports show that infants born to mothers, under similar conditions, were not infected. More information is needed to determine whether acute infection has any effect on the progress of gestation. Further information is also needed to determine whether the natural history of the acute infection is altered by pregnancy.

CHRONIC INFECTION

Currently available data *(18)* reveal that chronic HCV infection in the mother does not influence pregnancy outcomes or complications. Data *(19)* also suggest that pregnancy does not adversely affect the course of hepatitis. Several studies reveal that the majority of HCV antibody-positive mothers maintain normal AT levels during pregnancy.

The HCV PCR levels in blood of pregnant women appear to increase during the second and third trimesters. Ward et al. *(20)* found that, among pregnant women seeking medical attention in inner London, the prevalence of HCV antibody-positive is 0.8%, the rate of HCV PCR-positive is 0.6%, and 69% of cases were newly diagnosed during pregnancy. Baldo et al. *(21)*, in Padua, Italy, found that the characteristics independently associated with HCV antibody positivity in pregnant women were unmarried status, unemployed condition, and history of previous abortion.

Perinatal transmission of HCV has been extensively studied since serologic testing became available in 1990. Many studies show that, in the absence of human immunodeficiency virus (HIV) co-infection, perinatal transmission of HCV is uncommon. In Italy, Resti et al. *(22)* found that mothers with chronic HCV, who had previously delivered a HCV antibody-positive infant, were at no greater risk of infecting a subsequent infant. They also found that the chronicity of maternal infection is not a risk factor for perinatal transmission, and that each baby had an independently similar risk for contracting the infection. Zanetti et al. *(23)*, in Milan, Italy, found that there was no correlation between HCV genotype and risk of perinatal transmission. The rate of perinatal transmission is estimated to be 3.6–5%.

Studies of perinatal transmission, based solely on detection of HCV antibody, may just reflect the passive transfer of maternal antibody. It is estimated that up to 50% of neonates born to infected mothers have detectable antibodies that usually disappear by 6-24 mo postpartum. More accurate studies of perinatal transmission require the use of PCR for the detection of virus.

Maternal co-infection with HIV and HCV is associated with an increased risk for acquiring HCV infection at birth. A study conducted in Florence, Italy *(24)*, revealed that the risk of transmission increased as much as threefold, when mothers were co-infected with HIV, and had high levels of viremia. This increased risk of transmission is attributed to the increased HCV viremia found in HIV-infected persons, as the result of immunosuppression.

Available data suggest that the rate of perinatal transmission of HCV is not related to the route of infant delivery, i.e., vaginal delivery or cesarean section. In Germany, however, Hillemmans et al. *(25)* found that infants born by cesarean section, to mothers who were HCV antibody-positive, had a twofold risk of being antibody-positive after birth. Of this group of infants, 3.4% remained HCV PCR-positive 12 mo postpartum.

Concerning the possibility of HCV transmission via breast milk, a study conducted in Hamburg, Germany *(26)*, revealed that none of 76 samples of breast milk obtained from infected mothers contained HCV by PCR. Current reports reveal that infants breastfed by infected mothers, with high viral counts in blood, appear to be free of infection 12 mo postpartum. Delamare et al. *(27)* reported one case of possible HCV transmission via transplacental amniocentesis.

Mast et al. *(28)* found that mode of delivery and breastfeeding were not associated with HCV transmission. They also found that the overall risk of transmission was 4% for PCR-positive mothers, compared to 0% for PCR-negative mothers. Factors associated with an increased risk for transmission were prolonged duration of membrane rupture, use of internal fetal monitoring devices, and meconium-stained amniotic fluid. Obstetricians may be able to alter two of these factors to decrease the risk of perinatal transmission.

Current data reveal that, among 31 European medical centers, there were no uniform antenatal HCV-screening guidelines or breastfeeding recommendations *(29)*. Regarding to prevention of mother-to-infant transmission of HCV, immunoglobulin preparations have been ineffective against development of HCV infection, and HCV vaccines are not available.

Not much is known about the natural history of chronic HCV infection in infants infected during the perinatal period. The variability of infection factors, such as the genotype, level of viremia, and concomitant diseases, e.g., HIV, makes it difficult to interpret the results of available clinical studies. One study *(30)* revealed that up to 40% of HCV-infected children present evidence of mild-to-moderate chronic hepatitis after 3 yr of documented infection. Other small studies have not shown similar results. Given the paucity of long-term studies of HCV-infected infants, it is not possible to establish firm treatment guidelines at this time.

Hepatitis D

Hepatitis D virus (HDV) is a defective RNA virus that requires the presence of HBsAg for replication. Consequently, HDV infection occurs only in HBV-affected individuals. The predominant mode of viral transmission is parenteral, and cases of vertical transmission are uncommon. Prevention of vertical transmission is achieved by preventing maternal HBV infection with vaccination, or clearing the presence of HBV virus with interferon or LAM.

Data regarding HDV infection in pregnancy are scarce. There is currently no evidence that pregnancy has any impact on the natural course of the acute or chronic HDV infection. There is also no evidence of adverse effects of the viral infection on the course of gestation.

DIFFERENTIAL DIAGNOSIS OF LIVER DISEASE IN PREGNANCY

Viral hepatitis is common in pregnancy, but others causes of liver disease should be considered. This is a confusing area, because liver disease during pregnancy is not well-identified, and can lead to diagnostic errors. This subheading covers both liver diseases that are unique to pregnancy and liver diseases that do not have an infectious etiology, but may significantly affect the course of pregnancy.

Cholestasis of Pregnancy

Cholestasis of pregnancy is characterized by pruritus of the palms and soles, which often progresses to intolerable levels as the pregnancy progresses. It usually starts in the second semester, and resolves shortly after delivery. The biochemical changes are elevations of ATs up to 1000 U/L, elevated serum bile acids, and occasionally elevated bilirubin levels. The γ-glutamyl transpeptidase levels and prothrombin time are usually normal. Increases in rates of stillbirth and prematurity have been reported *(31)*.

HELLP Syndrome

The HELLP syndrome is a clinical entity that presents during the third trimester, or shortly after delivery, in pregnant women with pre-eclampsia or eclampsia, who have hemolysis, elevated liver enzyme (ATs) levels, and low platelet counts. It is estimated *(32)* that up to 20% of pregnant women with severe pre-eclampsia develop this syndrome.

Patients may develop severe epigastric or right-upper-quadrant abdominal pain. They may also present with pre-eclampsia symptoms, such as headache and excessive thirst. The majority of patients experience progressive worsening of the syndrome, which improves rapidly after delivery. Uncommon complications include hepatic hematoma, rupture, or infarction. Treatment consists of management of pre-eclampsia and prompt delivery.

Acute Fatty Liver of Pregnancy

AFLP develops during the third trimester. It presents with vague symptoms, such as malaise, nausea, and vomiting. Severe cases present with jaundice, coagulopathy, hypoglycemia, and hyperammonemia. When undiagnosed, AFLP may progressively worsen to coma and death. Biochemical changes include mildly to moderately elevated AT levels, prolonged prothrombin time, and decreased fibrinogen level. Liver histology reveals microvesicular fatty infiltration, predominantly in the central region. Most cases of AFLP are managed with supportive measures, including transfer to an intensive care unit, mechanical ventilation, and correction of abnormal coagulation times. Severe cases may require prompt termination of pregnancy. Some women have been reported to experience recurrent AFLP in subsequent pregnancies *(33)*.

The pathogenesis of AFLP remains unclear. Recent reports revealed that some women with AFLP are heterozygous for a defect in one of the enzymes (long-chain 3-hydroxyl-acyl CoA dehydrogenase [LCHAD]), involved in β oxidation of fatty acids in the mitochondria. These women remain asymptomatic until they become pregnant with a LCHAD homozygous fetus, and develop AFLP. Infants with LCHAD deficiency may develop a Reye's-like syndrome and possible death caused by nonketotic hypoglycemia. A DNA test is available to identify the gene defect involved in LCHAD deficiency. This test allows for identification of heterozygous mothers who should receive counseling regarding subsequent pregnancies *(34)*.

Budd-Chiari Syndrome

Pregnant women with an underlying procoagulant state, such as protein C deficiency, protein S deficiency, or the presence of anticardiolipin antibody, may develop spontaneous thrombosis of the major hepatic veins (Budd-Chiari syndrome). This may occur because of the relative hypercoagulable state present during late pregnancy. The Budd-Chiari syndrome occurs more frequently in late pregnancy or the immediate postpartum period. Unless treated with adequate systemic anticoagulation, or sometimes liver transplantation *(35)*, the development of this syndrome may have catastrophic results for the mother and/or the fetus.

Hepatic Masses

Hepatic masses may result in complications leading to fulminant hepatic failure during pregnancy, but would probably not be confused for viral hepatitis. These masses include adenomas, focal nodular hyperplasias, hemangiomas, metastatic malignant neoplasias, or cystic parasites, such as echinocochal cysts. One potential complication from these masses is rupture and/or hemorrhage during pregnancy *(36)*. Regardless of time of onset, nonmalignant masses, discovered once pregnancy is underway in an asymptomatic patient, should be closely monitored with serial ultrasonography.

Drug-induced Hepatotoxicity

Many commonly used drugs may affect the liver in a dose-related or idiosyncratic fashion. Drug-induced hepatotoxicity is not more likely to develop during pregnancy. When it occurs, however, it may result in diagnostic confusion. The incidence of adverse drug effects during pregnancy may be lower than that outside of pregnancy, because pregnant women are encouraged to not take medications.

The spectrum of liver damage is widely variable. The clinical presentation is usually vague and nondiagnostic. Liver histology may show varying degrees of hepatocyte necrosis. Management is mainly withdrawal of the insulting agent, supportive care, and liver transplantation in severe cases.

CONCLUSION

Acute and chronic viral hepatitis are highly prevalent worldwide, and represent a potential threat to pregnant women and their newborns, alike. This chapter reviewed the risk of vertical transmission of viral hepatitis, the effect of liver disease on the course of pregnancy, the potential effects of pregnancy on the natural course of hepatitis, and the differential diagnosis of viral hepatitis in pregnancy. The clinician must be keenly aware of the manifestations of both acute and chronic viral hepatitis, in order to make the correct diagnosis and implement measures to potentially prevent transmission of infection.

REFERENCES

1. Watson JC, Fleming DW, Borella AJ, et al. Vertical transmission of hepatitis A resulting in an outbreak in a neonatal intensive care unit. J Infect Dis 1993; 163: 567–571.
2. Willner IR, Uhl MD, Howard SC, et al. Serious hepatitis A: an analysis of patients hospitalized during an urban epidemic in the United States. Ann Intern Med 1998; 128: 111–114.
3. Hamid S, Jafri SM, Kahn H, et al. Fulminant hepatic failure in pregnant women: acute fatty liver or acute viral hepatitis. J Hepatol 1996; 25: 20–27.
4. Rab MA, Bile MK, Muharik MM, et al. Water-borne hepatitis E virus epidemic in Islamabad, Pakistan: a common source outbreak traced to the malfunction of a modern water treatment plant. Am J Trop Med Hyg 1997; 57: 151–157.
5. Klein NA, Mabie WC, Shaver DC, et al. Herpes simplex virus hepatitis in pregnancy. Gastroenterology 1991; 109: 239–244.
6. Johnson MA, Moore KH, Yuen GJ, et al. Clinical pharmacokinetics of lamivudine. Clin Pharmacokinet 1999; 36: 41–66.
7. Lorenzi P, Spicher VM, Laubereau G, et al. Antiretroviral therapies in pregnancy: maternal, fetal and neonatal effects. AIDS 1998; 12: F241–F247.
8. Lok AS. Natural history and control of perinatally acquired hepatitis B virus infection. Dig Dis 1992; 10: 46–52.
9. Margolis HS, Alter MJ, Hadler SC. Hepatitis B: evolving epidemiology and implications for control. Semin Liver Dis 1991; 11: 84–92.
10. Beasley RP, Trepo C, Stevens CE, et al. The e antigen and vertical transmission of hepatitis B surface antigen. Am J Epidemiol 1977; 105: 94–98.
11. Beath SV, Boxall EH, Watson RM, et al. Fulminant hepatitis B in infants born to anti-HBe hepatitis B carrier mothers. Br Med J 1992; 304: 1169–1170.
12. Milich DR, Jones JE, Hughes JL, et al. Is a function of the secreted hepatitis B e antigen to induce immunologic tolerance in utero? Proc Natl Acad Sci USA 1990; 87: 6599–6603.
13. Poovorawan Y, Sanpavat S, Pongpunlert W, et al. Comparison of a recombinant DNA hepatitis B vaccine alone or in combination with hepatitis B immune globulin for the prevention of perinatal acquisition of hepatitis B carriage. Vaccine 1990; 8(Suppl S): 56–59.
14. Yao FB, Li XX, Du YX, et al. Combined intramuscular-intradermal protocol of universal neonate HB vaccination irrespective of mother's status of HBsAg. Vaccine 1998; 16: 586–589.
15. Ruff TA, Gertig DM, Otto BF, et al. Lombok Hepatitis B Model Immunization Project; toward universal infant hepatitis B immunization in Indonesia. J Infect Dis 1995; 17: 290–296.
16. American Academy of Pediatrics Committee on Infectious Diseases. Universal hepatitis B immunization. Pediatrics 1992; 89: 795–800.
17. Stajich GV, Lopez GP, Harry S, et al. Iatrogenic exposure to mercury after hepatitis B vaccination in preterm infants. J Pediatr 2000; 136: 679-681.
18. Silverman NS, Jenkin BK, Wu C, et al. Hepatitis C virus in pregnancy: seroprevalence and risk factors for infection. Am J Obstet Gynecol 1993; 169: 583–587.
19. Floreani A, Paternoster D, Zappala F, et al. Hepatitis C virus infection in pregnancy. Br J Obstet Gynaecol 1996; 103: 325–329.
20. Ward C, Tudor-Williams G, Coteins T, et al. Prevalence of hepatitis C among pregnant women attending an inner London obstetric department: uptake and acceptability of named antenatal testing. Gut 2000; 47: 277–280.
21. Baldo V, Floreani A, Menegon T, et al. Hepatitis C virus, hepatitis B virus and human immunodeficiency virus infection in pregnant women in North-East Italy: a seroepidemiological study. Eur J Epidemiol 2000; 16: 87–91.

22. Resti M, Bortolotti F, Azzari C, et al. Transmission of hepatitis C virus from infected mother to offspring during subsequent pregnancies. J Pediatr Gastroenterol Nutr 2000; 30: 491–493.
23. Zanetti AR, Tanzi E, Newell ML. Mother-to-infant transmission of hepatitis C virus. J Hepatol 1999; 31(Suppl 1): 96–100.
24. La Torre A, Biadaioli R, Capobianco T, et al. Vertical transmission of HCV. Acta Obstet Gynecol Scand 1998; 77: 889–892.
25. Hillemmans P, Dannecker C, Kimmig R, et al. Obstetric risks and veritcal transmission of hepatitis C virus infection in pregnancy. Acta Obstet Gynecol Scand 2000; 79: 543–547.
26. Polywka S, Schroter M, Feucht HH, et al. Low risk of vertical transmission of hepatitis C virus by breast milk. Clin Infect Dis 1999; 29: 1327–1329.
27. Delamare C, Carbonne B, Heim N, et al. Detection of hepatitis C virus RNA (HCV RNA) in amniotic fluid: a prospective study. J Hepatol 1999; 31: 416–420.
28. Mast EE, Hwang LY, Seto D, et al. Perinatal hepatitis C virus transmission: maternal risk factors and optimal timing of diagnosis. Hepatology 1999; 30: 499A.
29. Pembrey L, Newell ML, Toro PA. European pediatric hepatitis C network. Antenatal hepatitis C virus screening and management of infected women and their children. Eur J Pediatr 1999; 158: 842–846.
30. Bortolotti F, Jara P, Diaz C, et al. Posttransfusion and community-acquired hepatitis C in childhood. J Pediatr Gastroenterol Nutr 1994; 18: 279–283.
31. Rioseco AJ, Ivankovic MB, Manzur A, et al. Intrahepatic cholestasis of pregnancy: a retrospective case control of perinatal outcome. Am J Obstet Gynecol 1994; 170: 890–895.
32. Sibai BM, Ramadan MK, Usta I, et al. Maternal morbidity and mortality in 4 pregnancies with hemolysis, elevated liver enzymes, and low platelets. Am J Obstet Gynecol 1993; 169: 1000–1006.
33. Barton JR, Sibai BM, Mabie WC, et al. Recurrent fatty liver of pregnancy. Am J Obstet Gynecol 1990; 163: 534–538.
34. Ibdah J, Bennett M. Fetal fatty-acid oxidation disorder as a cause of liver disease in pregnant women. N Engl M Med 1999; 340: 1723–1731.
35. Fickert P, Ramschak H, Kenner L, et al. Acute Budd-Chiari syndrome with fulminant hepatic failure in a pregnant woman with factor V Leiden mutation. Gastroenterology 1996; 111: 1670–1673.
36. Athanassiou AM, Craigo SD. Liver masses in pregnancy. Semin Perinatol 1998; 22: 166–177.

16 Prevention and Immunoprophylaxis of Chronic Viral Hepatitis

Raymond S. Koff, MD

CONTENTS

INTRODUCTION
PREVENTION BY MODIFYING EXPOSURE RISKS
IMMUNOPROPHYLAXIS OF HEPATITIS B
IMMUNOPROPHYLAXIS OF HEPATITIS D
IMMUNOPROPHYLAXIS OF HEPATITIS C
REFERENCES

INTRODUCTION

Despite the recent advances reflected in this book, therapeutic approaches in chronic viral hepatitis are still less than perfect. Furthermore, recent increases in understanding of the epidemiology and natural history of these persistent infections have been matched only partially by advances in prevention and immunoprophylaxis. In this chapter, current state-of-the-art prevention and immunoprophylaxis is reviewed, and future potential strategies are outlined. Primary prevention of chronic viral hepatitis involves reducing the risk of infection by decreasing exposure opportunities to the responsible viruses, or by reducing susceptibility to infection by passive or active immunization. Although considerable success has been achieved through immunization against hepatitis B virus (HBV) and HBV/hepatitis D virus (HDV) co-infections, with HBV vaccines and hepatitis B immunoglobulins, vaccines directed against HDV and hepatitis C virus (HCV) are not yet available. Similarly, neither HDV-specific nor HCV-specific immunoglobulins are in use. Recent advances in recombinant technology, immunization with DNA vaccines, and improved adjuvants hold promise that effective vaccines can be

From: *Clinical Gastroenterology: Diagnosis and Therapeutics*
Edited by: R. S. Koff and G. Y. Wu © Humana Press Inc., Totowa, NJ

developed. However, registration trials for HCV and HDV vaccines are possibly a decade away from initiation. Hence, nonimmunization-based efforts are necessary to reduce the risk of exposure and chronic infection, and for many years will continue to be an important component in the prevention of these bloodborne infections. Even when vaccines are available, complete vaccine coverage of the population will probably be difficult to achieve.

Another form of prevention, directed toward reducing the risk of disease exacerbation in those with chronic viral hepatitis, is also briefly described in this chapter, but is focused on the use of hepatitis A virus (HAV) vaccine and HBV vaccines in preventing super-infection of patients with established chronic viral hepatitis.

PREVENTION BY MODIFYING EXPOSURE RISKS

Nonimmunization-based prevention efforts require understanding of risk factors associated with infection, and implementation of strategies to reduce such exposures. Currently, more critical for the control of HCV infection than for HBV, given the absence of a vaccine for the former, prevention, without the use of immunization biologicals, applies to both infections, and are discussed together.

Hepatitis Caused by Injecting Illicit Drugs and Intranasal Cocaine Use

The sharing of needles, syringes, and other equipment for the injection of illicit drugs is responsible for a substantial proportion of both HBV and HCV infections. Prevention efforts may be instituted by primary care physicians through routine inquiry about the use of injection illicit drugs by their patients. Advice to discontinue drug use, discussion of substance abuse treatment, and, where available, participation in needle-exchange programs may be effective. If the latter are not available, education concerning appropriate sterilization techniques may be implemented. Unfortunately, because percutaneous transmission through shared injection equipment is highly efficient for both HBV and HCV, these approaches are likely to be effective only if instituted very early after drug use begins *(1)*. Current evidence suggests that needle-exchange programs reduce the risk of HIV infection, but their role in the control of HCV is more enigmatic. Higher concentrations of HCV and a higher prevalence of HCV infection in injection drug users may be responsible for this difference. Whether educational efforts describing the risk of sharing plastic straws or similar equipment for the intranasal snorting of cocaine would be effective is unknown, but seems rational. Reduction or elimination of illicit drug-injection behavior and illicit snorting of cocaine, by school-based early educational approaches that inform students about the risks, remains a goal. Providing routine HBV vaccination for drug-injection or snorting individuals at risk is highly appropriate, and, because injection drug users have an increased risk of acquisition of HAV, HAV vaccination also should be offered *(2)*.

Blood and Blood-Product-Associated Hepatitis

In the early 1970s, blood-donor screening for (hepatitis B surface antigen [HBsAg]) was introduced. Subsequently, in 1986, after considerable discussion, surrogate testing for non-A, non-B hepatitis was implemented, by screening for the presence of antibody to the hepatitis B core antigen, and by identifying donors with elevated levels of serum alanine aminotransferase. These hepatitis-screening techniques, together with changes in blood-donor selection criteria, resulted in a major decline in the frequency of posttransfusion HBV and HCV infection. The introduction of successive generations of anti-HCV screening of blood donors, beginning a decade ago, dramatically reduced the risk of transfusion-associated HCV infection. The estimated risk of HBV and HCV infection by transfusion, based on studies of repeat blood donors *(3)*, is about 1/65,000 U transfused for the former, and 1/100,000 U transfused for the latter. Currently, transfusion-associated HBV or HCV infection is either the result of human error (e.g., errors in transcription of test results) or a result of collection of blood during the diagnostic window period in acutely infected donors. This is the usually brief period in which asymptomatic donors may have circulating hepatitis viruses, without detectable antigen or antibodies. The newest screening approach, designed to reduce the serological window, and thereby to further decrease the risk of viral transmission, is routine screening of donors by highly sensitive nucleic acid tests. Initial studies *(4)*, using polymerase chain reaction testing of pooled plasma samples for HBV, HCV, and human immune deficiency virus (HIV), indicate that such donor screening can be achieved rapidly, and is feasible in routine practice. Other approaches to reducing the risk of transfusion-associated hepatitis are listed in Table 1.

Sexual Transmission of HBV and HCV

Both HBV and HCV may be spread by sexual contact, although the efficiency of sexual transmission is thought to be much lower for HCV. Primary care physicians should routinely inquire about high-risk sexual practices, such as failure to use condoms, multiple sex partners, and a past history or the presence of sexually transmitted diseases. If answered

Table 1
Strategies for Reducing
Transfusion-associated Bloodborne Hepatitis Virus Infection

Increased use of transfusion practice guidelines
Routine monitoring of compliance with transfusion practice guidelines
Increased use of stored, autologous blood for elective surgery
Increased use of perioperative blood recovery techniques
Acute normovolemic hemodilution
Appropriate use of erythropoietin
Use of virally inactivated or recombinant blood products
Development of red-cell substitutes

in the affirmative, advice is appropriate about changing behavior and the use of condoms to protect their partners and themselves. Vaccination against HBV should be undertaken in those susceptibles engaged in high-risk sex, and, if the individual is a male homosexual, vaccination against HAV is also reasonable. HBV vaccine should also be offered to as many of the sexual contacts of individuals found to be HBsAg-positive as logistically possible. Potential strategies for reducing sexual transmission are listed in Table 2. Long-term and monogamous sexual partners of HBV- or HCV-infected individuals should be tested for evidence of infection. If the index case has HBV, vaccination is recommended for the susceptible sexual partner. For the sexual partner of the index case with HCV, recommendations have been more equivocal and mostly limited to testing the partner for evidence of infection and providing information about the potential risks, so that an educated decision about the use of condoms can be made.

Maternal–Neonatal Transmission of HBV and HCV

Other than identification of the HBV-infected mother and immunization of her newborn infant, realistic methods for reducing the risk of maternal–neonatal transmission of the bloodborne hepatitis viruses are unknown. Breastfeeding has not been definitively implicated in transmission of HBV or HCV to the infant, even in HIV-positive women with high hepatitis virus titers *(5)*. For the nonpregnant HBV- or HCV-infected woman considering beginning a family or enlarging an established one, effective preconception antiviral treatment, leading to clearance of the responsible virus, would seem likely to eliminate or reduce the risk of transmission to the infant.

Table 2
Strategies for Reducing Sexual
Transmission of Bloodborne Hepatitis Viruses

Delaying the onset of sexual behavior
Consistent use of condoms
Limiting the number of sexual partners
Avoidance of other sexually transmitted diseases
Avoidance of trauma during sexual activity

Needlestick Injury and Mucosal Exposure to HBV and HCV in Health Care Workers

The risk of needlestick injury leading to bloodborne hepatitis virus infections in health care personnel has been studied for many years. Prevention efforts directed at health care workers have focused on the development of safer injection devices, the use of personal protective equipment, continuing education about the handling and disposal of used equipment, acceptance of the principles of universal precautions, and the prompt reporting of critical exposures. Infected patients with either HBV or HCV require education about the potential infectivity of their blood and body fluids, and the risks of sharing razor blades, tooth brushes, and other personal hygiene equipment. Blood spills in the house should be cleaned by the responsible patient, or, if undertaken by another member of the household, protective rubber or latex gloves should be worn. The risk of hepatitis virus transmission, resulting from tattooing, body-piercing, acupuncture, electrolysis, manicures, pedicures, and the barbershop shave, is poorly understood. Appropriate cleaning and sterilization procedures, if followed, should eliminate any risk from contaminated equipment.

IMMUNOPROPHYLAXIS OF HEPATITIS B

Hepatitis B virus (HBV) infection is the most common vaccine-preventable liver disease in the world. Over 300 million are chronically infected, and as many as 1 million deaths are attributed to the sequelae of this infection annually. The extraordinary protective efficacy of HBV vaccines, combined with their ability to provide prolonged protection in most individuals, strongly suggests that, despite concerns about the emergence of mutant HBV strains, universal use of the vaccines will eventually markedly reduce, if not eliminate, this infection. Although routine infant immunization against HBV has been adopted in many nations, coverage is still limited, particularly in developing countries where the infection may be endemic.

HBV Vaccines and Regimens

Plasma-derived vaccines comprise about 80% of worldwide HBV vaccine production, but are no longer available in the United States. Recombinant HBV vaccines were approved for use in the United States in 1986 and 1989. The two commercially available vaccines are produced by cloning the gene encoding the HBsAg, through use of a plasmid vector inserted into common baker's yeast. The yeast-derived HBsAg particles induce immunity by stimulating the endogenous production of neutralizing antibody to HBsAg (anti-HBs). Seroprotection is thought to be achieved when anti-HBs levels are 10 mIU/mL or higher. Antibody to the hepatitis B core antigen (anti-HBc) is not induced by the recombinant HBV vaccines. Rarely, transiently positive tests for HBsAg in serum may be found within 24 h following vaccine administration. The HBV vaccines are highly immunogenic, and are conventionally given in a three-dose schedule utilizing a deltoid injection site, or, in infants, the anterolateral muscle of the thigh. Recombivax hepatitis B (Merck), the first-approved recombinant HBV vaccine, is formulated to contain a 10-mcg adult dose of HBsAg protein, given in a three-dose schedule at 0, 1, and 6 mo. For children ages 0–19 yr, Recombivax hepatitis B is given in a 5-mcg, three-dose schedule. However, an optional regimen for children, ages 11–15 yr is a 10-mcg, two-dose, schedule (0 and 4–6 mo). Engerix-B (SmithKline Beecham), the second recombinant HBV vaccine approved in the United States, is formulated to contain a 20-mcg dose of HBsAg protein for older children and adults, given in a three-dose schedule. In children, ages 5–16 yr, the 10-mcg dose of Engerix-B is also approved for a three-dose regimen, in which the injection are spaced 1 yr apart (0, 12, and 24 mo), in order to improve compliance. A two-dose regimen is also under study *(6)*.

HBV vaccines containing the pre-S (middle and large surface) proteins, in addition to HBsAg, have been developed, but are not approved for use in the United States. These vaccines may eventually find a role in the revaccination of nonresponders to the conventional HBsAg-containing vaccines *(7)*. Further studies of their immunogenicity, reactogenicity, and the immunogenetic factors involved in the vaccine-induced immune response, are needed.

Vaccination Strategies

Current vaccination strategies in the United States call for screening all pregnant women for HBsAg, and rapid immunization with both vaccine and hepatitis B immunoglobulins of the neonates of those women found to be HBsAg-positive. Other infants, children, and adolescents through 18 yr of age, and high-risk groups are also candidates for HBV vaccine.

High-risk groups are generally defined as individuals with more than one sexual partner in a 6-mo period, and homosexual or bisexual males. Attendees at sexually transmitted disease clinics or public health clinics, and adolescents living in areas with a high frequency of teenage pregnancy, should be vaccinated. Intimate or household contacts of individuals who are HBsAg-positive also are vaccine candidates. Illicit injection drug users and patients with bleeding disorders, who are likely to receive nonrecombinant clotting factor preparations, should receive HBV vaccine. Patients with chronic renal failure are routinely vaccinated, and individuals who reside in institutions for the mentally retarded, and employees of such institutions, have been targeted for vaccination. Inmates in correctional institutions, in which injection drug use and homosexual behavior may occur, also are candidates. Health care or public safety workers (first-responders), and trainees in these fields, who are at risk because of occupational contact with blood or body fluids, should be vaccinated early in their careers. Travelers to regions of the world that are hyperendemic for HBV, and to which visits are prolonged, also should be considered for vaccination. Alaskan natives, Pacific Islanders, and the children of immigrants from hyperendemic regions are candidates for vaccination.

In a small proportion of otherwise healthy individuals, pre-vaccination testing for markers of past HBV infection has revealed the presence of isolated anti-HBc. Many of these (particularly those with low anti-HBc titers) appear to be false-positive results. Hence, the response to vaccination in these individuals is typical of the response in a previously unexposed person. Less than 5% of individuals with isolated anti-HBc may have detectable HBV DNA in serum, indicating continuing viral replication and no need for vaccination *(8)*. Because the cost of testing for HBV DNA is high, it may be more reasonable to simply administer all three doses of vaccine, and test for anti-HBs after the third dose.

Patients with chronic liver disease, e.g., chronic hepatitis C (CHC), are also candidates for the HBV vaccine, if serologic markers of HBV infection are absent, since super-infection by HBV may result in increased morbidity and high case-fatality rates. Limited data *(9)* indicate that vaccine responsiveness may decline with advancing disease, and that patients with cirrhosis awaiting transplantation are among the least responsive. Hence, early immunization, after the diagnosis of chronic liver disease, seems appropriate. Although, in a recently reported European study *(10)*, patients with CHC were less responsive to a non-U.S.-approved recombinant vaccine than were healthy controls, conflicting data *(11)* have been reported in the United States, about the commercially available U.S.-approved recombinant vaccines.

Protective Efficacy

Protective efficacy rates are close to 95% in the general population of vaccinated persons. Older individuals, the obese, smokers, and immunosuppressed patients are less responsive to vaccination. In these groups, peak titers of anti-HBs after a full course of vaccine, may be just above or below the seroprotective level, in as many as one-third of vaccinees. Patients with chronic cardiac and pulmonary disorders, hemodialysis and organ transplant patients, and HIV-positive patients with low CD4+ counts, are also less responsive. Use of higher doses of vaccine may augment antibody response in some of these patient groups, e.g., those on hemodialysis. In a small portion of vaccinated individuals, vaccine non-responsiveness appears to be genetically based. In these individuals, the absence of a dominant immune response gene, capable of mediating anti-HBs production, is thought to be responsible.

Testing for anti-HBs has been recommended, after the third vaccine dose in the immunocompromised, and may be appropriate for persons at occupational risk of infection, such as health care workers, in whom continued exposure to blood or body fluids is anticipated. Post-vaccination anti-HBs levels reach their peak later in older subjects, compared to the young *(12)*. As a consequence, post-vaccination testing should not be undertaken until at least 70–80 d after the final vaccine dose. Non-responders should probably be revaccinated with three additional doses of vaccines, if they are at increased risk. Testing for anti-HBs may also be appropriate for vaccinated infants born to HBsAg-positive mothers, and for the vaccinated sex partners of HBsAg-positive individuals.

HBV vaccine-induced immunity prevents subclinical HBV infection, clinically apparent hepatitis B, and chronic HBV infection. In immunized individuals in whom anti-HBs is induced, the duration of protection is prolonged for over 15 yr *(13)*, and possibly longer. In fact, it would not be surprising to learn that immunity is life-long. Immunity persists despite the observation that levels of anti-HBs may fall below the seroprotective threshold over time, and, in many vaccinees, become undetectable. The phenomenon of immunologic memory, dependent on the presence of memory cells, appears to be responsible for this persistence of immunity. There is some evidence that, in addition to immunologic memory following all three doses of the vaccine, immunologic memory may be retained, after even a single dose, for a few years *(14,15)*.

EFFECTIVENESS OF HBV VACCINATION PROGRAMS

Vaccine-induced eradication of HBV infection has yet to be achieved in any nation. In the less-affluent countries, high vaccine cost, difficulties in vaccine delivery, and other competing high-priority public health issues have impeded implementation of national HBV vaccination programs. Among the countries that have incorporated HBV vaccine into their pediatric immunization programs, Taiwan is a remarkably successful example. In just over a decade of universal infant vaccination, the rate of HBV chronic infection among young children has fallen by more than 85% *(16)*, and the incidence of HBV-associated hepatocellular carcinoma in children has been halved *(17)*.

In the United States, recommendations for universal infant, child, and adolescent HBV immunization were delayed until the 1990s, despite the earlier availability of vaccines. As a consequence, HBV prevalence did not decline in the period between 1976 and 1980, compared to that between 1988 and 1994 *(18)*. A reduction in reported cases of acute hepatitis B since 1987 has been identified, but appears to be mostly unrelated to vaccine usage.

Prevention of HAV Super-infection in Chronic Hepatitis B and CHC

HAV super-infection of individuals with chronic hepatitis B virus and chronic hepatitis C virus infection may exacerbate the liver disease, and, in some instances, may lead to acute liver failure *(19,20)*. This concept has not been accepted by all workers in the field *(21)*, but the recommendation that HAV-susceptible patients with chronic liver disease should be targeted for vaccination with one of the inactivated, whole HAV vaccines seems reasonable, and has become standard practice in many hepatology centers. HAV vaccination of patients who have received liver transplants is also reasonable. Information about the immunogenicity of HAV vaccines in patients with chronic liver disease remains limited, but, in general, the immune response to the vaccines appear to be adequate in those with mild to moderately severe disease. In one study, the immune response to inactivated HAV vaccine among Chinese HBV-carrier children appeared to be reduced, compared to that in noncarrier children, but the differences were not statistically significant through 5 yr of follow-up *(22)*. Furthermore, all vaccinated children had detectable antibodies to HAV at yr 5. In another study *(23)*, this one from Italy, inactivated HAV vaccine was reported to be highly immunogenic in young HBsAg carriers, as well as in those with chronic hepatitis B. In a study of adult patients with chronic liver disease in the United States, HAV vaccine

Table 3
Anti-HAV Seroconversion Rates
and Anti-HAV Titers in Healthy Adults and Patients
with Compensated Chronic Liver Diseases, Measured
1 Mo After Second Dose of Inactivated Hepatitis A Vaccine

Subjects studied	Seroconversion rate (%)	Geometric mean anti-HAV titer (mIU/mL)
Healthy adults	98.2	1315
Chronic hepatitis B	97.7	749
Chronic hepatitis C	94.3	467
Other liver diseases	95.2	562

appeared to be slightly less immunogenic than in healthy controls (11), and this seemed to be more pronounced in patients with CHC. Despite these findings, the antibody response after completion of the two-dose regimen appeared adequate to provide protection from infection. Nearly 95% of all vaccinated patients were seropositive for antibody to HAV, at the completion of the course (see Table 3).

The immunogenicity of the inactivated HAV vaccines appears to decline as the liver disease advances in severity. In patients with decompensated chronic liver disease, seroconversion rates and titers of postvaccination antibody to HAV are low (24). Based on these findings, early immunization should be considered for HAV-susceptible patients, following the diagnosis of chronic liver disease.

For chronic liver disease patients susceptible to both HBV and HAV, a combination HBV and HAV vaccine, called "Twinrix" (SmithKline Beecham), is now available. Although extensive studies are not yet available, immunogenicity is likely to be good in this patient group, if immunization is begun early after diagnosis.

Future Problems in HBV Immunoprophylaxis

The emergence of transmissable HBV escape mutants, which may lead to chronic infection, is a major concern, since these have been reported from many parts of the world, albeit in low frequency. They appear to be responsible for instances of breakthrough infections in immunized infants, but also have been reported in liver transplant patients who have been treated with hepatitis B immunoglobulins. The most common mutations found to date affect the common "a" determinant of HBsAg, and result in less binding of HBsAg to anti-HBs. Thus, the mutant HBV evades the protective ability of anti-HBs (25). The mutant HBV virus may arise *de novo* in infected infants, or can be transmitted from the mother *(26)*. Available information *(27)* suggests that spread of these escape mutants may be slow, but modeling studies *(28)* suggest that they may become the predominant form of HBV by late in the twenty-first century. If this is correct, it will be necessary to incorporate mutant-strain antigens into future versions of HBV vaccines.

IMMUNOPROPHYLAXIS OF HEPATITIS D

Although pre-exposure administration of HBV vaccines will protect against HBV–HDV co-infections, HDV super-infection of individuals with established HBV infection remains a problem. HBsAg-positive hemodialysis patients, injection drug users, recipients of multiple blood products, individuals with multiple sexual contacts, and others at increased risk for HDV acquisition, would be potential candidates for immunoprophylaxis. Neither a HDV vaccine nor a high-titer anti-HDV immunoglobulin preparation are commercially available. Preliminary studies *(29)* of the immune response to HDV antigens, and to synthetic HDV peptides, have been less than promising, and progress in this field has been slow. As a result, the development of a HDV vaccine is not likely for some time.

IMMUNOPROPHYLAXIS OF HEPATITIS C

Neither passive immunization with conventional or HCV hyperimmune globulin preparations nor active immunization with an HCV vaccine are currently recommended or available. Immunity to HCV infection is thought to be weak, and neutralizing, protective antibodies can be detected in only a small proportion of infected individuals, and seem to be isolate-specific. One consequence of this limited response is that superinfection by another HCV genotype may be identified in some patients chronically infected with one HCV genotype *(30)*. The high frequency of mutations, in that portion of the viral genome encoding the HCV envelope proteins, may be responsible for the escape of the virus from antibody-mediated clearance. Early studies *(31)* suggested that primary infection with HCV did not induce protective immunity in the chimpanzee model of infection. However, there is evidence *(32)* that the immune response of chimpanzees to HCV may not be analogous to that seen in infected patients.

Mechanisms of Protection

The immunodominant epitopes of HCV are likely to be localized to the structural, rather than the nonstructural proteins, of the virus. The

HCV envelope glycoproteins (GP), designated E1 and E2, are the putative sites of the immunodominant epitope. Antibodies to the envelope proteins are present in low titer in most HCV-infected individuals. At the N-terminal portion of E2, a hypervariable region I (HVR I) is present, and may play a key role in the emergence of HCV variants that escape immune recognition by neutralizing antibody activity. Antibodies to HVR I may have neutralizing ability, since they have been shown to block the attachment of HCV to human fibroblasts in tissue culture *(33)*. Despite these observations, it remains uncertain whether HVR I is the principal target of the neutralizing immune response to HCV. In studies of HCV infection in both chimpanzees and human beings, antibodies to E2 could not be correlated with self-limited infection *(34)*. In fact, persistence of these antibodies correlated with chronic infection. Other immune epitopes, in other portions of the structural proteins, also may function in the neutralization of the virus. The critical immune epitopes, their sites on the genome, and their specific sequences need to be identified.

Theoretically, if circulating neutralizing antibodies, directed to the immunodominant epitopes of HCV, are present prior to infection (as a consequence of vaccination or passive administration of antibodies), they may serve to protect susceptible hepatocytes from HCV infection during the initial viremic phase, by interfering with viral attachment and/or entry. Additionally, they may protect uninfected hepatocytes during the likely secondary viremia or contiguous exposure to virus that results from production and release of virus from infected, injured cells, early in infection. However, if HCV is capable of evading neutralizing antibodies, a HCV vaccine that simultaneously elicited cell-mediated immunity might prove more effective than one that only evokes antibodies, because cell-mediated immune responses may detect and destroy the initially infected cells, resulting in self-limited infection. This remains speculative, since the role of cell-mediated immunity in preventing HCV infection is still uncertain.

Passive Immunization with Immunoglobulin

Passive immunization, with conventionally prepared immunoglobulin, was studied prior to the availability of serological tests for antibodies to HCV, and prior to the characterization of HCV as an RNA virus. Attempts to reduce the risk of transfusion-associated non-A, non-B hepatitis (now known to have been mostly HCV infection) were undertaken in the hope that neutralizing antibodies might be present in immunoglobulin preparations in sufficient concentrations to reduce the severity or completely abort infection in the recipients. Prospective, randomized clinical trials of conventional immunoglobulin in the United States and in Spain *(35–*

38), provided conflicting results. Because HCV infection rates could not be accurately determined at that time, and measurement of neutralizing antibodies was impossible, the studies are difficult to interpret. Nonetheless, prophylactic of transfusion-associated hepatitis C with immunoglobulin has not been recommended, and the extraordinary effectiveness of current donor-screening techniques limits the need to consider passive immunization in this setting.

In the early 1990s, the U.S. Food and Drug Administration recommended that human plasma, collected for fractionation, be screened for anti-HCV. Hence, immunoglobulin preparations prepared in the United States are now likely to have no anti-HCV or HCV-neutralizing antibodies. Conventional immunoglobulin is therefore unlikely to have any efficacy in HCV immunoprophylaxis. immunoglobulin, made from unscreened plasma in Switzerland in 1991, has been reported to have high titers of neutralizing antibodies to HCV. This material was utilized, in an Italian study *(39)*, to assess the efficacy of repeated injection of large doses in preventing sexual transmission among heterosexual partners. Although, in this randomized, controlled trial, the risk of infection appeared to be reduced in recipients of this immunoglobulin, the study was terminated when testing of immunoglobulin for anti-HCV became mandatory in Italy in 1993. These observations suggest that there might be a role for HCV hyperimmune globulin in immunoprophylaxis.

Hyperimmune Anti-HCV Immunoglobulin

In a study *(40)* utilizing the chimpanzee model of HCV infection, the plasma of a patient with CHC was shown to contain antibodies to HCV, capable of neutralizing the virus in vitro. Challenge of animals with this inoculum did not produce infection, indicating that the virus had been neutralized. In addition to supporting the existence of neutralizing antibodies in HCV infection, that study also indicated that cell-based immunity was not essential for HCV neutralization in vitro. Neutralizing antibodies to HCV are thought to inhibit the replicative cycle of HCV *(41)*. Unfortunately, HCV-neutralizing antibody are isolate-specific, and may change as a consequence of the emergence of escape HCV mutants.

Utilizing a synthetic peptide derived from HVR I as the inducing antigen, a HCV hyperimmune serum has been developed *(42)*. When mixed with HCV in vitro, this material appeared to neutralize the virus, since, when the mixture was inoculated into chimpanzees, infection was prevented. HCV RNA-negative hyperimmune globulin prepared from anti-HCV positive human plasma containing antibodies to HCV core, NS3 and NS4 proteins also has been studied in the chimpanzee model *(43)*. In one animal, the hyperimmune globulin was infused intravenously 1 hr after intravenous challenge with an infectious dose of HCV. A second chimpanzee received anti-HCV-negative intravenous immunoglobulin 1 hr after identical challenge with HCV. The third animal was challenged with HCV, but was untreated. Acute HCV infection occurred in all three animals, as demonstrated by the rapid appearance of HCV RNA in serum, and the presence of HCV antigens in hepatocytes. In the chimpanzee that had received the hyperimmune globulin, the development of both elevated serum alanine aminotransferase levels and histopathological features of acute hepatitis were delayed. This suggested that, although the neutralizing antibodies in this HCV hyperimmune globulin did not prevent infection, they may have restricted the extent of intrahepatic replication.

Can a HCV human hyperimmune globulin, negative for HCV RNA, but containing sufficient neutralizing activity to prevent in vivo infection when administered either pre- or postexposure, be prepared? Would it be necessary to utilize anti-HCV-positive plasma as the starting material, or could synthetic peptides be utilized to induce antibodies in human volunteers, who would be plasma donors for preparation of the globulin? How large an inoculum would be needed to achieve protection, rather than delaying the onset of infection? Would such a preparation protect against more than one HCV genotype? How long would protection last? These are some of the questions that would need to be answered to pursue the notion of passive immunization.

Active Immunization

Major obstacles to the development of active immunization against HCV include failure to consistently propagate the virus in tissue culture systems, the absence of susceptible small animals, and the multitude of genotypes and subtypes of HCV that have been identified. Additionally, limited information about the immunodominant, neutralization epitopes, the range of reactivity of antibodies induced by these epitopes, and the existence of few assays for the quantitation of HCV neutralizing antibodies have impeded progress in vaccine development. Furthermore, the potential contributory role of cellular immune responses, in inducing protection and immunological memory, remains uncertain. Hence, it is not clear whether or not T-cell-inducing epitopes should be identified and incorporated into a prototype HCV vaccine. For a HCV vaccine to achieve approval, it will be essential to demonstrate acceptable protective efficacy rates, a good safety profile, a reasonably prolonged duration of protection, and the compatibility of such a vaccine co-administered with other commonly used vaccines. A number of approaches to the devel-

Table 4
Potential Approaches to Development of HCV Vaccine

Immunization with recombinant envelope GPs
Immunization with DNA, encoding HCV envelope proteins
Immunization with DNA, encoding nucleocapsid protein
Immunization with live virus vector expressing recombinant HCV proteins
Immunization with HCV anti-idiotypic antibodies

opment of a HCV are possible (Table 4), but information is limited to just a few.

PROTOTYPE ENVELOPE GP VACCINE

In one of the earliest attempts to develop a HCV vaccine *(44)*, envelope GPs (gpE1/E2), expressed in a recombinant vaccinia virus vector from one strain of HCV, were used to infect HeLa cells. After extraction, the GPs were combined with a potent adjuvant (MF59) and inoculated into seven chimpanzees. The animals were then challenged, at the peak of their antibody response to the envelope GPs, with low doses of the same HCV strain. Five of the seven chimpanzees appeared to be protected. In a subsequent report *(45)*, 2/3 chimpanzees, similarly vaccinated, were protected against both viremia and acute hepatitis, after challenge with a larger inoculum, containing a heterologous HCV 1a strain. High titers of neutralizing antibodies, measured by a "neutralization of binding" assay *(46)*, were observed in vaccinated chimpanzees, and a correlation of antibody levels with protection from infection was reported. The immunogenicity, safety, and protective efficacy of this prototype vaccine in human beings has yet to be reported. Phase 1 and 2 trials have been initiated.

GENETIC VACCINES AGAINST HCV

Vaccines made from of genetic material, either DNA or RNA, can encode specific viral antigens, such as those of the HCV envelope or its nucleocapsid, have received attention for their future potential in the immunoprophylaxis of HCV. Because DNA is more stable than RNA, DNA vaccines have been more extensively studied, and early work on the development of a genetic vaccine against HCV has concentrated on DNA. DNA vaccines, or "naked-DNA vaccines," as they are sometimes called, can be injected directly into the cells of host tissues (muscle, skin, or others), which express the viral gene producing the encoded protein. Through a complex process involving antigen-presenting cells, and costimulatory molecules, the expressed intracellular viral protein is taken up by the major histocompatibility complex (MHC) class I pathway, stimulating cell-mediated immunity. The humoral immune response is also primed, through the MHC-II pathway, helper T-cells, and co-stimulatory molecules.

Use of a genetic HCV vaccine, expressing the HCV nucleocapsid has been an area of investigation. The HCV nucleocapsid is antigenic, and well-conserved within and between HCV genotypes and subtypes at the amino acid level, and both B-cell and cytotoxic T-lymphocyte determinants have been mapped to this site in infected patients. Thus, a DNA vaccine encoding the nucleocapsid, and capable of inducing neutralizing humoral and T-cell immunity, may provide protection against the different HCV genotypes. Current studies have been limited to mice.

In one early study *(47)*, animals immunized with a DNA vaccine, in the form of chimeric constructs from the HCV nucleocapsid, expressing the first 58 amino acids of the nucleocapsid, and HBV surface antigen proteins, developed immune responses to both viruses. In other studies *(48,49)*, DNA encoding the HCV nucleocapsid was shown to induce humoral immune responses to the nucleocapsid protein and strong cytotoxic T-lymphocyte activity in vivo and in vitro. In immunized mice, protection against HCV nucleocapsid gene/transfected tumor cells was observed *(48)*. An IgM antibody response to the nucleocapsid without IgG has been observed in mice immunized with a plasmid containing the gene encoding the nucleocapsid *(50)*. IgG levels did rise after the mice were boosted with recombinant HCV nucleocapsid protein. The possible protective role of these antibodies was not addressed.

If a DNA vaccine against HCV can be developed, which induces neutralizing activity that is of prolonged duration, and protects against each genotype, it will be a major breakthrough in this field. The notion of a therapeutic vaccine would follow. Concerns about the safety of DNA vaccines, including development of antibodies to DNA, the triggering of autoimmune disease, the development of tolerance, and insertional mutagenesis, remain hypothetical and unsupported in trials of experimental DNA vaccines for other disorders (HIV, influenza).

OTHER VACCINE APPROACHES

A replication-deficient recombinant adenovirus vector system has been developed, which combines HCV envelope and nucleocapsid proteins into a live virus vaccine *(51)*. Immunized mice developed antibodies to E1, E2, and the nucleocapsid, but neutralizing activity was not assessed. The use of HCV anti-idiotypic antibodies mimicking the envelope or nucleocapsid antigens, to induce immunity, remains a fascinating but futuristic approach.

Candidates for HCV Vaccine

Appropriate candidates for a HCV vaccine may include newly identified injection drug users or intranasal cocaine users, renal failure patients at risk for hemodialysis, patients with blood-clotting disorders, and other recipients of multiple blood products, the sex partners of HCV-infected individuals, and possibly sex workers. Patients with other chronic liver diseases would be targeted, as well. Although the prevalence of infection appears to be low in health care personnel, those regularly exposed to blood and body fluids might be considered for immunization. If early administration, e.g., shortly after birth, of a HCV vaccine to the neonates of infected women could protect the neonates, then identification pre-delivery of pregnant HCV-infected women would become critically important. Because vaccine delivery to injection drug users early in their careers remains problematic, it seems likely that a targeted approach to high-risk individuals is likely to fail. If this concept is valid, only universal childhood vaccination against HCV is likely to reduce the rate of infection.

REFERENCES

1. Garfein RS, Vlahov D, Galai N, et al. Viral infections in short-term injection drug users: the prevalence of the hepatitis C, hepatitis B, human immunodeficiency, and human T-lymphotropic viruses. Am J Public Health 1996; 86: 655–661.
2. Koff RS. Hepatitis A. Lancet 1998; 341: 1643–1649.
3. Schreiber GB, Busch MP, Kleinman SH, et al. Risk of transfusion-transmitted viral infections. N Engl J Med 1996; 334: 1685–1690.
4. Roth WK, Weber M, Seifried E. Feasibility and efficacy of routine PCR screening of blood donations for hepatitis C virus, hepatitis B virus, and HIV-1 in a blood-bank setting. Lancet 1999; 353: 359–363.
5. Manzini P, Saracco G, Cerchier A, et al. Human immunodeficiency virus infection as risk factor for mother-to-child hepatitis C virus transmission; persistence of anti-hepatitis C virus in children is associated with the mother's anti-hepatitis C virus immunoblotting pattern. Hepatology 1995; 21: 328–332.
6. Gellin BG, Greenberg RN, Hart RH, et al. Immunogenicity of two doses of yeast recombinant hepatitis B vaccine in healthy older adults. J Infect Dis 1997; 175: 1494–1497.
7. McDermott AB, Cohen SB, Zuckerman JN, et al. Human leukocyte antigens influence the immune response to a pre-S/S hepatitis B vaccine. Vaccine 1999; 17: 330–339.
8. Silva AE, McMahon BJ, Parkinson AJ, et al. Hepatitis B DNA in persons with isolated antibody to hepatitis B core antigen who subsequently received hepatitis B vaccine. Clin Infect Dis 1998; 26: 895–897.
9. Horlander JC, Boyle N, Manam R, et al. Vaccination against hepatitis B in patients with chronic liver disease awaiting liver transplantation. Am J Med Sci 1999; 318: 304–307.
10. Wiedmann M, Liebert UG, Oesen U, et al. Decreased immunogenicity of recombinant hepatitis B vaccine in chronic hepatitis C. Hepatology 2000; 31: 230–234.

11. Keeffe EB, Iwarson S, McMahon BJ, et al. Safety and immunogenicity of hepatitis A vaccine in patients with chronic liver disease. Hepatology 1998; 27: 881–886.
12. Honorati MC, Palareti A, Dolzani P, et al. Mathematical model predicting anti-hepatitis B virus surface antigen (HBs) decay after vaccination against hepatitis B. Clin Exp Immunol 1999; 116: 121–126.
13. Liao S-S, Li R-C, Li H, et al. Long-term efficacy of plasma-derived hepatitis B vaccine: a 15-year follow-up study among Chinese children. Vaccine 1999; 17: 2661–2666.
14. Marsano LS, West DJ, Chan J, et al. Two-dose hepatitis B vaccine regimen: proof of priming and memory responses in young adults. Vaccine 1998; 16: 624–629.
15. Wistrom J, Ahlm C, Lundberg S, et al. Booster vaccination with recombinant hepatitis B vaccine four years after priming with one single dose. Vaccine 1999; 17: 2162–2165.
16. Chen H-L, Chang M-H, Ni Y-H, et al. Seroepidemiology of hepatitis B virus infection in children. Ten years of mass vaccination in Taiwan. JAMA 1996; 276: 906–908.
17. Chang M-H, Chen C-J, Lai M-S, et al. Universal hepatitis B vaccination in Taiwan and the incidence of hepatocellular carcinoma in children. N Engl J Med 1997; 336: 1855–1859.
18. McQuillan GM, Coleman PJ, Kruszon-Moran D, et al. Prevalence of hepatitis B virus infection in the United States: the National Health and Nutrition Examination Surveys, 1976 through 1994. Am J Public Health 1999; 89: 14–18.
19. Vento S, Garofano T, Renzini C, et al. Fulminant hepatitis associated with hepatitis A virus superinfection in patients with chronic hepatitis C. N Engl J Med 1998; 338: 286–290.
20. Keeffe EB. Is hepatitis A more severe in patients with chronic hepatitis B and other chronic liver diseases? Am J Gastroenterol 1995; 90: 201–205.
21. Asselah T, Bernuau J, Marcellin P. Prevalence of hepatitis C virus infection in patients hospitalized for hepatitis A. Ann Intern Med 1999; 130: 451.
22. Chan C-Y, Lee S-D, Yu M-I, et al. Long-term followup of hepatitis A vaccination in children. Vaccine 1999; 17: 369–372.
23. Nebbia G, Giacchino R, Soncini R, et al. Hepatitis A vaccination in chronic carriers of hepatitis B virus. J Pediatr 1999; 134: 784–785.
24. Dumot JA, Barnes DS, Younossi Z, et al. Immunogenicity of hepatitis A vaccine in decompensated liver disease. Am J Gastroenterol 1999; 94: 1601–1604.
25. Waters JA, Kennedy M, Voet P, et al. Loss of the common "A" determinant of hepatitis B surface antigen by a vaccine-induced escape mutant. J Clin Invest 1992; 90: 2543–2547.
26. Ngui SL, O'Connell S, Eglin RP, et al. Low detection rate and maternal provenance of hepatitis B virus S gene mutants in cases of failed postnatal immunoprophylaxis in England and Wales. J Infect Dis 1997; 176: 1360–1365.
27. Gunther S, Fischer L, Pult I, et al. Naturally occurring variants of hepatitis B virus. Adv Virus Res 1999; 52: 25–137.
28. Zuckerman AJ, Zuckerman JN. Molecular epidemiology of hepatitis B virus mutants. J Med Virol 1999; 58: 193–195.
29. Gerin JL, Casey JL, Bergmann KF. Molecular biology of hepatitis delta virus: recent advances. In: *Viral Hepatitis and Liver Disease* (Nishioka K, Suzuki H, Mishiro S, et al., eds.), Tokyo: Springer-Verlag, 1994, pp. 38–41.
30. Kao J-H, Chen P-J, Lai M-Y, et al. Superinfection of heterologous hepatitis C virus in a patient with chronic type C hepatitis. Gastroenterology 1993; 105: 583–587.

31. Farci P, Alter HJ, Govindarajan S, et al. Lack of protective immunity against reinfection with hepatitis C virus. Science 1992; 258: 135–140.
32. Wang Y-F, Brotman B, Andrus L, et al. Immune response to epitopes of hepatitis C virus (HCV) structural proteins in HCV-infected human and chimpanzees. J Infect Dis 1996; 173: 808–821.
33. Zibert A, Schreier E, Roggendorf M. Antibodies in human sera specific to the hypervariable region I of hepatitis C virus can block viral attachment. Virology 1995; 208: 653–661.
34. Prince AM, Brotman B, Lee D-H, et al. Significance of the anti-E2 response in self-limited and chronic hepatitis C virus infections in chimpanzees and humans. J Infect Dis 1999; 180: 987–991.
35. Kuhns WJ, Prince AM, Brotman B, et al. Clinical and laboratory evaluation of immune serum globulin from donors with a history of hepatitis: attempted prevention of posttransfusion hepatitis. Am J Med Sci 1976; 272: 255–261.
36. Knodell RG, Conrad ME, Ginsberg AL, et al. Efficacy of prophylactic gamma-globulin in preventing non-A, non-B post-transfusion hepatitis. Lancet 1976; 1: 557–561.
37. Seeff LB, Zimmerman HJ, Wright EC, et al. Randomized double-blinded controlled trial of the efficacy of immune serum globulin for the prevention of post-transfusion hepatitis: a Veterans Administration cooperative study. Gastroenterology 1977; 72: 111–121.
38. Sanchez-Quijano A, Pineda JA, Lissen E, et al. Prevention of post-transfusion non-A, non-B hepatitis by non-specific immunoglobulin in heart surgery patients. Lancet 1988; 1: 1245–1249.
39. Piazza M, Sagliocca L, Tosone G, et al. Sexual transmission of the hepatitis C virus and efficacy of prophylaxis with intramuscular immune serum globulin. A randomized controlled trial. Arch Intern Med 1997; 157: 1537–1544.
40. Farci P, Alter HJ, Wong DC, et al. Prevention of hepatitis C virus infection in chimpanzees after antibody-mediated in vitro neutralization. Proc Natl Acad Sci 1994; 91: 7792–7796.
41. Shimizu YK, Hijikata M, Iwamoto A, et al. Neutralizing antibodies against hepatitis C virus and the emergence of neutralization escape mutant viruses. J Virol 1994; 68: 1494–1500.
42. Farci P, Shimoda A, Wong D, et al. Prevention of HCV infection in chimpanzees by hyperimmune serum against the hypervariable region I (HVRI): emergence of neutralization escape mutants in vivo. Hepatology 1995; 22: 220A.
43. Krawczynski K, Alter MJ, Tankersley DL, et al. Effect of immune globulin on the prevention of experimental hepatitis C virus infection. J Infect Dis 1996; 173: 822–828.
44. Choo QL, Kuo G, Ralston R, et al. Vaccination of chimpanzees against infection by the hepatitis C virus. Proc Natl Acad Sci 1994; 91: 1294–1298.
45. Houghton M, Choo QL, Kuo G, et al. HCV vaccine: interim report. IX Triennial International Symposium on Viral Hepatitis and Liver Disease, Rome. 1996, pp. 21–25.
46. Rosa D, Campagnoli S, Moretto C, et al. Quantitative test to estimate neutralizing antibodies to the hepatitis C virus: cytofluorimetric assessment of envelope glycoprotein 2 binding to target cells. Proc Natl Acad Sci 1996; 93: 1759–1763.
47. Major ME, Vitvitski L, Mink MA, et al. DNA-based immunization with chimeric vectors for the induction of immune responses against the hepatitis C virus nucleocapsid. J Virol 1995; 69: 5798–5805.
48. Tokushiga K, Wakita T, Pachuk C, et al. Expression and immune response to hepatitis C virus core DNA-based vaccine constructs. Hepatology 1996; 24: 14–20.

49. Lagging LM, Meyer K, Hoft D, et al. Immune response to plasmid DNA encoding the hepatitis C virus core protein. J Virol 1995; 69: 5859–5863.
50. Hu G-J, Wang R Y-H, Han D-S, et al. Characterization of the humoral and cellular immune response against hepatitis C virus core induced by DNA-based immunization. Vaccine 1999; 17: 3160–3170.
51. Makimura M, Miyaka S, Akino N, et al. Induction of antibodies against structural proteins of hepatitis C virus in mice using recombinant adenovirus. Vaccine 1996; 14: 28–34.

Index

A

Abacavir
  mitochondrial affinity, 99
Acetaminophen toxicity
  ethanol, 258, 259
Active drug users
  therapeutic plan, 203
Active immunization
  hepatitis C, 318–320
Acupuncture, 234, 235, 238
Acute fatty liver of pregnancy
    (AFLP), 291
  pregnancy
    differential diagnosis, 300
Acute hepatitis A
  pregnancy, 292
Acute hepatitis B
  natural history, 42–44
  perinatal transmission, 42–45
  pregnancy, 294
Acute hepatitis C, 64
  pregnancy, 297
Acute hepatitis E
  pregnancy, 292, 293
Addison's disease
  interferon, 180
Adefovir
  chronic hepatitis B, 137
AFLP, 291
  pregnancy
    differential diagnosis, 300
Age
  CHC
    progression, 74
  chronic HBV, 43

  hepatitis B risk, 27
  HVC prevalence, 27
AIDS
  interferon-alpha, 183, 184
Alcohol, 257–261
  abstinence, 216, 217
  CHC, 261
    progression, 77
  chronic liver disease, 263
  interferon, 213
  intravenous drugs, 213
  ribavirin, 213
Alcoholic patient
  therapeutic plan, 202, 203
Allergic hepatotoxicity, 257,
    263, 264
Allopathic medicine, 234
Alopecia
  minoxidil, 223
Alpha-interferon
  HCV-HIV co-infection,
    100, 101
Alpha-interferon-ribavirin com-
    bination therapy, 102, 103
  adverse effects, 104
ALT
  normal
    therapeutic plan, 206
Alternative medicine
  historical development,
    234, 235
  traditions, 237–242
Alternative therapy
  evaluation
    Congressional mandate,
      236

literature, 236, 237
rationale
    resurgent interest, 235
    surveys, 235, 236
Ambien, 227
American Board of Homeotherapeutics competency examination, 241
Anemia
    ribavirin, 267
Anorexia
    management, 220
Antimycobacterial drugs, 267
Antioxidant therapy, 217
Antisense oligonucleotide/ribozymes
    chronic hepatitis B, 139, 140
Antiviral therapy
    chronic HBV, 54, 55
    HCV
        HIV, 100–105
    hepatotoxicity, 99
Anxiety
    patient education, 215
Ascites, 82–83
Assembly
    hepatitis C virus, 21
Asthma
    interferon, 180, 181
Atopic dermatitis
    interferon, 181
Autoimmune disease
    antiviral therapy, 174–186
    chronic viral hepatitis, 169–184
Ayurveda, 238–240
    training, 240

B

BDNA test, 194
Benzodiazepine, 227
Bloodborne hepatitis
    blood transfusion
        reduction, 308

Blood transfusion, 29, 30
    bloodborne hepatitis virus infection
        reduction, 308
    jaundice, 29
Body piercing, 32
Botanical healing, 234
Breastfeeding
    HCV, 298
Breast milk
    HCV, 298
Budd-Chiari syndrome
    pregnancy
        differential diagnosis, 300, 301

C

CBC, 195, 196
CccDNA
    hepatitis B virus, 3, 4
Cellular entry
    hepatitis B virus, 2, 3
CHC. *see* Chronic hepatitis C
Chi, 238
Children
    CHC
        progression, 75, 76
        therapeutic plan, 206
Child's A cirrhosis
    decompensation, 79–83
    outcome, 81–83
Chinese medicine
    traditional, 237, 238
Chiropractic, 235
Cholestasis
    pregnancy
        differential diagnosis, 299
Cholestatic hepatitis C, 283, 284
Christian Science, 234
Chronic hepatitis B, 44–46
    adefovir, 137
    age, 43
    algorithm, 200

Index

antisense oligonucleotide/
  ribozymes, 139, 140
antiviral therapy, 54, 55
co-infection
  HCV, 49
emtricitabine, 137
entecavir, 137
extrahepatic manifestation,
  48, 49
famciclovir, 136, 137
HCC, 50, 51, 275
immunomodulatory therapy,
  137–139
interferon therapy, 124–130
lamivudine, 130–135
lamivudine-interferon combination therapy, 135, 136
liver transplantation, 276
molecular approaches, 139, 140
pregnancy, 293–299
prognosis, 49, 50
progression, 51
serologic diagnosis, 191
survival, 49, 50
thymosin, 138
treatment, 123–142
  plan, 197–200
vaccines, 138, 139
Chronic hepatitis C (CHC), 64–70
  alcohol, 261
  algorithm, 201
  co-infection
    HBV, 78, 79
    HIV, 79
  interferon, 147, 148
  interferon relapse
    retreatment, 154–158
  interferon-ribavirin combination therapy, 149–158
  normal ALT, 70, 71
  pregnancy, 297–299
  progression, 65, 71, 72
  extraneous factors, 77, 78
  risk factors, 73–79
  viral factors, 77
  quality of life, 213, 214
  risk factors, 212, 213
  therapeutic plan, 200–202
  treatment, 145–162
    assessing response, 159–161
    future, 161
    patient selection, 146, 147
Chronic liver disease
  alcohol, 263
  dose-dependent drug-induced
    toxicity, 262
Chronic viral hepatitis
  autoimmune disease, 169–184
    treatment, 172–182
  initial evaluation, 192, 193
Cirrhosis
  HBV
    survival, 52
  HBV-HCV co-infection, 114
  histologic progression, 197
  interferon-ribavirin combination, 205
  primary biliary, 176, 177
  therapeutic plan, 205
Clathrates, 241
Cocaine
  hepatitis C, 61
  intranasal, 31, 306, 307
Competency examination
  homeopathy, 241
Complete blood count (CBC),
  195, 196
Coumadin
  interferon alpha, 266
Council on Homeopathic Education
  training program accreditation, 241
Crohn's disease
  interferon, 174–176

Cryoglobulinemia, 221
CTL, 9, 17, 42, 43
Cytochrome P-450, 253, 254
   nitric oxide, 266
Cytokines, 47
Cytotoxic T lymphocyte (CTL), 9, 17, 42, 43

D

Decision making, 214
Decompensation
   Child's A cirrhosis, 79–83
      outcome, 81–83
Dehydroepiandrosterone (DHEA)
   variability, 242, 243
Depression
   interferon, 213, 227
   late-onset, 229
   ribavirin, 267
Dermatologic complications, 221, 222
DHEA
   variability, 242, 243
Diabetes mellitus
   interferon, 224
Dialysis patients, 36, 37
Dideoxycytidine
   mitochondrial affinity, 99
Dideoxyinosine
   mitochondrial affinity, 99
Dietary Supplement Health and Education Act, 242
DNA
   oxidant stress, 258
DNA-based vaccines
   chronic hepatitis B, 139
Dose-dependent hepatotoxicity, 261–263
   factors influencing, 262, 263
Doshas, 239
Drug-induced hepatic injury, 254–257
   vs. toxicity, 255

Drug-induced hepatotoxicity
   dose-dependent
      chronic liver disease, 262
   pregnancy
      differential diagnosis, 301
Drug-induced liver disease, 254
Drugs
   doses
      adjustments, 267–269
      injectable illicit, 306, 307
      intravenous, 60, 61, 213
      metabolism, 253–255
         interferon, 264–266
Drug users, 35
   therapeutic plan, 203

E

Eddy, Mary Baker, 234
Elderly
   therapeutic plan, 206
Emtricitabine
   chronic hepatitis B, 137
Encapsidation
   hepatitis B virus, 5
Engerix-B, 310
Entecavir
   chronic hepatitis B, 137
Erythema multiforme, 221
Erythema nodosum, 221
Ethanol
   acetaminophen toxicity, 258, 259
   iron overload, 260, 261
   metabolism, 257
   methotrexate toxicity, 259, 260
Ethnic groups
   CHC progression, 75
   HVC prevalence, 27
Exposure risks
   modification, 306–309
Eye problems
   management, 221

Index

F

Famciclovir
   chronic hepatitis B, 136, 137
Fatigue
   exercise-tolerance program, 219, 220
Fialuridine
   hepatotoxicity, 99
Flu-like symptoms
   Tylenol, 219
Food supplements, 242
Fulminant hepatitis
   hepatitis C, 64
   risk
      HBV-HCV co-infection, 113

G

Gender
   CHC
      progression, 75
Genetic vaccines
   HCV, 319, 320
Genome
   hepatitis B virus, 4
Ginseng products
   variability, 242, 243
Glucose metabolism
   interferon, 224
Glycyrrhizin, 245
Grave's disease
   interferon, 223, 224

H

HAART, 95, 267
Hahnemann, Samuel, 234, 240
Hashimoto's thyroiditis
   interferon, 223
HBeAg, 293
HBsAG, 293, 295
   spontaneous seroconversion
      HBV-HCV co-infection, 112
HBV. *see* Hepatitis B virus

HCC. *see* Hepatocellular carcinoma
HCV. *see* Hepatitis C virus
HDV
   genotypes, 194
Headaches
   mydrin, 219
   trazadone, 219
Health care workers, 311
   exposure reduction, 309
   prevalence, 37
   transmission, 37
HELLP, 291
   pregnancy
      differential diagnosis, 299, 300
Hemodialysis patients, 36, 37
Hemolysis elevated liver enzymes low platelet count (HELLP), 291
   pregnancy
      differential diagnosis, 299, 300
Hemolytic anemia
   ribavirin, 225
Hemophiliacs, 34, 35
Hepatic fibrosis, 71, 72
Hepatic inflammation
   CHC
      progression, 76
Hepatic masses
   pregnancy
      differential diagnosis, 301
Hepatitis
   autoimmune manifestations, 170
   blood associated, 307
   chronic
      autoimmune disease, 169–184
      initial evaluation, 192, 193

Hepatitis A
  acute
    pregnancy, 292
Hepatitis B
  acute. see Acute hepatitis B
  alternating dominance, 112
  blood transfusion, 29, 30
  chronic. see Chronic
    hepatitis B
  cirrhosis
    survival, 52
  dialysis patients, 36, 37
  epidemiology, 25–38
  geographical distribution, 26
  HCV
    latency, 111, 112
    replication, 111
  health care workers, 37
  hemophiliacs, 34, 35
  household contacts, 33
  immune globulin prophylaxis
    HBV re-infection, 276–278
  immunopathogenetic mechanisms, 46–48
  immunoprophylaxis, 309–315
    future problems, 314, 315
  injection drug use, 31
  injection drug users, 35
  liver transplant, 55, 56
  military veterans, 36
  natural history, 41–56
  pregnancy
    prophylactic treatment, 295, 296
    vertical transmission, 294, 295
  prevalence, 26, 27
  prisoners, 36
  recurrent
    LAM, 280, 281
  re-infection
    LAM, 278, 279
  risk
    chronic infection, 27, 28
    sequelae, 27, 28
  transmission, 28–34
    maternal-fetal transmission, 32
    nosocomial, 31, 32
    sexual, 33, 34
    transplantation, 30
    recipients, 35
  vaccine, 54, 308, 310–312
    effectiveness, 313
Hepatitis B e antigen (HBeAg), 293
Hepatitis B immunoglobulins
  LAM, 279, 280
Hepatitis B immunoglobulins-LAM, 279, 280
Hepatitis B surface antigen (HBsAG), 293, 295
  spontaneous seroconversion
    HBV-HCV co-infection, 112
Hepatitis B virus (HBV)
  cccDNA, 3, 4
  cellular entry, 2, 3
  encapsidation, 5
  genomic organization, 4
  hepatocarcinogenesis, 7, 8
  immune-escape mutants, 10, 11
  immune system evasion, 9
  integration, 6, 7
  molecular virology, 2–12
  mutants, 53, 54
    polymerase, 11, 12
  re-infection
    immune globulin prophylaxis, 276–278
  replication
    HCV, 110, 111
  replication cycle, 2, 3

reverse transcription, 5, 6
transcription, 4, 5
translation, 5
usurpation
   HCV, 112
vaccine
   pregnancy, 295, 296
viral mutation, 10
virion production, 8, 9
X protein, 7, 8, 48
Hepatitis B virus-HCV co-infection, 109–118
  cirrhosis, 114
  clinical presentation, 113–115
  fulminant hepatitis risk, 113
  HbsAG
    spontaneous seroconversion, 112
  HCC, 114, 115
    surgical resection, 115
  histologic presentation, 113–115
  interferon therapy, 116
  liver transplant, 116, 117
  therapeutic plan, 206
  viral replication, 110–113
Hepatitis B virus-hepatitis D virus co-infection
  liver transplantation, 275
Hepatitis C
  active immunization, 318–320
  acute, 64, 297
  blood transfusion, 29, 30
  chronic. *see* Chronic hepatitis C
  co-infection
    HBV, 62
  dialysis patients, 36, 37
  epidemiology, 25–38
  HCC
    risk, 83–86
  health care workers, 37
  hemophiliacs, 34, 35
  household contacts, 33
  immunoglobulin, 316, 317
  immunoprophylaxis, 315–321
  incidence, 63
  injection drug use, 31
  injection drug users, 35
  intravenous drugs, 60, 61
  maternal-fetal transmission, 62
  military veterans, 36
  natural history, 59–86
  nosocomial transmission, 31, 32
  passive immunization, 316, 317
  prevalence, 26, 27, 60
  prisoners, 36
  risk factors, 60–63
  serologic diagnosis, 191, 194
  transmission, 28–34
    maternal-fetal transmission, 32
    nosocomial, 31, 32
    sexual, 33, 34
    transplantation, 30
    recipients, 35
  vertical transmission, 62
Hepatitis C virus (HCV)
  alternating dominance, 112
  antiviral therapy
    HIV, 100–105
  assembly, 21
  autoimmune manifestations, 170
  breastfeeding, 298
  breast milk, 298
  genetic vaccines, 319, 320
  HBV
    replication, 110, 111
    usurpation, 112
  hepatocarcinogenesis, 19

immune system evasion, 16–18
intracellular antiviral
    response, 18, 19
latency
    HBV, 111, 112
liver transplantation, 281, 282
molecular virology, 12–22
perinatal transmission, 297, 298
proteins, 19
    processing, 15, 16
replication
    HBV, 111
    HIV protease inhibitors, 99
replication cycle, 12–14
RNA replication, 19, 21
secretion, 21
translation, 14, 15
transmission
    parenteral, 96, 97
    sexual, 96, 97
    vertical, 97
vaccine, 316–320
    candidates, 321
    development, 319
viral entry, 14
Hepatitis C virus-HIV co-infection, 95–105
    alpha-interferon, 100, 101
    natural history, 97, 98
    therapeutic plan, 206
Hepatitis D
    immunoprophylaxis, 315
    pregnancy, 299
Hepatitis D virus (HDV)
    genotypes, 194
Hepatitis E
    acute
        pregnancy, 292, 293
Hepatocarcinogenesis
    hepatitis B virus, 7, 8
    hepatitis C virus, 19

Hepatocellular carcinoma (HCC)
    chronic HBV, 50, 51
    chronic hepatitis B, 275
    HBV-HCV co-infection, 114, 115
    hepatitis C
        risk, 83–86
    surgical resection
        HBV-HCV co-infection, 115
Hepatotoxicity
    allergic, 257, 263, 264
    dose-dependent, 261–263
        factors influencing, 262, 263
        toxicity-type, 256
    dose-independent, 257
    drug-induced
        dose-dependent, 262
        pregnancy, 301
    idiosyncratic, 263, 264
    unpredictable, 263, 264
Herbal therapy, 242–247
    hepatotoxicity, 246, 247
Herpes simplex virus
    pregnancy, 293
Highly active antiretroviral
    therapy (HAART), 95, 267
High-risk groups, 311
HIV. see Human immunodeficiency virus
Homeopathy, 234, 240, 241
    competency examination, 241
    training program accreditation, 241
Host factors
    CHC
        progression, 73–76
Human immunodeficiency virus (HIV)
    anti-HCV therapy, 100–105
    hepatitis C co-infection, 95–105
    mitochondrial toxicity, 99, 100

protease inhibitors
  HCV replication, 99
HVR1, 17
Hydration, 220
Hydrotherapy, 234
Hyperimmune anti-hepatitis C
    virus immunoglobulin,
    317, 318
Hypersplenism, 82
Hyperthyroidism
  interferon, 223
Hypervariable region-1 (HVR1),
    17
Hypothyroidism
  interferon, 223

I

IBD
  interferon, 174–176
Idiosyncratic drug toxicity, 257
Idiosyncratic hepatotoxicity,
    263, 264
IFN-alpha. *see* Interferon-alpha
Illicit drugs
  injectable, 306, 307
Immune-escape mutants
  hepatitis B virus, 10, 11
Immune globulin prophylaxis
  hepatitis B
    HBV re-infection, 276–278
Immune response
  CHC
    progression, 76
  HBV, 46–48
Immune system evasion
  hepatitis B virus, 9
  hepatitis C virus, 16–18
Immune thrombocytopenia (ITP)
  interferon, 177, 178
Immunization. *see also* Vaccines
  hepatitis C, 316–320
Immunoglobulin
  hepatitis C, 316, 317

Immunoprophylaxis, 305–321
  HBV
    future problems, 314, 315
    hepatitis B, 309–315
    hepatitis C, 315–321
    hepatitis D, 315
Income
  hepatitis C, 62
Inflammatory bowel disease
    (IBD)
  interferon, 174–176
Influenza vaccines
  interferon, 266
Injectable illicit drugs, 306, 307
Injection drug use, 31, 35
Insomnia
  ribavirin, 227
Integration
  hepatitis B virus, 6, 7
Interferon
  Addison's disease, 180
  alcohol, 213
  asthma, 180, 181
  atopic dermatitis, 181
  bone marrow toxicity, 226
  CHC, 147, 148, 202
  chronic hepatitis B, 124–130,
      198, 199
    adverse effects, 128
    long-term outcome, 129, 130
    patient selection, 124–127
    prednisone priming, 128
    response factors, 127
  Crohn's disease, 174–176
  depression, 213, 227
  diabetes mellitus, 224
  drug interactions, 266
  drug metabolism, 264–266
  glucose metabolism, 224
  HBV-HCV co-infection, 116
  IBD, 174–176

immune thrombocytopenia, 177, 178
influenza vaccination, 266
irritability, 213, 227
liver transplantation
  recurrent HCV, 284
multiple sclerosis, 179
myasthenia gravis, 178, 179
positive autoantibodies
  without AIDS symptoms, 173, 174
primary biliary cirrhosis, 176, 177
psoriasis, 177
respiratory tract symptoms
  management, 220, 221
rheumatologic disease, 181, 182
sarcoidosis, 179, 180
side effects, 103, 104
  management, 217–228
  neuropsychiatric, 203, 204
  systemic lupus erythematosus, 181, 182
  thyroid dysfunction, 223, 224
  ulcerative colitis, 174–176
Interferon-alpha (IFN-alpha)
  AIDS, 183, 184
  autoimmune effects, 170, 171
  chronic HBV, 54, 55
  theophylline, 266
  warfarin, 266
Interferon dementia syndrome, 227, 228
Interferon-ribavirin combination therapy
  CHC, 149–158
    previously untreated patients, 152–154
    side effects, 267
    treatment-naive patients, 149, 150

cirrhosis, 205
liver transplantation
  recurrent HCV, 284, 285
  safety, 158, 159
  side effects, 218
Interleukin-12, 47
Internet, 214
Intracellular antiviral response
  hepatitis C virus, 18, 19
Intranasal cocaine, 31, 306, 307
Intravenous
  alcohol, 60, 61, 213
Intravenous drugs
  hepatitis C, 60, 61
  ribavirin, 213
Iron overload
  CHC
    progression, 77, 78
    ethanol, 260, 261
    ribavirin, 266, 267
Irritability
  interferon, 213, 227
Ischemic retinopathy, 221
ITP
  interferon, 177, 178

J–L

Jaundice
  transfusion, 29
Kapha, 239
Laboratory evaluation, 190, 191, 194
  baseline, 195, 196
LAM. see Lamivudine
Lamivudine-interferon combination therapy
  chronic hepatitis B, 135, 136
Lamivudine (LAM)
  chronic HBV, 54, 55
  chronic hepatitis B, 130–135, 199, 200
    adverse effects, 133, 134
    dose regimen, 132, 133
    efficacy, 130

long-term outcome, 134, 135
patient selection, 130–132
resistance, 134, 135
response factors, 133
HBV
re-infection, 278, 279
hepatitis B immunoglobulins, 279, 280
liver transplantation, 278
mitochondrial affinity, 99
recurrent HBV
posttransplant, 280, 281
Late-onset depression, 229
Leukocytoclastic vasculitis, 221
Lichen planus, 221, 222
Licorice, 245
Literature
alternative therapy, 236, 237
Livedo reticularis, 221
Liver
fibrosis, 71, 72
inflammation
CHC, 76
masses
pregnancy, 301
Liver biopsy, 196
Liver disease
chronic
alcohol, 263
dose-dependent drug-induced toxicity, 262
pregnancy
differential diagnosis, 299, 301
Liver function tests, 195, 196
Liver transplantation, 273–286
chronic hepatitis B, 275–281
chronic viral co-infection, 274, 275
HCV, 281, 282
hepatitis B, 55, 56
indications, 274
LAM, 278
recurrent HCV
risk factors, 282, 283
treatment, 283–285
Lust, Benedict, 234

M

Maintenance therapy, 229
Manipulation, 234
Marijuana
hepatitis C, 61
Marital status
hepatitis C, 62
Massage, 235
Maternal-fetal transmission, 32
hepatitis C, 62
Maternal-neonatal transmission, 308
Medications. see Drugs
MEOS, 257
Mesmerism, 234
METAVIR fibrosis score, 72
Methotrexate toxicity
ethanol, 259, 260
Microsomal ethanol-oxidizing system (MEOS), 257
Military veterans, 36
Milk thistle, 217, 242–245
Minoxidil
alopecia, 223
Molecular memory, 240, 241
Multiple sclerosis
interferon, 179
Myasthenia gravis
interferon, 178, 179
Mydrin
headaches, 219

N

NADPH, 253
National Center for Complementary and Alternative Medicine (NICAM), 234
Naturopathy, 234, 241, 242

training, 242
Nausea
  management, 220
Needle exchange programs, 35, 306, 307
Needlestick injuries
  reduction, 309
NICAM, 234
Nicotinamide adenine dinucleotide phosphate (NADPH), 253
Nitric oxide
  cytochrome P-450, 266
Nonsteroidal antiinflammatory drugs (NSAIDs), 217
NSAIDs, 217

O

OAM, 233, 234
Office of Alternative Medicine (OAM), 233, 234
OLT
  HBV-HCV co-infection, 116, 117
Orthotopic liver transplantation (OLT)
  HBV-HCV co-infection, 116, 117
Oxidant stress
  DNA, 258

P

Palmer, Daniel David, 234
Parenteral transmission
  HCV, 96, 97
Passive immunization
  hepatitis C, 316, 317
Patients
  data analysis, 197
  education, 196, 197, 214–217
    anxiety, 215
    self-injection, 152
    therapy effects, 215, 216

evaluation, 190–196
history, 190
selection, 212–217
PBC
  interferon, 176, 177
PBMCs, 14
PCR, 194, 228
PEG-Intron
  maintenance therapy, 229
Perinatal transmission
  HBV, 42–45
  HCV, 297, 298
Peripheral blood mononuclear cells (PBMCs), 14
Physical examination, 190
Pitta, 239
PKR, 18
Polyarteritis nodosa, 221
Polyethylene glycol interferon, 104
Polymerase chain reaction (PCR), 194, 228
Polymerase mutants
  hepatitis B virus, 11, 12
Porphyria cutanea tarda, 221
Positive autoantibodies
  without AIDS symptoms
    treatment, 173, 174
Pregnancy, 291–301
  CHC, 297–299
  differential diagnosis
    AFLP, 300
    Budd-Chiari syndrome, 300, 301
    cholesteatosis, 299
    drug-induced hepatotoxicity, 301
    HELLP, 299, 300
    hepatic masses, 301
  hepatitis A
    acute, 292

hepatitis B
  acute, 294
  chronic, 293–299
  prophylactic treatment,
    295, 296
  vaccine, 295, 296
  vertical transmission,
    294, 295
hepatitis C
  acute, 297
hepatitis D, 299
hepatitis E
  acute, 292, 293
herpes simplex virus, 293
liver disease
  differential diagnosis,
    299–301
rebetron, 224
ribavirin, 224, 225
Pretreatment evaluation, 214–217
Primary biliary cirrhosis (PBC)
  interferon, 176, 177
Prisoners, 36
Protease inhibitors
  hepatotoxicity, 100
Protective efficacy, 312, 313
Proteins
  hepatitis C virus, 15, 16, 19
Prototype envelope GP vaccines, 319
Pruritus
  rebetron, 222
Psoriasis, 222
  interferon, 177
Psychiatric patients
  therapeutic plan, 203, 204
Psychosocial issues
  treatment plan, 204
Pyrazinamide, 267

Q, R

Quality of life
  CHC, 213, 214
Race
  CHC progression, 75
  HVC prevalence, 27
Rebetron
  pregnancy, 224
  pruritus, 222
  side effects
    management, 216
    therapeutic monitoring, 228
Recombinant immunoblot assay
  (RIBA), 194
Recombivax hepatitis B, 310
Recurrent hepatitis B
  posttransplant
    LAM, 280, 281
Recurrent hepatitis C virus
  liver transplantation
    risk factors, 282, 283
    treatment, 283–285
Replication cycle
  hepatitis B virus, 2, 3
  hepatitis C virus, 12–14
Retinopathy
  ischemic, 221
Reverse transcription
  hepatitis B virus, 5, 6
Rheumatologic disease
  interferon, 181, 182
RIBA, 194
Ribavirin. *see also* Interferon-
    ribavirin combination
    therapy
  alcohol, 213
  anemia, 267
  depression, 267
  hemolytic anemia, 225
  insomnia, 227
  intravenous drugs, 213
  iron overload, 266, 267

maintenance therapy, 229
pregnancy, 224, 225
Rifampin, 267
Risk
   CHC, 212, 213
   progression, 73–79
   HCC
      hepatitis C, 83–86
      hepatitis C, 60–63
RNA-activated protein kinase (PKR), 18
RNA replication
   hepatitis C virus, 19–21

S

Sarcoidosis
   interferon, 179, 180
Secretion
   hepatitis C virus, 21
Selective serotonin transport inhibitors (SSRIs), 227, 228
Self-injection
   patient instruction, 152
Sexual transmission, 33, 34, 307, 308
   HCV, 96, 97
   reduction, 309
Silybum marianum, 217, 242–245
Silymarin. *see* Milk thistle
Sinusitis, 221
Skin rash, 222
Sleeping pills, 227
Smoking
   CHC
      progression, 79
Snakebites, 242, 243
Sonata, 227
SSRIs, 227, 228
St. John's Wort
   unwanted pregnancy, 247

Steatosis
   CHC
      progression, 78
Still, Andrew Taylor, 234
Suicide, 229
Surveys
   alternative therapy, 235, 236
Systemic lupus erythematosus
   interferon, 181, 182

T

Tattoos, 32
T-cell vaccines
   chronic hepatitis B, 139
Theophylline
   interferon alpha, 266
Therapeutic monitoring, 228, 229
Thompson, Samuel, 234
Thrombocytopenia
   interferon, 226
Thymic gland extract, 245, 246
Thymosin, 245, 246
   chronic hepatitis B, 138
T-lymphocytes, 47
Toxicity-type hepatotoxicity
   dose-dependent, 256
Traditional Chinese medicine, 237, 238
Training
   naturopathy, 242
Training program accreditation
   homeopathy, 241
Transcription
   hepatitis B virus, 4, 5
Transfusion, 29, 30
Transfusion-associated bloodborne
   reduction, 308
Translation
   hepatitis B virus, 5

hepatitis C virus, 14, 15
Transmission
  CHC
    progression, 74, 75
  maternal-fetal, 32, 62
  maternal-neonatal, 308
  parenteral, 96, 97
  perinatal, 42–45, 297, 298
  sexual, 33, 34, 96, 97, 307, 308
  reduction, 309
  vertical, 62, 97, 294, 295
Transplantation, 30
  recipients, 35
Travelers, 311
Trazadone, 227
  headaches, 219
Tylenol, 217
  flu-like symptoms, 219

U, V

UC
  interferon, 174–176
Ulcerative colitis (UC)
  interferon, 174–176
Unpredictable hepatotoxicity, 263, 264
Vaccine escape mutants, 53, 54
Vaccines
  chronic hepatitis B, 138, 139
  DNA-based
    chronic hepatitis B, 139
  HAV, 313, 314
  HBV, 54, 308, 310–312
    effectiveness, 313
    pregnancy, 295, 296
  HCV, 316–320
    candidates, 321
    development, 319
    genetic, 319, 320

influenza
  interferon, 266
  prototype envelope GP, 319
  T-cell
    chronic hepatitis B, 139
Valium, 227
Vasculitis
  leukocytoclastic, 221
Vata, 239
Vedas, 238, 239
Vertical transmission
  HBV
    pregnancy, 294, 295
  HCV, 97
  hepatitis C, 62
Veterans
  military, 36
Viral entry
  hepatitis C virus, 14
Viral factors
  CHC
    progression, 77
Viral mutation
  hepatitis B virus, 10
Viral replication
  HBV-HCV co-infection, 110–113
Virion
  hepatitis B virus, 8, 9
Vitamin A, 217
Vitamin E, 217
Vomiting
  management, 220

W–Y

Warfarin
  interferon alpha, 266
Websites, 214
X protein
  hepatitis B virus, 7, 8, 48
Yin and yang, 237